Psychological Assessment and Therapy with Older Adults

Psychological Assessment and Therapy with Older Adults

Bob G. Knight and Nancy A. Pachana

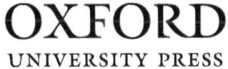

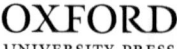
UNIVERSITY PRESS

Great Clarendon Street, Oxford, OX2 6DP,
United Kingdom

Oxford University Press is a department of the University of Oxford.
It furthers the University's objective of excellence in research, scholarship,
and education by publishing worldwide. Oxford is a registered trade mark of
Oxford University Press in the UK and in certain other countries

© Oxford University Press 2015

The moral rights of the authors have been asserted

All rights reserved. No part of this publication may be reproduced, stored in
a retrieval system, or transmitted, in any form or by any means, without the
prior permission in writing of Oxford University Press, or as expressly permitted
by law, by licence or under terms agreed with the appropriate reprographics
rights organization. Enquiries concerning reproduction outside the scope of the
above should be sent to the Rights Department, Oxford University Press, at the
address above

You must not circulate this work in any other form
and you must impose this same condition on any acquirer

Published in the United States of America by Oxford University Press
198 Madison Avenue, New York, NY 10016, United States of America

British Library Cataloguing in Publication Data
Data available

Library of Congress Control Number: 2014948876

ISBN 978–0–19–965253–2

Oxford University Press makes no representation, express or implied, that the
drug dosages in this book are correct. Readers must therefore always check
the product information and clinical procedures with the most up-to-date
published product information and data sheets provided by the manufacturers
and the most recent codes of conduct and safety regulations. The authors and
the publishers do not accept responsibility or legal liability for any errors in the
text or for the misuse or misapplication of material in this work. Except where
otherwise stated, drug dosages and recommendations are for the non-pregnant
adult who is not breast-feeding

Links to third party websites are provided by Oxford in good faith and
for information only. Oxford disclaims any responsibility for the materials
contained in any third party website referenced in this work.

Foreword

As many readers of this book well know, there is a growing need for behavioral and mental health services for older adults worldwide as our population ages. Geropsychology—the application of "the knowledge and methods of psychology to understanding and helping older persons and their families to maintain well-being, overcome problems and achieve maximum potential during late life" (American Psychological Association, 2010; see <http://www.apa.org/ed/graduate/specialize/gero.aspx>)—is a growing specialty area of practice within professional psychology (Knight et al., 2009). However, even without specialized geropsychology training, most practicing psychologists and other mental health professionals will be seeing increasing numbers of older adults in their practices due to demographic trends, shifts to integrated models of care and, perhaps, increased receptivity of the Baby Boomer generation to mental health services compared with earlier-born cohorts.

Bob Knight and Nancy Pachana, leading scholars of clinical geropsychology, have made an important contribution to the growing literature in the field (e.g., see <http://gerocentral.org/>). The major influence of this volume is to provide a unifying framework that will help readers to consider the question, "What's age got to do with it?" when conducting psychological assessment and psychotherapy with older adults. The CALTAP model—Contextual, Adult Life Span Theory for Adapting Psychotherapy—helps us to consider the meaning of "age," from maturational, generational, social and cultural contextual, and late-life specific challenge perspectives. They apply the CALTAP model to the assessment and treatment of behavioral and mental health issues common among older adults.

An important theme throughout this volume is that both older adults and therapists are often at risk of misattributing distressing symptoms, functional difficulties, or social changes to "old age," rather than to specific illnesses or other conditions that can be helped, leading to a sense of hopelessness. How often do we hear our older relatives, friends, *ourselves*, and many health care professionals say things like "of course you're [fill in the blank—e.g., in pain, depressed, isolated, unable to do what you want to do . . .], you're getting old, what do you expect?!?" Drs. Knight and Pachana ask readers to collaborate with their patients in considering carefully what experiences may or may not be attributable to "normal aging" and to be clear that often much can be done to alleviate distress, and improve functioning and quality of life, even if certain aging-related changes (e.g., hearing loss) or chronic illnesses cannot be "cured."

The authors' discussion of the impact of cohort, social contexts, and cultural issues throughout this book is so very helpful in providing therapists a lens through which to appreciate the wide variety of lived experiences of older people, and the implications of these diverse experiences for psychological assessment, treatment, and the therapeutic relationship. Culturally competent practice with older adults entails understanding the historical time and place in which individuals came of age, and how life experiences at different points of history varied significantly for people depending upon gender, sexual orientation, ethnicity, socioeconomic status, immigrant status, and so forth. These components of diversity affect health beliefs, understanding of and attitudes toward conditions such as depression or dementia, and receptivity to a range of health and mental health services. Likewise, the social context of aging varies widely, depending upon the extent of family and social support, whether an individual lives in the community versus one of many types of residential care facilities, and extent of engagement with the health care system and aging services network. Drs. Knight and Pachana's international perspectives enrich the discussion, together with case examples illustrating the impact of cultural background, immigration and assimilation, and intergenerational relationships on geropsychology practice.

The specific-challenges of late life are framed in a patient-centered way that encourages clinicians to consider how late-in-life challenges specifically affect the individual, based upon her conceptions of quality of life and valued aspects of functioning. They encourage an individualized approach that aims to discourage older adults from overgeneralizing aged peers' experiences to their own.

Finally, Drs. Knight and Pachana address the therapist's experience of work with older adults in a validating manner that encourages us all to be aware of our attitudes, feelings, and potential assumptions/stereotypes about aging and older people. In the chapter on geropsychology supervision and consultation, they discuss specifically the importance of addressing attitude competencies when supervising trainees, including risk for both unrealistically negative and positive attitudes towards older adults that can affect the therapeutic process.

For psychologists and other mental health professionals working with older adults, and geropsychology teachers, supervisors, and students, this volume will be a welcome addition to one's library.

Michele J. Karel, PhD
Psychogeriatrics Coordinator
Mental Health Services
Office of Patient Care Services
Veterans Health Administration
Washington, DC, USA

Preface

We have been thinking about assessment and treatment of older adults for a long time—these topics form the basis of our teaching, research, and interactions with colleagues and students. Often the topics of assessment and treatment are handled separately, but in the case of older adults specifically, this frequently does not make sense. From a clinical perspective, embarking on any therapeutic work with an older person necessitates understanding that age-related changes in later life may affect a client's presenting problems. Measurement of aspects of emotional, cognitive or functional performance may therefore be important to ascertain before embarking on a course of therapy. Similarly, cognitive and emotional functioning are intimately tied together at all ages. However, given the greater risk—with increasing age—of both age-expected as well as abnormal changes in functioning, particularly with respect to cognition, the clinician who chooses to work with older adults needs to be familiar with the instruments and specific therapeutic techniques that may be required to successfully treat an older person suffering such changes.

In order to approach the tasks of assessment and treatment with older adults in a systematic way, it helps to have an organizing model to offer guidance. The CALTAP model serves such a function in this text. CALTAP serves here as a meta-theoretical framework in guiding an integrated approach to both assessment and psychotherapy with older adults, and Chapters 1 and 2 offer overviews of our thinking with respect to this.

In the remaining, diagnostic-specific chapters, assessment issues for that diagnosis are explored, then the CALTAP themes of developmental aging, social context, cohort differences, and cultural issues frame discussions of psychotherapy with older adults with that diagnosis. Chapters 3 and 4 cover Depression and Anxiety; comorbidities between these two disorders, as well as implications of later versus earlier onsets of these conditions are also considered. Chapter 5 deals with neurocognitive disorders and their impact on individuals, as well as caregivers, in both community and nursing home contexts. Psychological factors of chronic illness are covered in Chapter 6. Substance abuse and sleep disorders, which may be comorbid with and exacerbate other conditions, as well as greatly affect quality of life in later years, are discussed in Chapters 7 and 8, respectively. Psychoses and personality disorders in later life, which often pose significant assessment and treatment dilemmas, are covered in Chapters 9 and 10. Chapter 11, the final chapter in the book, contains a discussion of supervision and peer consultation, as they relate to assessment and treatment of older clients. In each of these later chapters, case examples for illustrative purposes are provided; these appear as boxed text.

We have ended with a chapter on supervision because we both felt strongly that thoughtful and supportive supervision forms the basis of both skill, as well as confidence as a therapist. Seeking supervision and consultation on cases is familiar as a requirement for ethical and effective clinical practice during one's career. However, the importance of attention paid to the development of attitudinal competencies as a key component of effective therapy has not been emphasized enough. Attitudes are important in working with older adults, where cohort, cultural, and age gaps may lead to ageist attitudes affecting the therapeutic relationship, as well as the process of therapy itself.

We hope that this text will be viewed as useful both to psychology trainees embarking on work with older adults or those wishing to increase their competence in working with this population. Equally, we hope that practicing therapists in the area or new to the area of geropsychology find this text helpful to approaching assessment and therapy with older adults.

Contents

1 The CALTAP model and working with the older adult client *1*
2 CALTAP in assessment approaches and strategies *19*
3 Depression in late life *38*
4 Anxiety in later life *62*
5 Dementia *83*
6 Psychological issues affecting medical conditions *112*
7 Substance misuse and abuse *133*
8 Sleep disorders and complaints in later life *153*
9 Psychosis and bipolar disorder *172*
10 Personality disorders in older adults *191*
11 Supervision and consultation in clinical geropsychology *207*

   References *223*
   Author Index *261*
   Subject Index *267*

Chapter 1

The CALTAP model and working with the older adult client

Introduction to the CALTAP model and working with the older client

A psychologist with years of experience saw a client over 70 years of age for the first time. The client was brought in by her daughter, who had made the appointment. The daughter had indicated that her mother was not as able as she used to be, a bit forgetful, and needed to accept that she is older now and should let her daughter do more things for her. The client appeared depressed, and told the psychologist that she was more forgetful than she used to be, that her eyesight was failing, and she found it harder to walk than it used to be. She said she was sad that her life was not what it once was and was getting worse all the time as she grew older. She felt that her daughter did too much for her, worried too much about her, and that she was depressed, in part because she didn't want to be a burden to her daughter. The psychologist took her word and the daughter's as realistic assessments of the client's condition, since it was consistent with what he knows about aging. He worked with the client for a few months on accepting her lower level of functioning and relying more on her daughter without blaming herself for this. The client said she appreciated having someone to talk to and his perspective on her problems, and seemed a bit less depressed at the last session they had together. *But was this outcome as successful as it could have been?*

If the psychologist had more knowledge and skills, and fewer ageist stereotypes, he could have done a more accurate assessment. He would have discovered that the client was depressed and anxious, but did not have any significant memory impairment. He could have discovered, with more incisive questioning, that while her declining eyesight was clearly a problem, her difficulty in walking was nearly entirely due to depression interfering with her motivation to exercise and with anxiety leading to an unrealistic fear of falling. With reduction in depressed and anxious mood using the psychologist's usual methods to achieve the improvement in mood, she became more active physically and felt more energetic. With these successes and the client's confidence that the therapist understands and likes older people, she opened up more about conflicts with her daughter. The psychologist was able to help her understand that some of these were due to her and her daughter being from different generational cohorts; they have different attitudes toward some of the daily issues in their lives, while others are individual disagreements that the client could be more assertive in resolving. The psychologist saw the mother and daughter together a few times to help them work out a different way of talking and settling disagreements, which increased the mother's independence and sense of control over her life. This reduced the daughter's perceived need to take care of her mother and her feeling of being overwhelmed by that care. *In this scenario, both the client and her daughter were afforded the chance to improve their relationship and perhaps be better able to face challenges that may occur in the future, for example, if the daughter needs to move due to work commitments, or if the mother loses functionality and must consider entering a nursing home.*

For psychologists starting to work with older adults, as well as more experienced psychologists who may be just beginning to work with older adults, a common question is how different it is to work with older clients than with young or middle-aged adults. Our answer to this question is framed in our clinical experience, and within the context of lifespan developmental psychology and the science of gerontology. It may be more or less the same as working with younger clients, but the potential for lifespan issues to significantly affect the client, the therapist, or the progress of the work in therapy should be kept in mind. The basic principles and techniques of assessment and psychotherapy are largely transferable when working with older adults, even in more advanced old age, with or without the presence of major health or cognitive concerns. Older adults, as NP likes to remind her students, are not a different species.

On the other hand, the much higher base rates of neurological disorders (especially the dementias) and of medical comorbidities, can make working with older clients different to working with younger adults. Normal aging changes may make working with very old clients different. The pervasiveness of stereotypes of older adults in our society can also lead psychologists to perceive differences that are not present. Paradoxically, it seems that a moderately high level of expertise in geropsychology may be needed to treat older clients the way one would treat a younger client. It can certainly require some expertise to know whether specialized knowledge and skills are needed with an older client.

Thus, while the basic tenets of psychological assessment and treatment remain valid in this population, it is also considered important that they be augmented by knowledge of, and sensitivity to, the experience of aging, with its many changes for the individual and the context in which older adults live, work, and play. This perspective led to the creation of the Contextual, Adult

Lifespan Theory for Adapting Psychotherapy (CALTAP) model (Figure 1.1) as a way of conceptualizing applied psychological work with clients within a lifespan perspective. The model has been described and placed in the context of the research literature elsewhere (Knight and Lee 2008; Knight and Poon 2008), but in brief, the model is transdiagnostic, as well as transtheoretical in nature. It was designed to be useful in providing a perspective from which to view potentially puzzling aspects of the client's, or indeed the therapist's, behaviors and reactions, rather than relying on a prescriptive method to guide the therapeutic encounter.

In this chapter, our main focus is to describe the implications of the CALTAP model in clinical practice, with a focus on how it can guide both the psychologist and the client in how they think about aging. This is useful because, in our experience, although psychological assessment and intervention principles are similar to those used in younger cohorts, the aging process can affect, often in a subtle manner, the nature and reaction of the patient to the presenting problem, and may also impact the therapeutic process itself. Therapists may have unexamined feelings about their own aging, which can affect their ability to work effectively with an older client. Irrespective of the therapist's knowledge and comfort with aging, it can often be the case that the client has not worked out how their own experience and reactions to aging may be affecting their feelings,

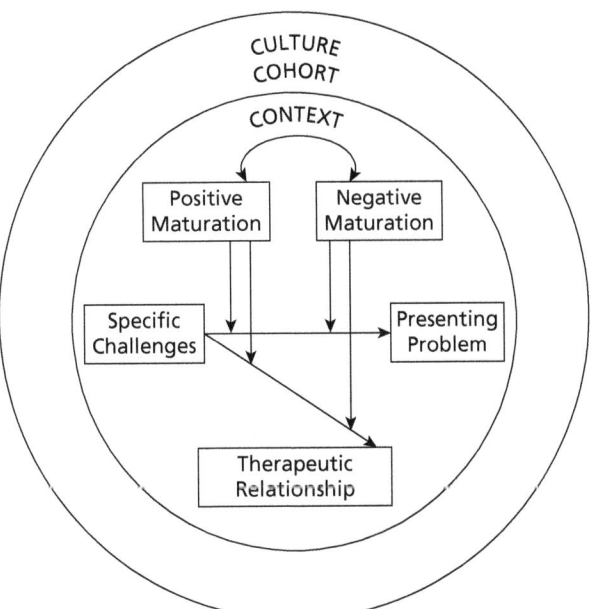

Fig. 1.1 CALTAP—Contextual Lifespan Theory for Adapting Psychotherapy.

thoughts, and behaviors. We will begin by explaining how the CALTAP model can guide the psychologist's thinking when approaching work with the client. Later in the chapter, we will explore how the model can be used to help foster relevant self-reflection on the aging process by the older clients themselves.

CALTAP and developmental aging

Starting from the center of Figure 1.1, one assertion of CALTAP is that the major differences between psychological work with older adults and younger age-groups arise in the assessment process and understanding the presenting problem, on the one hand, and on the therapeutic relationship itself, on the other. The techniques and principles of therapy with older adults differ little from work with younger clients when the problems and their contexts are similar. Accurate understanding of older adults' presenting problems, however, is complex for many reasons, including the need to have an accurate understanding of normal developmental aging and other sources of age differences, as well as the ability to identify effects of specific challenges, including late life illnesses, side effects of treatments, and to recognize the neurocognitive impairments common at older ages. Without such an understanding, one may gain only a superficial understanding of the problem, or one may underestimate the complexity of the interplay between important factors. For example, lack of recognition of how medication side effects or mild cognitive impairment (MCI) might affect mood, or how activities of daily living impairments can lead to inaccurate assessment, which might derail not only rapport with the older adult, but also the development of effective intervention strategies.

On the whole, we think that changes in cognitive and emotional functioning due to developmental aging have a relatively minor influence on assessment and therapy with older adults. The need for tools that take account of age differences and the need for appropriate normative data from which to interpret test data have more of an impact on what might be conceived of as the more technical aspects of assessment and the meaningful interpretation of the data obtained. As we will begin to explore in this chapter, these age differences are typically more related to social context, cohort differences, and interacting influences of culture and cohort, rather than to developmental aging per se.

With respect to negative aspects of developmental aging, normal changes with cognitive aging may require some slowing of the pace of the therapeutic conversation. Changes in both the speed of processing and working memory may move the introduction of new ideas to a slower pace as well—one or two at a time, rather than multiple parts of complex ideas at once. When doing an assessment, it is better to tell patients directly and unambiguously what assessment data are for and who will receive reports. In undertaking treatment, it is probably also better to tell clients what you want them to know, rather than relying on inferential reasoning on their part. That said, these effects of cognitive aging are small (albeit generally noticeable at more advanced ages), and individual differences among older adults are generally larger. As always, one needs to be attentive to specific needs of the individual client.

On the positive side of developmental aging, most older adults benefit from experience and develop expertise in multiple life domains. They develop skills in their work, in the tasks of living, in their avocations, in relationships with friends, rivals, and lovers, as well as some expertise in the workings of the families that they are part of and the ones they know through friends. Many older adults develop implicit psychologies of interpersonal relationships and of family life that are quite helpful in therapy. As people age, they also accumulate multiple examples of how a situation may develop or how a person may react, and so generally have wider, richer experiential schema that can be used in therapy to solve current problems or reawaken coping strategies.

Emotional changes with aging also tend to work in favor of therapy. Older adults tend to be better at emotion regulation and to have better coping skills, resources that can be tapped during the therapy process. When seeking help from psychologists, older persons are often overwhelmed by the specific challenges of later life—chronic illness and disability, grief, and caregiving for frail family members. Therapists, especially those with knowledge and skills in working with clients who are facing these challenges, can greatly assist their clients' understanding of these issues, and their ability to use the coping skills and emotional regulation strategies acquired over several decades of adult life.

There are, of course, exceptions, for example, people who have never coped well or regulated their emotions well, and have not benefited greatly from experience as they have aged. Enduring problems with coping and integrating experience are often associated with personality disorders (see Chapter 10). For these clients, the process of therapy may move more slowly and involve more new skill acquisition, rather than reawakening of prior skills and experiences. It is also worth noting that some older adults with psychological disorders experience problems for the first time in late life, but people with ongoing or recurring psychological problems also grow older. The distinction between late and earlier life onset disorders is of importance with all of the diagnoses considered in this book.

One observation about the effects of developmental aging on the therapy relationship is that both negative and positive effects of aging can affect the usual practice of psychology. In our view, these effects are mostly in the influence they have on the therapist or the therapeutic relationship, rather than the effects of developmental aging on the client. This lifespan developmental view can also be used in therapy to give the client a clearer view of what aspects of their life are, and are not, due to growing older. Separating the effects of aging, cohort differences, social context, illness, and anxiety and depression, for example, provides a more accurate and optimistic understanding of a client's life than either the client or the therapist attributing it all to the client just being old.

On the other hand, being faced with a client who has much greater life experience than the psychologist and who has better coping skills (although they may currently be overwhelmed by challenges that are more common in later life) is also daunting. This positive side of aging compels the psychologist to consider what they have to offer the client. The obvious answer is psychological expertise and skills, but many fall into the trap of assuming, at least implicitly, that we are offering clients our own life experience. Working with older clients is a useful corrective to this unhelpful stance, which is dangerous with clients of any age, since the client's needs are rarely a match for the psychologist's specific individual life experience.

Specific challenges of later life

The generally positive view of aging alluded to in "CALTAP and developmental aging" is based on normal to successful aging and does not take into account diseases that are age-linked or simply more common in later life. In the CALTAP model, "specific challenges" refers to problems that arise more frequently in later life than in earlier adulthood, such as chronic illness and disability, bereavement, caregiving. These problems are not only found with older adults, but are more common in later life, and a psychologist who sees a lot of older adults will need the necessary knowledge and skills in working with these problems. A key concept here is the specificity of the challenges and the assumption that change, rehabilitation, or adaptation are always possible. This view of the challenges of later life is in contrast to the traditional adaptation to generic losses stance that used to characterize work with older adults.

Neurocognitive disorders are much more common in late life and have serious to eventually devastating effects on cognition in those who are affected. Chronic physical illnesses of all kinds are more common in late life. They range from the asymptomatic through the annoying, which require some changes in lifestyle, to the disabling. In some cases, these late life diseases are life-altering for both the older adult, and their family and friends, and some are terminal with predictable prognoses.

Issues in working with chronic illness and disability are addressed in Chapter 6 on psychological aspects of physical illness. Bereavement is addressed in

Chapter 3 on depression, since depression is the common psychological disorder associated with complicated bereavement, and caregiving issues are addressed in Chapter 5 on dementia, since much work with dementia caregivers involves helping them gain the knowledge and skills related to caring for the person with dementia. The rest of psychological interventions with caregivers would generally be addressing depression and anxiety arising from the stresses of the caregiving experience for some caregivers.

In general, while differences due to developmental aging alone are important to understand, we find that other aspects of the CALTAP model, particularly the influences of social contexts and cohort differences, are typically even more influential. Cohort differences often also interact with cultural differences in complex ways. In the next section, we explore the influence of social context on making psychological work with older clients distinctive.

Social contexts

Moving to the innermost of the background context effects in the CALTAP model (Figure 1.1), we note that one source of age differences among clients that lies outside the client is the social context in which the client is living. Lawton (1980) noted early in the development of clinical geropsychology that the environment is a major influence on much of the behavior that we think of as specific to old age. Thus, context is an important aspect of the CALTAP model and is depicted in Figure 1.1 as the next ring of influence out from the center in the model. Context is also an important element of training to work with older adults (or gaining experience to help work with older clients in the case of experienced therapists), in that it is useful for the psychologist to have some direct observer experience of the social ecology of programs and living situations for older adults in the area in which they work, whether it occurs within a program of formal study or is self-directed.

Age-segregated environments are especially pervasive in their influence on older adults' behavior and emotions. Understanding the levels of care in the 24-hour care system for older adults, their entrance and exit requirements, based on functional ability and behavior, the organization of the staff, the shared rules of operation, and so forth is one important aspect of this knowledge. It is also important to understand that each specific organization will have its own social flavor and organizational culture. Staff may be friendly and flexible, or reserved and authoritarian. Residents may have significant input into decision making or only a token input. Persons with severe neurocognitive impairment may be in a separate section or may be integrated with cognitively intact residents.

Age-segregated independent living for older adults can be even more diverse, with many of the distinctions among places dependent on the residents who are living there at any one time. Organizationally, such residences vary across several dimensions including:

- whether or not they are part of a larger facility that includes assisted living and/or nursing home level care;
- whether they provide subsidized rents based on income;
- whether they are intentionally age segregated;
- whether they are naturally occurring senior communities, i.e., some neighborhoods, housing developments, apartment buildings, and mobile home parks may not be age segregated by design and policy, but simply have become senior communities with the aging of residents. Sometimes this is maintained by natural selection, but can be influenced artificially to maintain age-based selection of newcomers.

These communities each have their own social ecology as well. Some are tolerant of residents' increasing functional impairments over time, while others may encourage more disabled residents to move elsewhere. Some provide emotional support for residents who have lost a loved one or who are caring for a disabled family member; others ignore problems in their community in order to hold onto an image of a community comprised of active, successfully aging seniors. Some welcome young visitors, whereas others have rules against extended visits by younger family members, including children and grandchildren. Some enforce a rigid rule that older adults must divest themselves of their pets upon entry, while others are more welcoming of animal companions.

Understanding these environments is important in comprehending their influence on clients, and their role in shaping clients' behavior and emotions. Clients living in age-segregated environments are often wrestling with adjusting to life in them and understanding their place in the social milieu there. The older adult may not have anticipated the impact of this shift in living environment on their sense of self, as well as their feelings and behaviors. Showing some understanding of what the environment is like is helpful in building a rapport with the client. Understanding the nature of the environment and its effects on the client is also important in considering assessment approaches and feedback to staff in such institutions (Pachana et al. 2010a). Being able to offer sound advice about how best to maneuver in the environment, and about what is changeable and what is not likely to change can be helpful in therapy. At times, clients will be actively trying to understand what level of care they need now and in the near future. A good sense of what the levels of care are and what an individual client may want to focus on in choosing an individual facility can be very useful in providing support in the client's decision-making process.

Bringing this understanding to family consultations on issues of appropriate levels of care for the older client is also a useful skill. The older adult's family members often have misunderstandings about the nature of care and of the social ecology of age-segregated living environments. This can lead to trying out facilities that are either more restrictive than the client needs or wants, or to trying out places that do not provide as much supportive care as is needed. Even moving to an age-segregated independent living community may be somewhat perplexing to family and friends, and may lead to inaccurate assumptions about the person's motivations for doing so. A rather common error with respect to relocation to assisted living centers is assuming that moving an older family member into a care environment will solve issues related to social isolation and loneliness. Whether this works or not is likely to depend on the programs and organizational culture of the specific facility, and also on how outgoing the older family member is or might like to be. Family members may also have different levels of comfort in discussing residential care needs and issues, and this may have particularly deleterious consequences in terms of care planning when dysfunction has characterized family relationships in the past.

Older clients living in age-segregated settings are likely to draw upon their experience of that environment and what is happening with other residents in it to understand their own aging process, both what has happened to date and what to expect in the future. It can be a helpful corrective to distressing perceptions to help the client understand the selection factors that brought the residents together in that setting—level of functional ability, desire or need for assistance, etc. Then, the client can be guided to explore both how they are like, and unlike, other residents. It can also be useful to discuss the organizational characteristics of the setting and how they influence their experience. What is the management style of key administrators? How much input do residents have in shaping activities? All of these elements shape a perception of day-to-day life experience there, which is partly independent of aging.

A common issue in living in age-segregated communities is the relatively greater frequency of hospitalizations and deaths. Clients can find this distressing, of course. It helps to explore these feelings, acknowledge them as part of living in that setting, and help the client think clearly and realistically about their individual level of risk for serious illness and probable life expectancy.

The extent to which the psychologist's practice focuses on clients who live in age-segregated environments and/or in consulting with the staff of those facilities shapes the nature of the practice, and of the knowledge and skills that will be needed. Working in long-term care facilities requires detailed knowledge of the organizational structure of the facilities and skills in consultation in those environments. It will, in general, also mean working with a specific subpopulation of older adults, typically, those who are less functional physically and cognitively than those in independent living settings. It is useful to maintain awareness of the distinctive nature of this work and it is important to realize that the clients seen in these settings are not representative of aging as a whole. When the professional working with older adults loses sight of this distinction, they are likely to start assuming that all older adults end up with severe impairments and so develop a negative view of the aging process, including of their own aging. This negativity is likely to affect both work with older clients and the professional's job satisfaction and attitude toward their own aging.

Community-based programs for older adults also have their own social ecologies and shape the aging experience of those who are active participants in them. Senior recreation centers, senior multipurpose centers, meal sites, and clubs that focus on older adults all have their own rules, social cliques, and somewhat shared attitudes toward what aging is like. Knowing something about the local range of what is available in the community and being able to help older clients think through how they match with such groups, and what is important to them in seeking out such social settings, is also useful in working with older clients.

An important element of this thinking through the social context of their living situation starts with helping clients weigh the pros and cons of whether they want to be in age-segregated or age-integrated environments. Society in general, and younger family members in particular, can either automatically encourage or discourage older adults to think of community activities and living environments that are age segregated (based perhaps on their perceptions of the older adult in question, as well as anxieties about their own aging). Many older adults will prefer settings that involve a wider age range and may be biased against age-segregated settings. Others will flourish in such environments. An active exploration of these decisions is useful in working with older clients, regardless of the final decision made.

With regard to such decisions, and many others involving older adults, the emphasis of the CALTAP model, and our approach, is on attention to individual differences, which are at least as large in older as in young adulthood, and on careful consideration of the person–environment fit. In principle, this focus should come naturally to psychologists, but society as a whole engages in considerable stereotypical thinking about older adults as a relatively homogenous category of people. Unfortunately, psychologists themselves may fall prey to negative stereotypes and biases with respect to aging, particularly with respect to work with specific populations and in specific settings such as nursing homes (James and Haley 1995; Koder and Helmes 2006). Supervision can play a vital role in pointing out such attitudes (see Chapter 11 for more details about the role of supervision in working with older clients).

Cohort influences

The larger contextual background influences in the CALTAP model are cohort and culture. They are in the same circle of the model (Figure 1.1) because of their roughly equivalent and pervasive influences, and because, as we will see throughout the book, they often interact with one another in setting the background historical–cultural influences in the client's life and the ways that the older client differs from those clients born into a later era with differing cultural influences.

Within lifespan developmental psychology and gerontology, *cohort* refers to a group of people born within a certain time span who share a sense of group identity. Thus, the term is roughly similar to the way that generation is used by the popular media in referring to the Baby Boomer generation, Generation X, Millennials, etc. Cohort distinctions will vary across cultures and countries, based on their individual socio-historical histories. In several East Asian countries (e.g., Japan, South Korea, Taiwan, Hong Kong), a key cohort difference is between those earlier born cohorts who remember when the country was still a developing, poor, and more agricultural society, and those later borns who only know the country as a wealthy, high tech society. In Spain, a key distinction is between cohorts who experienced the Franco years and those later borns with no direct memory or experience of those years. It is important not to think of cohorts only along national lines, but also important historical lines; across cultures, gay and lesbian individuals of different cohorts will have various experiences with the process of coming out; earlier cohorts will have vivid memories of when their attraction to same sex partners was illegal and had repercussions that later born cohorts will not fully appreciate (Kimmel 2014).

In this context, the emphasis is on the concept that when we make age comparisons at any one point in time, we are typically confusing differences due to developmental aging with differences between cohorts. In clinical geropsychology, it can be useful to take the client's birth year and add 20 as a rough indicator of when they became an adult and formed their sense of identity, which was shaped in some large part by cohort experiences. The therapist can then consider what cohort that is and what the socio-historical influences were on young adults of that era. It is also useful to think and speak of differences between people of different ages that are due to cohort influences as distinctions between "earlier born" and "later born" cohorts, since saying "older" and "younger" cohort perpetuates the focus on age as the key dimension of difference.

One way of emphasizing the importance of the distinction is to consider that changes due to aging mean that when you reach the age your parents are now, you will be like your parents in those ways. On the other hand, if the differences between you and your parents are cohort differences, when you reach your parents' age, you will be like you are now, only older. As Baby Boomers become older, they will process information more slowly and have more trouble ignoring distracting noises in the environment. They are, however, unlikely to develop a fondness for Big Band swing, World War II era music, or to take on the World War II generation's social and moral values. Thus, within the CALTAP model, a clear idea of potential cohort influences is highlighted as important in working effectively with older adults.

There are cohort differences in many areas of importance to psychologists working with older clients. Across birth cohorts from the early twentieth century to the latter part of it, successive cohorts tend to be better at inferential reasoning and in visuospatial functions (Schaie 2013). Mathematical abilities rise and fall across cohorts, demonstrating that not all cohort effects are linear, nor do they all favor later born cohorts (Schaie 2013). Similarly, there are cohort, as well as age differences in personality (McCrae et al. 1999; Smits et al. 2011). Finally, there are some cohort differences in the incidence and prevalence of specific mental health disorders. For example, cohorts born after World War II have higher levels of depression and of most other mental disorders (Koenig et al. 1994), but this has appeared to level out somewhat over time (Spiers et al. 2011; Kessler et al. 2005a).

There tend to be cohort effects in political orientations, and in social and moral values as well. There are also generally cohort differences in response to new developments in technology and new social changes. These differences can shape an individual's sense of being old and also shape the perception that later born cohorts have of the earlier born. In the USA, attitudes toward gay rights and the legalization of marijuana show strong cohort effects, for example. In Europe, attitudes toward migrant populations show strong cohort effects, while in Australia and New Zealand, it is the attitudes toward indigenous peoples that show strong cohort effects. In Asia, cohorts are sometimes divided by their embrace of Western ways of thinking or behaving, particularly in family matters. While new digital technologies are transforming the way that everyone communicates and tracks information, later born cohorts have a native fluency and acceptance of these technologies, whereas earlier born cohorts may range from non-participants, through "second language" awkwardness, to "non-native fluency."

Being able to understand older clients from their own cohort perspective is similar in many ways to being able to understand other clients who are different from us—people of the other gender, people with a different sexual orientation, different social class, different cultural backgrounds, different work experiences, and so forth. As in other cases, it is equally important with cohort differences to understand the client's own perspective on the influence of these larger social effects on them, rather than relying only on one's knowledge or stereotypes about persons from that cohort. For example, Baby Boomers tend to be portrayed in the popular media in the USA as having all opposed the Vietnam War, but clearly there are also members of that generation who supported the war. Exploring the client's sense of how they fit into and may have rebelled against, the socially constructed general experience of their cohort is an important aspect of understanding the whole person. Thus, among other things, working with earlier born clients requires that the psychologist be able to rise above their own cohort perspective. Without that ability, people working with earlier born clients often have a tendency to side with relatives of clients from their own cohort, whose values and perspectives they may more easily share.

In psychological assessment and therapy, there may well be a need to adapt materials used with earlier born clients to employ simpler language and to avoid psychological jargon due to lower educational levels in general and to less likelihood of having had exposure to psychology constructs or coursework in particular. This adaptation is expected to be less needed as the Baby Boomers move into the older adult years than it has been in the last few decades. Of course, as with any group-based recommendation, one needs to consider the individual client's educational level. It would be pointless and might damage rapport to simplify conversation and materials with an earlier born client who has advanced education, for example.

Similarly, it may be useful to adapt aspects of therapy to the older client. For example, if homework is given as part of therapy it may be useful *not* to refer to it as homework, as this may unintentionally imply a power or knowledge differential between therapist and patient that in an older client may interfere with good rapport (Kazantzis et al. 2003). Careful attention to the process of therapy is warranted, for example, taking extra time if needed to explain the rationale and structures employed in cognitive-behavioral approaches (e.g., agenda setting; Secker et al. 2004). This also will afford the therapist the chance to discuss any potential resistance or uncertainty about aspects of the therapy early on, potentially heading off problems before they have a chance to develop.

In a case used (with the client's permission) in teaching psychotherapy with older adults, the client was living with her daughter and granddaughters, and was uncomfortable with them having boyfriends staying overnight at times. Discussions of the case involved having the students explore whose side they were inclined to take in this difference of moral viewpoints and why. The client herself understood her viewpoint as old fashioned, and as having been developed decades ago in the context of a small town in a more conservative state in the USA. She was still uncomfortable, however, with the later born family members' behavior. Students were asked to consider who should decide what the house rules should be about overnight stays of boyfriends. The discussions helped students think through their own cohort-based biases and the psychopolitical aspects of working out such differences in values within a family. In fact, some of the change in the client's feeling about the situation grew out of the therapist taking her viewpoint on the difference and exploring whether she wanted to ask for changes in what the others were doing.

Indeed, part of working with older clients is helping them understand their own aging. This understanding, in turn, often depends on sorting out what is due to aging and what is due to cohort effects. The client in this teaching case felt better about seeing her viewpoint as due to cohort effects, rather than as more evidence of being an old woman. In time, she came to decide that, actually, she was envious of the freedom that women in later cohorts had to divorce and that she wished she had felt able to divorce her husband (who had died before she became a client in our clinic). Such self-reflection is useful in therapy; the CALTAP model can help therapists facilitate such self-reflection in their clients.

Families are always comprised of people from different cohorts, of course. The cohort perspective is often helpful in giving family members a different way to think about their differences than age- and relationship-based attributes. Interpreting differences among family members in the way they see current family issues, as well as differences in their social, moral, and political views, as cohort differences is often helpful in taking the conversation out of an old versus young framework and also in separating the disagreements from family relationship issues. One woman in her 80s was seen with her daughter from time to time to help with conflict in their relationship. Both found some relief from the tension in their disagreements from seeing them as partly rooted in being from different cohorts with distinct ideas about how women handle problems, the importance of career, and differing ideas about health and how to relate to doctors. The disagreements continued, but the broader context for why they were happening took away some of the emotional impact of feeling that the mother/daughter did not respect the other's viewpoint. As lifespans continue to increase and increasing numbers of generations interact, perhaps at times under one roof, opportunities for both conflict and increased understanding will grow.

Cultural context

Cultural beliefs and values shape the way all of us see our worlds and construct our relationships with others. While we have some consciously held ideas about our own culture and those of others, many of these ideas are stereotypes and can lead us astray in developing an understanding of individual clients. In many ways, the essence of cultural differences is one person assuming "Of course you'd do X this way," while it would never occur to the other to do X that way.

Specific influences of culture in psychological work with older adults focus, in part, on the meaning of being older. Is aging viewed as mainly positive or negative? How much respect is due to older adults and how is it expressed? How much authority do older adults have over their adult (and often middle-aged to young-old (people aged 65-75)) children? In some cultures, the oldest male makes decisions about key family issues and may also act as a judge in settling disputes within the family. Psychologists may become involved when the oldest male has severe neurocognitive impairment, and the family is still obeying and bringing disputes to him, with resulting family dysfunction.

Family structures are shaped by culture as well. Is the basic concept of family the nuclear family, or is it extended and multigenerational? Is family determined mainly by genetic and legal ties or does it include fictive kin? When older members need help and care, who is the culturally designated care provider? Is that care seen as an automatic seamless part of life, or do individual needs and goals of family members take priority? In much of Western White culture, the expected order of probable primary caregivers is spouse, daughter, then daughter-in-law. In East Asian cultures with Confucian values, the oldest son's wife is the primary caregiver, and the designation is so clear that secondary support is unlikely. Among African Americans, there is more likelihood of secondary and tertiary caregivers, and of flexible changing of these roles over time. In Australian Aboriginal cultures, care is the responsibility of the extended family and, to a certain extent, the community as a whole, although this may break down if the older person is forced by circumstance to move away from traditional living spaces and familiar lines of support. If a family has been transplanted to a different cultural context, there may be differences in accommodation and assimilation among family members within the new cultural context, which can also cause tension; this will be discussed further.

Some clients' understanding of respect for older persons includes not being able to acknowledge the severe cognitive decline resulting from neurocognitive impairment and resulting changes in the parent's role in the family. A sensitive discussion of the medical and neuroscience view of what is happening, with ample time for the client to absorb the information and explain to the therapist what is acceptable in the medical view, and what is unacceptable and why, is an important element of working through this dilemma. It is important to see if it is conceivable in the client's culture that an older person with an illness can still be respected. Then, can an older person with an illness of the brain still be respected? Is there a stigma associated with having such a disorder in the person's culture? The therapist may realize in such discussions that their own culture treats older family members with brain impairments in disrespectful ways, perhaps, by ignoring their presence and talking about them as if they were not there, or otherwise treating them as non-persons.

In general, a good working stance for the psychologist is to assume ignorance of the client's culture and explore their understanding of the client's culture and the role of those cultural influences in shaping the focal problem of therapy, as well as their feelings about it. In most cases, the therapist will work within the client's cultural framework to resolve the client's problems. Instances may arise when there could be a direct conflict between the psychological understanding of what to do and the client's culture. It may be appropriate to explore that conflict in terms such as "Psychologists in general would say that you really need to talk directly with your mother about this" and so enlist the client in sorting out how to communicate about difficult or taboo issues, or find another workable solution.

It is worth noting that culture and cohort differences interact. Over time, societal views about what constitutes a distinctive minority culture change. In the USA in the early to mid-twentieth century, many European immigrant groups had very distinct cultural identities and several suffered from active discrimination. In much of the USA in the late twentieth to early twenty-first centuries, these groups have merged into being generically White. Although still a distinct minority, African Americans born early enough to remember segregation and the more pervasive openly hostile racism of the mid-twentieth century and earlier have a different sense of their culture than those born later, who only know the post-civil rights era USA. Shifting demographics in the USA mean that what is the "dominant" culture, either in terms of power or numbers of influence, may shift significantly over the next decade.

These interactions of cohort and culture play out in more intimate relationships within recently immigrated families in which cohort differences overlap with the cultural differences as the later born generations in the family acculturate within the adopted country. Helping members of the family place their parent–child disagreements in the context of the different experiences each of them has had in acculturation within the new country and how their different cohort background shaped their acculturation can reduce the felt conflict, and the more nuanced understanding can lead to compromise solutions.

For example, recently immigrated families (i.e., where the older adults are immigrants) can have conflicts over expectations regarding who provides care that also involves the value of respect for the elders and of family unity. It can be helpful to review, with older family members, what their own experience of caring for older family members was like and how they felt about it. Fairly often, the remembered reality was difficult, rooted in obligation, and resented. It is also useful to explore the history of immigration and their hopes for the younger members of the family. Much of the time there is considerable pride in the success and in some of the aspects of the younger family members' acculturation. This, at least, places the current conflicts in a context of "you wanted them to be successful here, and maybe they changed in more ways than you planned." For the younger members, it can remove the differences with the parent from the parent–child conflict framework to an understanding of how the parent's world view is distinct from their own due to their differing experiences with both the nation of origin and the new nation that they have moved into. Both generations can then consider how to negotiate these cultural differences.

Summary

In brief, CALTAP argues that there are a number of ways that psychological work with older adults is different from work with younger adults. The theme is, however, that relatively few of these differences are due to developmental aging. Most of the differences are due to the specific social contexts in which some older adults live, to the fact that they were born earlier and grew up in a different era and so a distinct sociocultural context, that they and their family may also have been shaped by a different cultural context.

In general, BK suggests that psychologists working with an older client pose the question "What would I do if this client were 40 rather than 70?" and then consider why one would do anything differently with the older client. There are sometimes reasons to do something differently, but the reasons are seldom due to age. They may relate to the social context, to cohort differences, to interactions of culture and cohort. They may be due to the presence of comorbid medical disorders or to the presence of a dementia. One would also treat a younger adult with these disorders differently than one without them.

In the Chapter 2, the complexity of the assessment process with older persons is considered in more detail. This complexity is affected by the CALTAP influences discussed in this chapter and is especially driven by the specific challenges of later life. The much higher prevalence of neurocognitive disorders in later life makes some skill in recognizing the late-life dementias essential to work with older clients. The very high prevalence of chronic illnesses and disability in later life make comorbidity of medical and mental health problems the rule, rather than the exception, which also complicates assessment, as well as interpretation of results. The manner in which results are shared with family members, other health care professionals, and the client is an important skill, and may influence coping and care plans going forward.

Chapter 2

CALTAP in assessment approaches and strategies

Introduction to CALTAP in assessment approaches and strategies

Clinical practice with older persons, including clinical assessment of older patients, requires a lifespan approach (Donders and Hunter 2010; Laidlaw and Pachana 2009). For the clinical psychologist, it will be important in their work with older clients to ascertain which instruments best reflect what they want to get out of an initial assessment or what may be most helpful to the client in monitoring progress over time. For a psychologist with more of a neuropsychological specialization, working with older patients necessitates knowing the full spectrum of tests available to assist with referral questions that may be more specific to this age group, including particular tests for conditions such as dementia.

Often assessment, whether in the course of general psychological assessment and intervention, or in the context of a more extensive and focused neuropsychological evaluation, is relatively similar between older and younger clients, as has been suggested in Chapter 1 with respect to interventions. For example, the tests given to ascertain the extent and nature of memory difficulties, or to understand the patient's experience of low mood, may not differ between a 35-year-old and a 75-year-old person. However, there are some aspects of the older client and their context, which might trigger an assessment approach that includes more geriatric-specific tests, selection of specific tests to augment a more routine screening battery, or test result interpretations that are more explicitly guided by the age of the client. This is particularly true of older persons of advanced age, or where the state of the person's cognition, physical health, and/or mental health is such that assessment must be brief and targeted. Specific contextual issues (such as low educational attainment or very advanced age), as well as particular diagnoses or disorders may favor the use of a test specifically developed for older adults with that disorder or diagnosis. The better normative data and potentially superior psychometric properties such a test offers over a test with less specific normative data, or one originally designed and evaluated with younger adults, means that it will have greater utility. In longer neuropsychological examinations, careful consideration may also need to be given to how the neuropsychological assessment is structured, and how feedback is presented to the older client, their family, and to the referral source. Again, this is particularly true for clients of more advanced age, and with more severe or complex physical health concerns or multiple comorbidities of a medical and/or psychiatric nature. In all cases, in order to be able to meaningfully interpret test results from older persons, attention must be paid to past levels of performance, and relevant social and developmental history.

This chapter aims to present an overview of important issues with respect to testing approaches and choices in the context of working with older clients. We do this in order to meld together the assessment and therapy aspects of working with older clients. Working with older adults simultaneously necessitates a greater appreciation for the potential for cognitive dysfunction to appear, as well as a strong recognition that aging per se is not usually accompanied by significant cognitive decline. Furthermore, the geropsychologist is aware that cognitive declines later in life, as is the case in younger clients, may reflect psychiatric or medical conditions, or may signal the presence of a progressive neurocognitive disorder. With the greater prevalence of neurocognitive disorders in late life, assessment may frequently develop along more neuropsychological lines in older adult clients. Given this, we have pulled from both neuropsychotherapy approaches and from the CALTAP model in order to suggest sound assessment approaches to working with older adults in clinical practice.

Specifically, we explore how the incorporation of a systematic lifespan contextual approach (CALTAP; Knight and Poon 2008) can enhance all aspects of assessment approaches with older adults, in a similar way to that of therapeutic interventions with this population, as covered in Chapter 1. Adopting an approach like CALTAP can positively influence a range of potential aspects of the assessment process, including:

- conceptualizing the case;
- test selection and administration;
- interpretation of results;
- feedback to the patient, family, and referral sources;
- constructing a report;
- follow through on rehabilitation recommendations and referrals to other health professionals.

In particular, the influence of context, cohort group, and culture are highlighted where appropriate below; the potential influence of the client's own view of their maturational processes, as well as the therapist's views of the aging process, are also discussed. This lifespan approach to assessment processes and practices has the capacity to improve the clinician's working relationship with older patients, their families, and formal and informal caregivers, as well as their own experience in the role of assessor (see Figure 1.1 for a graphical representation of the CALTAP model).

Adopting CALTAP as a conceptual framework works with a broad range of neuropsychological assessment frameworks and theoretical orientations (e.g., a hypothesis testing, process approach to testing or a more fixed battery approach to assessment). Indeed, within the specific contexts of assessment of older clients, CALTAP serves as an organizing principle of potential vital utility, particularly for trainee neuropsychologists and more experienced clinicians with limited experience in working with older adult populations.

The neuropsychotherapy approach

Clinical assessment practices have not necessarily been theory-driven with respect to the totality of the interaction with the patient, particularly in the case of older clients. In neuropsychology, there have been theory-driven approaches to the assessment of patients—for example, the Edith Kaplan process approach (Kaplan 1988) versus the Luria Nebraska battery approach (Golden and Freshwater 2001; James et al. 1983) to neuropsychological assessment, and specific rehabilitation strategies, for example, with respect to memory rehabilitation/enhancement approaches (e.g., Camp 2006).

Judd (1999) offered the closest to a melding of a lifespan clinical psychology and neuropsychology approach to assessment and intervention with patients. His theoretical approach, which he labeled neuropsychotherapy (Judd 1999), pointed out the need for clinical psychology knowledge about a broader formulation of cases and empirical intervention strategies to be paired with neuropsychological assessment and rehabilitation techniques for best outcomes. He offered numerous examples of this in action. With respect to older adults, he pointed to the high rates of comorbidity between psychiatric conditions, such as depression and cognitive decline, and progressive neurological conditions, and suggested that these needed to be assessed and treated in tandem, using best practices in geropsychology (e.g., multidisciplinary approaches wherever possible) in order to achieve good outcomes.

Similarly, the need for closer collaboration with patients in realizing the most efficacious, as well as satisfying outcomes for both the patient and the neuropsychologist have been explored by a variety of authors (Gorske 2008; Gorske and Smith 2009; Ruff 2003). The slight variation on neuropsychotherapy, known as therapeutic neuropsychotherapy (Finn 2007; Fischer and Finn 2008; Gorske 2008; Gorske and Smith 2009) is growing as an area of research and practice interest across a variety of settings and contexts. Therapeutic neuropsychology espouses the idea that neuropsychological assessment is a collaborative exercise between the patient and the psychologist, and that part of the goal of the assessment is always to answer the specific queries of the patient. This approach requires that the neuropsychologist consult more extensively about the patient's own goals, fears, and hopes, with respect to what could be achieved by such an assessment. This approach uncovers potential misgivings about both the testing and its outcomes, as well as assisting the neuropsychologist in structuring both the assessment and the feedback from the assessment to best match patient goals, which are sometimes lost in the service of "answering the referral."

This stance is perhaps of particular value when working with older clients requiring neuropsychological assessment. Older adults may inevitably feel judged during cognitive assessments; many in this cohort, particularly the generations born before and during World War II, are less well educated and, more importantly, less experienced with formal testing situations than later born cohorts, including the current Baby Boomer cohort. There is some literature to suggest that the experience of feeling evaluated and judged during assessment procedures directly and negatively affects scores on these tests (Abrams et al. 2006; Hess et al. 2003; Hess and Hinson 2006; Rahhal et al. 2001). Anxiety in general may translate into poorer performance on testing, at the very least, and can lead to considerable distress. However, it is likely that this reaction to testing will not be as strong in later born cohorts.

Age-specific fears and anxieties can magnify this effect. Similarly, older adults may legitimately wonder what their test results are being used for. Ideas about having their home, finances or other liberties curtailed as a result of testing are real possibilities, and the nature of testing and with whom results will be shared, as well as possible implications of testing (e.g., on driving), should be discussed before testing commences.

While researchers and practitioners writing about neuropsychotherapy and therapeutic neuropsychology have noted the particular importance of these approaches for the care of older adults, neither has attempted specifically to systematically incorporate a lifespan approach. Moreover, these approaches have been targeted primarily at neuropsychologists carrying out more extensive and targeted assessments on a broad range of clients, rather than clinical psychologists or neuropsychologists incorporating testing of older adults into their everyday practice.

The importance of the clinical interview

Most clinicians in practice have an interview format that may be more or less structured. Ideally, the clinical interview for clients at any age is a combination of structured or semi-structured instruments, paired with probes of pertinent information guided by clinical judgment and the client's presentation. A structured interview assists in making the picture of how the patient is experiencing their symptoms as clear as possible to both the patient and the therapist. Moreover, this picture now can be compared with subsequent therapy sessions in order to gauge progress in therapy, or lack thereof, and to aid in the recognition of the emergence of any new symptoms. Although in clinical practice many clinicians may choose not to use some of the more lengthy structured or semi-structured interviews, the basic notion that structure, completeness, and some reference to normative data are key components of best practice, should be borne in mind.

Often a clinician's primary assessment strategy is the initial clinical interview. There is no substitute for a careful interview, one which simultaneously gathers pertinent data, acquaints the clinician with the patient's unique circumstances, and ideally, forms a solid base for building rapport. A poorly executed clinical interview of an older adult, in contrast, can interfere with rapport building, miss critical information necessary for selecting (or possibly deleting) tests from the clinician's usual go-to instruments, as well as for interpreting said instruments. With older clients there is an increased risk of missing vital information, for example, important effects of medical conditions or medications that have not been asked about. An incomplete interview of an older client has the potential to steer the assessment and/or the intervention in the wrong direction.

There are a variety of structured and semi-structured diagnostic interview tools appropriate for use with older adults. These include the Structured Clinical Interview (SCID; First et al. 1996a), the Composite International Diagnostic Interview (CIDI; Kessler et al. 1994), and the MINI International Neuropsychiatric Interview (Lecrubier et al. 1997). The SCID and the CIDI provide comprehensive and clinically rich data, but can be relatively lengthy to administer, depending on the patient's presenting problems and history, and may therefore be more appropriate within clinical research settings. The MINI was developed as a short, structured, diagnostic interview, and is compatible with both DSM-IV and ICD-10 diagnostic systems; a version compatible with DSM-5 may be developed in the future. The MINI was validated against the longer SCID (Sheehan et al. 1998), but takes only 15–20 minutes to administer. Its response format is simple and makes its use with older patients with MCI less challenging than longer instruments with more abstract and protracted response set requirements. Busy clinicians can pick and choose among the modules for a tailored clinical tool. Structured or semi-structured interviews, such as the MINI (Lecrubier et al. 1997) have better reliability and validity than solely unstructured interviews (Edelstein and Semenchuk 1996). Structured interviews are superior in assessing the presence and severity of disorders, and in monitoring change in symptoms over time, as compared with self-report instruments (Dennis et al. 2007).

Both comorbid medical conditions and medication use are important issues to discuss in any clinical interview of older clients. It is useful to ask older clients to bring a list of current medical conditions, together with a list of prescribed and over-the-counter medications with them to the interview, so any potential important illnesses or medications are not overlooked.

Whatever interview format is followed, during the interview process the clinician should be alert to age-related changes that could affect information obtained, as well as rapport with the client. Clients with vision or hearing impairments, or other functional disabilities such as mobility problems, should have these accommodated by the clinician. Older adults may not signal if they are having difficulties hearing, for example, and the clinician should be proactive in this regard. In general, it is more helpful to be sure the client can see your face when you speak, to speak clearly, and to sit to the side of the ear with the best hearing ability. Talking loudly is not recommended as a general strategy. If one speaks more loudly, adjusting in steps to where the client can hear is better than just adopting a very loud voice. Asking the client what works best for him/her is, of course, a good strategy. A reminder before the interview about bringing glasses and other sensory aids, if relevant, will also be useful.

Done with care, the initial interview provides the best opportunity to learn about the client's cohort identity, social context, and cultural background.

The CALTAP model applied to assessment with older adults

Developmental aging and the assessment process

The psychologist who treats older adults needs to be cognizant of both reported and disclosed biopsychosocial events and milestones contained both within the referral and offered at interview. However, these must be placed within the context of an understanding of normal developmental trajectories in later life. Older adults experience minor physical, mental, and social changes, of both a positive and negative nature, as a matter of course as they age. Knowing what is normal and what appears abnormal, both with reference to population norms, as well as the individual's life history, is therefore key. This assists with both the specific tasks at hand (e.g., choosing an assessment strategy), as well as the overall clinical interviewing and testing process (e.g., establishing good rapport, knowing what to ask, knowing what tests to choose).

The way the referral of an older patient is interpreted and acted upon offers many opportunities to examine how CALTAP can guide practice. For example, the referral source may be ignorant or biased about changes in cognition or functioning with increasing age. A patient may be referred for cognitive testing simply because of advanced age. Changes in cognition may automatically be attributed to age and other potential etiologies ignored. The referral source may not disclose all information to the client if they feel a need to paternalistically "protect" the client from bad news.

This was the case with the referral of a client seen by NP in New Zealand. The 64-year-old woman was referred for neuropsychological testing. The referral read "declines in memory – strongly suspect dementia." However, when NP asked the client why she thought she had been referred for testing (a most useful question!), she replied, "I'm very worried about my memory, so I went to my GP [general practitioner]. I was concerned I might have Alzheimer's disease, but he assured me that it wasn't possibly that. So he sent me to you to figure out what it really is." The woman looked at least 10 years younger than her stated age, a career woman with a high level of education; it is possible that in the face of her fears her GP sought to reassure her, with potentially disastrous consequences (in the end she did not have a diagnosis of dementia).

CALTAP emphasizes the importance of specific age considerations in the interaction with patients. In neuropsychology, an awareness of the need for good age-based norms on which to base interpretation of test results is widely acknowledged (Attix and Welsh-Bohmer 2006; Owens et al. 2000). The need to potentially adapt our approaches to older persons, however, with regard to how the testing session is scheduled and carried out, as well as the sensitivities around how test results are fed back to older clients and their families, has been slower to develop (Pachana et al. 2010b). The neuropsychologist needs to be aware that the way the testing process proceeds may also influence results. For example, testing sessions should be clearly discussed as to their length, aims, and potential outcomes with the patient and their family. The testing room itself should be quiet, well-lit (but free from glare), and comfortable, and put the client at ease. Questions should be encouraged and answered openly by the neuropsychologist. Such steps can serve to minimize noise in test data and allow the clinician to gauge the best abilities of the person at hand.

How tests are administered and selected is a fundamental component to assessment, and with older adults various aspects of the characteristics of the older adult may influence test choice and administration. For example, sensory deficits may dictate test selection (or the decision to give a self-report measure verbally, for example). In older adults, aspects of normal aging may influence ones' senses and thus one's response to the test. For example, color discrimination errors increase with increasing age, and the ability to accurately make finer color distinctions in later life is influenced by both the intactness of the structures of the eye, the presence of age-related problems such as cataracts, and post-receptive processing changes in the visual cortex (for a more complete discussion of vision and aging, see Schieber 2006). Thus, if choosing to give a test such as the Stroop, which depends on the ability to distinguish reliably among colors, it would be prudent to consider giving a version of the test designed for older adults (e.g., the California Older Adult Stroop Test; Pachana et al. 2004). This example illustrates a core principle in testing with older adults—tests should be chosen that minimize noise in the data due to normal changes in sensory, cognitive, and interpersonal functioning due to increasing age, which may lead to false positives on testing.

Conceptualizing individuals in later life as having strengths and weaknesses, mirroring contemporary theories of maturation, which have moved away from deficit models, can usefully inform approaches to the interview (Baltes 1991; Laidlaw and Pachana 2009; Morris et al. 2000). This can also serve to orient the patient and any significant others to this way of viewing the presenting issues.

Such an approach has the potential to calm fears and allow explorations of possible therapeutic ways forward. Older adults themselves may have consciously or unconsciously incorporated ageist attitudes toward their own abilities, and this can affect every aspect of the assessment process and should be addressed. Thus, a focus on strengths and weaknesses in the face of aging can help both the patient, as well as the clinician, find their way through the assessment process. In particular, it can help the psychologist in thinking to the next steps of test selection and assessment structure. Tests might be chosen because they can illustrate a useful intact ability, not just to illuminate deficits. Decisions about the number and type of tests to be given, and the duration of testing sessions, depend equally on intact abilities, as well as deficits in the patient.

It is useful for psychologists to keep in mind that emotional, as well as cognitive changes in later life have an important bearing on the types of questions that evaluations attempt to answer. For example, capacity assessment depends not only on intact memory, judgment, and reasoning, but also awareness of the intentions and motivations of others, ability to operate within social networks and so forth. Cognitive complexity (Labouvie-Vief and Diehl 2000; Mascolo and Fischer 2010) and emotional complexity (Labouvie-Vief and Medler 2002; Ready et al. 2008) in later life have both been the subject of research in the last decade, and to some extent our existing tests may only capture a portion of this complexity. Usefully, research studies point to the fact that older adults' functioning in these realms is best understood by interpreting normative data on objective tests within the individual's social and cultural context, which fits in very well with CALTAP.

Social context and the assessment process

The context in which the work is done will affect the nature of the assessment and will also have a strong selection influence on the type of older clients seen for assessment. As a clinical geropsychologist, depending on the setting and client base, assessment may or may not prove a core part of practice. In some public health contexts, assessment may be a routine part of intake procedures or may be required for funding or auditing purposes. For example, in Australian aged care settings assessment of mood with the Cornell Scale for Depression in Dementia (Alexopoulos et al. 1988) is required at intake in commonwealth-funded nursing home settings, as mandated by funding bodies (e.g., Australian Institute of Health and Welfare 2013). In private practice settings, in contrast, assessments by clinicians may be confined to mood self-rating scales and the occasional mental status test. (For an excellent compilation of tests developed for geriatric patients, see Burns et al. 2004).

The reliability and validity of assessment scales are related in part to the settings in which they are administered. Just as not all test instruments have been validated on older adult samples, so too not all tests are validated for use in all settings. The psychologist would do well to investigate whether a particular test has been validated or is recommended (or perhaps not recommended) for use in a particular setting. For example, a practice setting of increasing importance to psychologists is primary care medicine, and many instruments are being validated and even developed for use in this setting (Brodaty et al. 2002; Mitchell et al. 2010).

Residential care for older adults

One setting in which test use should be carefully considered in terms of appropriateness is residential aged care. In such settings the purpose and nature of testing needs to be clear, and the tests used chosen carefully (Pachana et al. 2010a). Who gives the test and how it is interpreted in the nursing home setting must also be considered—it may, for example, be prudent for a consulting psychologist to suggest tests that may be given as part of routine care by a range of health professionals, and others that are best administered by the psychologist, or at least best administered by appropriately trained staff in the care facility. Even where and when the test is given in the nursing home (e.g., a quiet room, at a time of day to best capture the information one is after) are important considerations. For example, giving tests of mood or cognitive functioning later in the day, when energy is flagging or if sundowning is present, will not reflect functioning at other times of day.

Medical care settings and the geropsychologist

Many times it may be unclear to health professionals whether symptoms are indicative of physical or psychological phenomena, and so referral to the psychologist for testing, including personality testing, may help establish an etiology for at least a subset of presenting symptoms. In such cases testing combined with a careful history may prove invaluable in charting a way forward with respect to interventions. It is useful for clinicians to have a broad range of tests available to them if puzzling or complex cases present themselves, as such data may be quite useful in case conceptualization. For example, in a case where a past history of anxiety disorders is combined with recent diagnosis of COPD, establishing when and to what extent anxiety symptoms manifest may usefully guide treatment. In the case of sleep problems, self-reports of sleep patterns, as well as expectations regarding sleep outcomes may both be useful in guiding the clinician's treatment approach (see Chapter 8 on sleep disorders for further information).

Sometimes the psychologist is given the task of trying to unravel a set of puzzling or inconsistent symptoms, especially in cases where other health professionals have concluded that such symptoms reflect a psychological source. This may prove frustrating in terms of knowing where to start with assessment; here, the clinician would be wise to consider not giving or at least delaying testing in favor of a close exploration of the client's symptoms, history, and medical and psychological history. Often, knowledge of how, for example, multiple medications or past history of abuse play out with older adults may offer clues to the origin of current symptoms. An astute geriatric psychologist may recognize undetected substance abuse or complicated grief, which may have been missed by other professionals. Or the psychologist may be best placed to put together a jigsaw puzzle of test results, clinical observations and self-reports by the client, in a psychological framework, to arrive at potential hypotheses about what may be underlying current behaviors. In some instances, when no explanation is either obvious or likely, then moving the client forward in terms of coping, accommodating and adapting to the present situation may be the best way forward.

For example, in a case where multiple etiologies are causing pain and fatigue, resulting in impaired attention and concentration, as well as depression, the psychologist may prefer to organize the existing medical data and present this within a psychological context, with minimal to no additional test data. In such a case, moving the client forward to adopt enhanced coping strategies is probably more important than gathering more testing data.

Societal ageism

Another aspect of the social context for both the psychologist and the client is societal ageism. It is possible that if the test administrator is not familiar with older persons, then their approach to administering tests may be influenced by age stereotypes and bias. The clinician may erroneously assume that older adults will be adverse to testing (or homework, such as a mood rating scale, for that matter) and may refrain from giving mood ratings to older adults, thinking they won't be compliant or just will not "get it." There is no empirical support for such a stance, and much empirical support for the value of ratings and assessments given for screening or as part of homework (Kazantzis et al. 2003).

A clinician might believe that older adults in general suffer from impaired memory, and either not bother to test cognitive functioning (which could assist in planning intervention strategies) or believe that the tests, screens, and self-report measures will be too difficult for the older person to complete. The clinician may not be aware of the proliferation of tests designed and validated specifically on older adult populations, and so miss the opportunity to collect data of the greatest fidelity and perhaps most relevance to the older client.

Older adults themselves may hold such negative self-stereotypes about their own abilities, and there is a growing literature on the potential impact of such self-stereotyping on testing performance by older patients (Merckelbach et al. 2012). Such negative self-stereotypes can impede progress in both testing and therapy by making the client reluctant to give their best effort on tests or to make changes suggested in therapy.

Testing may also serve to allay fears in older persons about age-related changes. For example, if there is a discrepancy between observed behavior (such as ability to negotiate activities of daily living), and self-report of mood or cognitive symptoms, objective testing may help clarify the situation for both the client and the clinician. Often, older adults present with worries about changes in memory due to the increasing salience of minor cognitive slippage in light of increasing age. After age 65, losing one's car keys or forgetting where the car is parked may take on new and more sinister connotations. In such cases, even brief cognitive screening may serve to reassure the majority of clients that they are still functioning within the limits of their age-matched peers, and may denote the need for further assessment in a minority of instances.

Social network of the older client

In older patients the opportunity to gather collateral information may be limited if the patient has limited social or family networks. Another problem with information gathering while trying to chart a path forward from the referral involves unhelpful interactions with families. These unhelpful interactions may spread to staff at residential facilities. This can result in information about the resident's behaviors being couched in terms of either the family's or the staff's influence and biases, but rarely results in objective data. Less dramatic examples, where information gathering requires finesse, include cases of overly involved or anxious family members who may intentionally or unintentionally hinder information gathering.

Within the social network of the older client, there are often many "stakeholders" invested in the physical, cognitive, and emotional well-being of older adults. Indeed, the increasing lifespan of older adults may have had an unanticipated effect of lengthening the list of interested parties, since adult children are often joined by grandchildren, and possibly even great-grandchildren, in having an intense interest in what is happening with the older adult. This may be out of worry about the need for increased care, appropriate (or inappropriate) interest in the older adult's finances and/or health with respect to decision-making capacity, or may reflect simple affection and concern. Older persons are increasingly acting as primary caregivers for their grandchildren or potentially great-grandchildren, and so any loss of capacity may affect a wider range of persons very directly. Siblings of older adults involved in neuropsychological evaluations often express worry about the implications of results for their own cognitive functioning and potential future declines of their own mental faculties.

In addition to immediate family, interested parties may include friends, neighbors, concerned health professionals, and community support staff. Each of these may in turn be valued sources of collateral information, or perhaps persons who question results or recommendations based on personal agendas. Informants may be either potential facilitators or barriers to recommendations as well. For example, primary care physicians are very often the first port of call for health care over the lifespan, particularly in later life, and may be in an ideal position to offer valuable background data and medical history for older adults—assistance that is often invaluable if family members are not on the scene. However, such individuals with long-standing relationships with the older patient may themselves have biases or even blind spots with respect to a decline in functioning. In such scenarios diagnoses and/or recommendations may be questioned or ignored. In the situation where an older adult does not have a regular primary care physician or family, data gathering may be severely hampered, requiring instead a shift of focus to understanding the current context of the person as fully as possible.

Caregiving situations, whether it be that the caregiver is, in fact, the older person being tested (perhaps caring for a spouse, adult child with developmental disability, etc.) or the caregiver is a stakeholder in the results of testing (e.g., an adult child caring for an aging parent), should be carefully considered with respect to feedback. Consideration of how potential ethical issues around confidentiality should be best handled is important. How diagnoses will be received, whether additional supports are necessary, and even who should attend feedback sessions also should be carefully considered.

Cohort differences and assessment of older adults

An intriguing and largely unsettled question is how to think about older norms for established psychological tests. If a test was normed 20 years ago and the norms include people in their 60s then, do those norms now apply to current 60-year-olds or to current 80-year-olds? The answer will depend on whether the test results would be primarily affected by developmental aging or by cohort differences. To our knowledge, this question is not addressed in the current literature in any systematic way. However, it is worth considering the age and representativeness of a test's normative data when working with older clients.

Future cohorts may well be more familiar and comfortable with cognitive screening and neuropsychological testing, but earlier born cohorts may feel judged or intimidated by the testing process. Also individuals themselves may have a more anxious response to testing, and this should be factored into the giving of tests and feedback about results.

Cultural influences on assessment of older adults

As our communities become more culturally diverse, the importance of taking culture into consideration in clinical practice is increasingly important for psychologists. Older patients of culturally and linguistically diverse (CALD) backgrounds are increasingly common; for example, in Australia, Access Economics (2009) estimates that the prevalence of dementia will increase from 257,275 in 2010 to around 1.13 million people by 2050. At the same time, the numbers of people from a CALD background who have dementia will increase from 35,549 to 119,582. Demand for assessment and treatment approaches for neurological conditions in these groups is increasing, and according to a global study conducted by the World Health Organization, eight out of ten disorders in the three highest disability classes are neurological problems (Menken 2000). CALTAP facilitates systematic incorporation of cultural contexts into psychological assessment and treatment approaches.

Complications and issues in assessing older adults
Specific illnesses in later life and effects on assessment

The older adult is more likely to have chronic illnesses and disabilities, and these may have a direct impact on how testing sessions are structured. Breaking testing into multiple sessions may be more feasible, although there are risks of the older adult experiencing variation in levels of cognitive functioning that would require additional interpretation for scores across sessions. Physical limitations such as diabetes may require frequent breaks for food, for example. Sensory or physical limitations may influence test selection and even modality. It is also the wise psychologist who gives the most critical tests first, such that if the patient for whatever reason cannot continue testing, at least the main issues raised in the referral can be addressed. The need for rapid, clinically valid, and practical bedside testing is crucial in work with older adults, particularly older adults in nursing home settings (Pachana et al. 2010a).

In terms of assessment instruments given in the course of therapy, if the test taker has multiple medical issues, this could impact self-reporting of symptoms of both anxiety and depression (Byrne et al. 2010), potentially resulting in false positive results. In general, tests specifically designed for older persons, such as the Geriatric Depression Scale (GDS; Yesavage et al. 1982) and the Geriatric Anxiety Inventory (GAI; Pachana et al. 2007) ask minimally about symptoms that may be endorsed simply due to normal age-related changes (e.g., vegetative symptoms, lack of sleep, etc.), thereby minimizing the risk of false positives. Overly complex wording of items or complicated response sets in tests can also limit their usability and reliability in older cohorts (Pachana et al. 1994).

A client with an unusual presentation or history may warrant more focused instruments, or one developed for that particular subpopulation. For example, although many assessment tools, including the Montreal Cognitive Assessment (MoCA; Nasreddine et al. 2005) and the GDS (Yesavage et al. 1982) have been shown to work well with Parkinson's patients, a clinician working with such a patient may wish to gather some additional data to assist with treatment planning; here, the Parkinson Fatigue Scale (PFS-16; Brown et al. 2005) may be of use. This brief 16-item self-report instrument surveys aspects of fatigue and their impact on daily functioning. As fatigue is a common issue in persons with Parkinson's disease that can impact mood and quality of life, measuring this with a standardized tool helps assure both a baseline for later comparison purposes, as well as a more valid and systematic measure of a key area with treatment implications.

Of course, a major set of illnesses affecting older adults that are a common question for assessment are neurocognitive disorders. Cognitive decline and its expression across a range of cognitive abilities is well documented in the literature (Apostolova and Cummings 2008; Monastero et al. 2009; Park et al. 2003). It is this very state that often is the subject of the psychologist's assessment efforts. Here, an understanding of expected versus abnormal cognitive aging trajectories is key. This will affect both assessment considerations in terms of test selection and interpretation of results, as well as treatment recommendations.

Affective tests are an important part of testing, as depression and anxiety remain underdiagnosed in older adults (Pachana and Byrne 2012). Symptoms of anxiety and depression may mimic those of dementia, and in actual practice, particularly with frail elders or older adults with chronic mental illness, this may appear more daunting a distinction, perhaps one impossible to completely resolve. Therefore, establishing as much clarity as possible with respect to the emotional state of the older adult, and their emotional history, is invaluable to the clinician. Clinicians should note that older adults from different cultural or cohort backgrounds may use different words to describe emotional states, and have varying degrees of comfort in discussing such matters. As a final note on affect, grief over a lost spouse or other loved ones, including other sources of emotional support such as beloved pets, should not be overlooked as having an impact on test results and even motivation for testing.

Using cognitive screens

The Mini-Mental State Exam (MMSE; Folstein et al. 1975) is still the most widely used instrument for cognitive screening across a range of disciplines and circumstances, and is simple and easy to administer in clinical practice. Although limited in terms of the scope of information it provides to the clinician, it is a useful way to communicate results to other professionals in widely understood terms. MMSE scores should always be interpreted in light of age and education (Tombaugh et al. 1996), rather than simple cut-off scores (as unfortunately is widely practiced).

Cognitive screens such as the Modified Mini-Mental State Exam (3MS; Teng and Chui 1987) have good psychometric properties, have some advantages with respect to overcoming educational and cultural biases over the MMSE, and are appropriate for older populations (Ismail et al. 2010). The 3MS offers a more comprehensive survey of cognitive functioning, including executive functioning, with the added advantage of a more standardized administration than the MMSE while also yielding the original Folstein MMSE score as an option. The domains sampled include those of the MMSE (orientation, registration, mental reversal, recall, naming, repetition, reading, 3-stage command, and copying pentagons), with the addition of cueing prompts and multiple choice options to gauge cognitive limits, and additional items, such as similarities and language generativity (animal naming). The 3MS is useful in situations where a finer-grained picture of cognitive functioning is required.

The MoCA is a brief cognitive screening tool designed to assess attention and concentration, executive function, memory, language, visuoconstructional skills, conceptual thinking, calculations, and orientation (Nasreddine et al. 2005). It is in wide use, and has been tested and found effective for determining cognitive decline in a variety of populations including patients with Parkinson's Disease (Dalrymple-Alford et al. 2010), as well as in detecting MCI (McLennan et al. 2011). The MoCA is relatively brief and takes about 10 minutes to administer. Sensitivity and specificity are excellent for detection of MCI (90% and 87%, respectively) and Alzheimer's disease (100% and 87%, respectively) (Nasreddine et al. 2005). Two alternate forms of the MoCA are available, which is useful to avoid test-retest effects (Phillips et al. 2011).

If the clinician has not administered a cognitive screen, but notices during therapy sessions that the older client seems to not understand the homework assignment, misinterprets what the clinician is saying, or if their behavior or thinking changes for the worse over the course of treatment, cognitive screening might help shed some light on what is going on. It might be that the older adult had such preserved interpersonal skills that any cognitive deficits were hard to pick up initially. Thinking or behaviors changing over time could signal declines associated with MCI or dementia, but could also reflect a host of other etiologies of note, including changes in medication that have had cognitive side-effects as a consequence.

If the clinician suspects that some change warrants testing, it is important to share their concerns with the client, particularly clients who have been in therapy for a while, so that such testing does not negatively impact rapport and the therapeutic relationship. In some cases, the suggestion of such testing may, in fact, be welcomed, especially if the client has noticed and wondered about the changes themselves. In other cases, such a suggestion may be greeted with fear or anger. Testing always carries with it the possibility of revealing unwanted information to all parties involved, and so due consideration to its timing and best use is warranted.

With this in mind, the clinician may wish to be particularly wary of family members insisting on cognitive testing so that relatives can be shown to lack capacity. Undue influence and the potential for elder abuse may be behind such requests, and the clinician should be vigilant about being drawn into such a situation. There are specific tests and test approaches for older adults undergoing capacity assessment (Moye et al. 2013), as well as tests designed to detect the tendency to be susceptible to undue influence (Pinsker et al. 2006).

After the assessment

Assessments are often conceptualized as being primarily in the service of referral sources in search of diagnoses, rather than patients in search of ways forward through illness. In many cases reports can focus too much on test results and metrics at the expense of careful recommendations, and good liaison with all concerned parties to a case. The psychologist in possession of clinical and neuropsychological skills who is also attuned to the concerns of older adults can provide a unique and often crucial service to health professionals, multidisciplinary teams, and older adults in distress. Follow through, particularly on complex cases, goes beyond handing in a report and certainly encompasses feedback to all parties.

Effective follow through, particularly in complex cases, can be daunting, however. Sometimes the psychologist is cast in the role of assessor only, and other feedback or follow through may not be welcome from other parties, including other health professionals. Complex cases can evolve with dramatic shifts in the older person's health and acute admissions. In addition, changes in living situation, changes in care regime, and so forth, can be challenging for the clinician, who effectively can find themselves chasing a moving target. Large numbers of stakeholders with differing, and often competing opinions and agendas, can hinder appropriate or even sensible follow-through. In the case of nursing home residents, the maddeningly slow pace at which care sometimes moves can frustrate timely follow-through of cases. Reimbursements rarely cover the time and effort that may be involved in follow-through of complex geriatric patients.

The consulting clinical psychologist or neuropsychologist is often asked directly about the issue of follow up assessments. Whether requested or not, a statement about the potential need for repeat assessments is nearly always warranted. In other words, the psychologist should be very clear with the referral source about the potential value of follow-up assessment. In some cases this may be extremely valuable, particularly early in the course of cognitive decline, when a diagnosis may hinge on demonstrated declines over time. In other cases a follow up assessment may have little value, if a diagnosis is well-established in a person with advanced dementia, for example. Yet we have seen repeat referrals for testing of this latter category of patients, almost without thought on the part of the referrer. Assessment procedures, apart from their cost, are time-consuming and stressful for the individual, and unnecessary testing should be avoided at all costs.

Thus, if such a statement is not offered by the psychologist completing an assessment, the patient may be subject to needless and potentially stressful repeat assessments for little gain. Ideally, suggested situations in which such repeat testing is warranted (e.g., in the face of a major change in functioning), and/or a timeframe (in the next 6 months, but not longer than 1 year, for example), are of great utility and usually greatly appreciated. If possible, the goals of any future retesting, such as to confirm a downward trajectory in cognitive functioning, or to ascertain if a rehabilitation strategy is having the intended effect, are useful as well.

Sharing results and recommendations

It is discouraging to realize that in only about 70% of cases are the results of formal neuropsychological assessments given back to the patient in a feedback session; this includes patients across a wide range of ages and circumstances (Bennett-Levy et al. 1994; Smith et al. 2007). This is an important consideration as the lack of feedback may fuel anxiety in older patients. Sometimes barriers to giving timely feedback are cited—these can include difficulties in scheduling older clients in for follow-up sessions and institutional barriers (e.g., no allocated time by the hospital to give such feedback). However, ethical as well as practical difficulties may stem from not giving such feedback, including poorer treatment outcomes (Gass and Brown 1992).

In neuropsychotherapy approaches, which emphasize a shared agenda in testing between the test giver and the test-taker, the feedback session follows the outline of initial expectations, concerns, and goals of the patient and significant others as outlined in the initial contact session. The importance of constructing feedback that can be usefully utilized to work toward best treatment outcomes cannot be stressed enough. Feedback should also take place in a timely fashion; long delays may add to worry and stress, and allow potential windows of opportunity to close (Pope 1992). A straightforward approach to giving feedback is appreciated by all. Feedback can be tailored to different individuals, but it is best if all parties know who has received what information (Postal and Armstrong 2013).

Research and practice imperatives in geriatric assessment

The area of clinical assessment in older adults is receiving increasing attention, and several texts on the topic have appeared in recent years (e.g., Attix and Welsh-Bohmer 2006; Lichtenberg 2010). More attention, however, is required from an overarching theoretical perspective, to shed light on approaches to assessment that are most efficacious with older adults. Given the heterogeneity of this population, research should be carried out to ascertain approaches which might best serve older adults in different interpersonal circumstances and contexts, with particular attention to differences in cohort and culture, in addition to differing diagnoses, health contexts, and levels of social supports.

Thoughtful, structured approaches to assessment practice are particularly important when working with older clients. This is a group whose many challenges to the psychologist are the same challenges that make practice with this group so rewarding. Yet the challenges require psychologists to have a good network of colleagues with which to discuss cases, and potential ethical and legal issues. Keeping up with the burgeoning literature in this area is vital, as improved research methodologies, changes in diagnostic systems, and advances in health care itself make geriatrics a fast-changing discipline. Finally, self-care is important at all career stages when dealing with older clients. Practitioners whose practice is primarily assessment may not see the need for such care in the same way that psychotherapists might. Yet there is research on the toll that assessment can take, for example, research on neuropsychologists' personal reactions when called upon to make diagnoses or give feedback about dementia or other neurological disorders (Green 2006).

Summary

Assessment approaches with older adults, similar to psychotherapy, include a large degree of overlap with approaches used with younger adults. The CALTAP model offers a way for clinical interviews, test selection, interpretation, and feedback, as well as assessment approaches to specific cohorts or contexts (such as with residents of nursing home facilities) to be approached with an awareness and appreciation of how issues of cohorts, culture, and contexts might impact on the client (and their families), the therapist, and the work between these individuals. In subsequent chapters, diagnostic or symptom specific issues with regards to assessment and treatment of older clients are elaborated, illustrated with indicative case examples.

Chapter 3

Depression in late life

Introduction to depression in late life

In the next three chapters, we discuss depression, anxiety, and dementia with frequent cross-referencing with regard to both assessment and intervention. These are the most common psychological disorders of older adulthood, the most widely known among professionals (although awareness of anxiety disorders in late life lags behind the other two), and have the most extensive set of available screening instruments and the largest literatures. In principle, however, we think that professionals working with older adults should at least keep in mind the full set of disorders discussed in this book.

In their review, Fiske et al. (2009) put the general prevalence of major depressive disorder (MDD) in older adults at between 1 and 5%, with higher rates in medical outpatients, medical inpatients, hospice patients, and residents in long-term care facilities. They also note that while the prevalence of diagnosed MDD is lower in older adults than in midlife, depressive symptoms are higher, and there is evidence suggestive of either differences in the presentation of depression in later life (e.g., more minor depression) or of failures to diagnose depression accurately in older adults.

We would also note that, in the past, depression associated with bereavement was excluded from clinical diagnosis by the DSM manuals. DSM-5 (American Psychiatric Association 2013) has changed this exclusion and now recognizes the possibility of clinical depression occurring in response to bereavement as a severe stressor. The guidance in making the distinction is rooted in depressed mood and/or anhedonia, rather than only feelings of loss, and on the continuousness of the mood rather than the often more episodic nature of intense emotional distress during grief. Given the fairly common occurrence of bereavement and multiple bereavements in later life, the CALTAP model has considered bereavement as one of the specific challenges of later life, with attitudes, knowledge, and skills related to grief work oriented therapy an important component of working with older adults.

Depression is associated with significant burden among both younger and older adults. A 2000 report by the World Health Organization classified depression as fourth in terms of medical conditions with the greatest disease burden;

as operationalized by Disability-Adjusted Life Years, which represents years of life lost to premature death and years of life lived with a disability. Depression has been shown to detrimentally affect the course and outcome of a number of medical conditions, such as mortality due to coronary artery disease and cancer (Brown et al. 2003; Frasure-Smith and Lesperance 2010). Older adults with depression may face additional detrimental consequences and symptoms. Depression in the elderly has also been demonstrated to be a risk factor for long-term care admission, recurrent falls, and incident dementia (Blazer 2003b; Harris 2007).

Depression, although not the most common psychiatric disorder in later life, is one which often causes significant emotional distress and marked decreases in quality of life (Blazer 2003b). Depression is also linked in many people's minds, both within the health care professions, as well as members of the public, with aging. Among health professionals depression is still often erroneously associated with normal aging. Despite public health campaigns in many countries about depression as a treatable mental illness, many adults, including older adults, do not recognize depression as an illness and do not seek treatment. Much has been written about specific barriers to treatment of psychiatric illnesses, including depression in later life, but older adults themselves have reported that despite problems of access and cost, an additional barrier is finding a mental health professional who understands what they are talking about when they are describing emotions and thoughts which cause them distress (Woodward and Pachana 2009).

Late-onset depression (first episode after the age of 60) differs from chronic depression carried into later life in several ways, including reporting of increased hopelessness and cognitive dysfunction, including executive dysfunction, as well as increased likelihood of neurobiological symptoms, such as increased ventricular size (Blazer 2003a). Personality disorder and a family history of psychiatric illness are more common in early onset depression, while persons with early and late onset depression do not seem to differ on severity or neuropsychological performance (Brodaty et al. 2001). Putative subtypes of what might be termed "minor depressions" include "depression without sadness" (Gallo et al. 1994), "depletion syndrome" (Adams 2001), and "dysthymic disorder" (American Psychiatric Association 1994). The first two are purported to be more common in later life, while dysthymic disorder more commonly presents in middle age and may persist into later years (Blazer 1994). Subtypes of depression can be conceptualized along such lines (i.e., the severity or number of symptoms endorsed); others have suggested the balance between more psychological and more physical symptoms causing distress (Parker and Hadzi-Pavlovic 1996). Recent work into how later-life changes in the brain, such as vascular insults, might impact development of disturbed mood (e.g., Paranthaman et al. 2012), and the temporal relationship between late-onset depression and dementia (e.g., Li et al. 2011) are ongoing.

Assessment of depression in late life

In order for the initial assessment to best inform treatment approaches, careful consideration of the instruments chosen and an accurate diagnosis of depression are essential. For example, a psychologist not skilled in the assessment of older adults may mistake early stages of a progressive dementia for depression, or more commonly, attribute changes in memory and behavior associated with depression to an incipient dementia. In the latter case the client's age may consciously or unconsciously lend support to such a diagnosis. And of course an older person may present with both a mood disorder and dementia.

Clinical interview

The clinical interview is important for accurate diagnosis, and accurate diagnosis is generally more difficult to pin down in older patients. Older adults often present with complex health and psychiatric histories, coupled with the added confusion of medications or other medical interventions that may produce their own health and psychiatric symptoms as side effects. Depression in older adults may be difficult to diagnose, as symptoms of depression may mimic other medical illnesses, and depression is often comorbid with other health conditions (Blazer 2003a). Some symptoms associated with depression (i.e., lack of appetite) may reflect a medication side-effect, or an iatrogenic effect of a medication interaction. This may be of particular concern in older adults, who are often taking multiple medications (Little and Morley 2013). Thus, the use of a semi-structured or structured interview, with its systematic inquiry into a broad range of symptoms and functioning, as described in Chapter 2, may help overcome such difficulties. If possible the clinician can ask clients to bring relevant information such as a complete medical history and a list of current medications with them to the interview.

In addition to complex presenting problems in older adults, the diagnostic criteria for mental disorders themselves often do not adequately capture the experience of such conditions in later life, nor do they adequately guide diagnosis for this age group (Jeste et al. 2005). Recently, there has been increasing attention paid to subsyndromal depression and the adequacy of diagnostic criteria for older adults (see Bruce 2010, and the accompanying special issue of *The American Journal of Geriatric Psychiatry*, **18**(3)). Diagnosis in older adults is often complicated by a range of contextual factors (such as culture or cohort experiences, and wording choices), which can influence the reporting of symptoms.

Interview duration and how responses are presented may be particularly relevant parameters when interviewing depressed clients. Fatigue and motivation may make one continuous interview session unfeasible. Older adults with MCI may offer more reliable data with multiple, shorter interviews. Mohlman and colleagues (2012) in their excellent article on interviewing older adults, suggest giving clients a visual display of dimensional rating scales, as well as being vigilant for older clients misunderstanding response instructions, time periods in question, or being confused by language used in inventories. For example, if multiple questionnaires are given in succession, differing time periods for reporting symptoms (e.g., "in the last week" versus "in the last month") should be pointed out. If older adults are confused by any terminology in a questionnaire, even such apparently self-explanatory queries such as "I find it easy to dismiss worrisome thoughts" (from the Penn State Worry Questionnaire, Meyer et al. 1990), a rephrasing of the item verbally is probably useful. Inventories such as the Neuropsychiatric Inventory (NPI; Cummings et al. 1994) have had published manuals for administration and scoring that emphasize checking with older respondents to be sure that their responses accurately reflect what they think, to insure the most accurate picture is obtained (see Chapter 5 on dementia for more explication on scoring the NPI).

Older adults may have a different way of speaking about their depression due to cohort or cultural differences or simple individual idiosyncrasies. The clinician should be alert to the client's ways of expressing their experience of depression, whether it be expressions such as "down in the dumps," or through reference to physical symptoms of fatigue or bodily aches and pains. Zarit and Zarit (2007) point out the pitfalls of lapsing into jargon while interviewing older adults; it may be best to mirror as much as possible the way the client is speaking about their symptoms, or at the very least to not stray too far from layman's terms. Mapping of cultural norms for expressing depression have appeared in the literature (e.g., Yeung et al. 2004), but the proviso here is that such norms are often cohort-specific, and may be influenced by factors such as degree of acculturation and presence of cognitive impairment.

In today's increasingly global societies, in both the developed and the developing world, the clinician would be wise to note whether cultural factors may play a role in how the client experiences depressive symptoms, as well as how this influences disclosure. Older Chinese adults, for example, may view acknowledging mental illness as resulting in a loss of face (i.e., lian 臉 or mien-tzu 面子), which governs social interaction in Chinese societies (Hu 1944) and reflects the cultural dimensions of stigma in the Chinese context (Yang 2007).

Older adults generally may not understand their symptoms of depression as being part of an actual psychiatric disorder (Zarit and Zarit 2007); this appears to be even more pronounced among several cultural groups (Choi and Gonzalez 2005). However, it is interesting perhaps to note the relative resilience of ethnic minorities within the dominant culture, who most often demonstrate only marginally higher rates of psychiatric illness despite pronounced cultural stressors (Sakauye 2012).

Cognitive screening

Older adults with depression and particularly late-onset depression often cite memory problems as a significant symptom, more so than younger populations (Blazer 2003b). As such, a common referral question (in the minds of either the referral source and/or the clinician) may be whether the client is experiencing depression or the onset of a dementia (see Case Example 3.1A). Thus, use of a brief cognitive screen, such as the Montreal Cognitive Assessment (MoCA; Nasreddine et al.

Case Example 3.1A Martin: assessing depression and dementia

Martin was referred to Sue by his primary care physician for memory complaints. Martin was a robust 78-year-old who took great care in his appearance. He was accompanied by his wife, Louise, who in contrast looked tired and rather overwhelmed. Louise was Martin's second wife. She was in her late-fifties and owned her own small catering business. Martin explained that he had been seeing his physician for his annual physical, when the issue of memory was raised. In the course of completing "that silly set of questions—I never write checks anymore so why should I know the exact date? I'm retired!" the question of difficulties with memory arose. Martin seemed equivocal on the issue, stating that while his memory "was not what it used to be" he was nevertheless not concerned about it. Louise was silent through most of the initial interview—at one stage during the structured clinical interview she offered to correct a point, but was told in no uncertain terms by Martin that "that is just your memory of it—it isn't mine."

Sue decided to give Martin the 3MS as then she could compare Martin's current cognitive score on the Folstein MMSE items with the MMSE score of 23 obtained by his primary care physician two weeks earlier, but yet derive the extra information provided in the 3MS. Martin scored similarly on the recall and orientation items, again complaining about not needing to know the exact date. "Anyway, Louise can always tell me." On the 3MS, Martin seemed to have particular trouble with items tapping into executive functioning, and on the animal naming task he went completely off-track, beginning with farm animals, but then naming farm tools and crops. Martin's score of 82 was just above the cut-off of 80 for clinically significant cognitive decline.

Upon receiving feedback on his performance, Martin appeared quite annoyed at first, continuing to belittle the significance of "some minor slips—what is that in the grand scheme of things?" However, toward the end of the interview Martin lapsed into reminiscing about earlier times, his work as a professor of European history at the local university, and suddenly became tearful. Louise, who had not shown much emotion to this point, suddenly took his hand. "It will be OK, darling," she said, looking at Sue with a look of both concern and determination in her face.

2005), or the 3MS (Teng and Chui 1987), discussed in Chapter 2, could be useful in such circumstances to help the clinician to see how the client is faring with respect to cognition in the present moment, as well as offering data to compare with other administrations of cognitive screens, if available. (See Chapter 5 for more detail about administering cognitive tests if dementia is suspected.)

Assessing depressive symptoms

Research on the assessment of depression in geriatric populations, and on instrument development in depression in general and depression in later life in particular, has left clinicians with a relatively large array of tools from which to select measures to assist with diagnosis, as well as guide treatment. Clinicians can select measures developed for more general as opposed to more specific populations, and may also choose instruments aimed specifically at either symptom severity or more targeted diagnosis. Many of these tools come in longer or shorter versions, some have been developed for specific populations (e.g., cultural groups or neurological subpopulations). The individual characteristics of a specific client, in terms of sociodemographic characteristics, cognitive status, comorbid conditions, and their own stance toward assessment are important considerations guiding assessment.

The Geriatric Depression Scale (GDS; Yesavage et al. 1982) is the most widely used age-specific screening test for depression developed for older adults. Its original 30 items had the dual advantages of minimizing somatic items (and, therefore, false positives in older adults with comorbid health concerns), as well as offering a simple yes/no response format suitable for those patients with mild memory impairments. Since its initial development, the GDS has been used in many studies with a wide range of community, inpatient, outpatient, and institutionalized populations (e.g., Friedman et al. 2005). A website on the GDS and the various versions and translations of the scale is maintained at Stanford University (<http://www.stanford.edu/~yesavage/GDS.html>).

Many short forms for the GDS have also been developed and compared for efficacy (e.g., Chattat et al. 2001). The GDS is available in 30-, 15-, and 10-item versions (Izal et al. 2010); shorter versions are also available (e.g., Almeida and Almeida 1999). Some of these are developed for specific settings (e.g., nursing home version; Jongenelis et al. 2005); others are employing empirical methods to derive the most sensitive/specific item set either within or across settings (e.g., Izal et al. 2010). Generally, for gaining an initial understanding of presenting symptoms, longer versions of scales may be preferable. These may also have superior measurement characteristics, as is the case with the 10- or 15-item versus the 30- or 5-item versions of the GDS (Izal et al. 2010). The 15-item version has the most robust published evidence for solid psychometric properties combined with relative brevity (Almeida and Almeida 1999). Mitchell and colleagues (2010) also reported the 15-item version as being best suited for use in nursing home settings (see Case Example 3.1B). An informant version (both 30- and 15-item versions are available) may be useful when the patient is unable to self-report or self-report is unreliable (Brown and Schinka 2005).

> ### Case Example 3.1B Martin: assessing depression and dementia (continued)
>
> Given Martin's distress when his cognitive screening results were discussed with him, Sue decided to administer a depression screen on his next visit. However, his lack of insight into his cognitive symptoms, and general tendency to minimize his symptoms, limited his ability to report on affective symptoms. Louise had called her to say that she and Martin had argued on the way out of the clinic because, seeing he was upset, she had offered to drive them home; he had refused and become very angry. However, Louise also reported that Martin had appeared withdrawn during the week, and did not wish to take part in their weekly bridge game with close friends. Given this information, Sue decided to give Martin the 15-item GDS, but then also gave Louise the informant version of that scale, so that she could compare their views of Martin's mood. In the end Martin denied all symptoms of depression, while Louise's informant score of 9 indicated the presence of depressive symptomatology. When discussing these results with the couple, Martin's bravado broke down. He confessed to having had several near misses while driving his beloved Citroen around town. He was afraid that Louise would have to give up her business to care for him, and he did not want to be a burden. "I would feel terrible if it came to that."
>
> Although Martin's score on the 3MS was borderline normal, he was a highly educated man and Sue would have expected his performance to be higher. In this case, Sue was concerned about whether this was a presentation of depression or dementia.
>
> Sue referred Martin for a more extensive neuropsychological testing session, given his reports of his driving and other cognitive lapses. This decision was bolstered by the fact that Martin had a high level of education and his estimated premorbid functioning, given his history, was considerably higher than the current test results. Martin agreed to continue to see Sue for a few sessions, some with Louise and some on his own, to look at his mood and as a support while further testing was completed.
>
> In Martin's case, the assessment result was that both depression and dementia were suspected. Additional assessment was needed given the presumed early stage of the dementia and his high education level. Even if dementia was confirmed, intervention for the depression could improve his overall level of functioning.

In terms of measuring the severity of symptoms of depression in older adults, one frequent question is whether to use a tool designed more broadly for adults such as the Beck Depression Inventory II, or BDI-II, by Beck and colleagues (Beck, Steer, and Brown 1996), or to use a tool designed more specifically for use with older adults, such as the GDS. Here, the best answer is probably reflected in the tests themselves. If the older adult is high functioning and articulate, the BDI-II may give good information about level of distress and also allow the older adult to give a more nuanced picture of their current level of symptoms. In such cases, an older adult will often say that the more truncated yes/no response set of the GDS does not let them tell their story as well as they might like—they are afraid the nuances of their experience may be missed. They may be concerned also that the clinician is viewing things in a black or white manner, which mimics the yes/no response format on the test. This can be an important consideration. The BDI-II itself has been shown to have solid psychometric performance among community-dwelling older adults (O'Riley et al. 2005).

The question of assessing depression if cognitive impairment or dementia is present may also arise. The Cornell Scale for Depression in Dementia (Alexopoulos et al. 1988) is a widely used, informant-based scale appropriate in such instances. However, there may be notable gaps between informant ratings of mood and the patient's own assessment of mood; for example, Towsley et al. (2012) describe under-reporting of depressive symptoms in a nursing home sample compared with patient self-report, and urge attempting to inquire directly about mood from persons with dementia. See Chapter 5 for further information about assessing depression in persons with dementia.

As anxiety is often comorbid with depression in later life, a similar pair of tests, the Beck Anxiety Inventory (BAI; Beck et al. 1996) and the Geriatric Anxiety Inventory (GAI; Pachana et al. 2007), should be considered in the same light as the discussion of the BDI-II and the GDS in the preceding paragraphs. Again, the characteristics of the patient, as well as the particulars of the presenting problems can guide the clinician in instrument selection (see Chapter 4 for more information about screens for anxiety symptoms).

While the BDI-II and the GDS are the most widely used tests in clinical practice with older clients, a number of other tests are available to the clinician (e.g., various forms of the Patient Health Questionnaire screen for depression; see Kroenke et al. 2010 for discussion of validity in general populations, and Chunyu et al. 2007, for information about sensitivity and specificity in geriatric populations). An important component in instrument selection for any client, however, is selecting the test with the strongest evidence base that was designed, or had norms developed, for a population most closely resembling the current patient. If the patient has a progressive neurological condition or other medical issue such that the prime consideration is testing for depression *in a person with that condition*, rather than *in an older adult*, then a population-specific measure for that condition may be the most appropriate choice.

A few words may be appropriate with respect to other available choices for a depression screen for an older population. Both the Center for Epidemiologic Studies Depression Scale (CES-D; Hertzog et al. 1990) and the Zung Depression Rating Scale (ZDRS; Zung and Zung 1986) have been shown to be appropriate and efficacious for use in older populations, but have not been empirically demonstrated to be as good as, or superior to, the GDS. Similarly, the Patient Health Questionnaire (PHQ-9; Kroenke et al. 2001; Pinto-Meza et al. 2005) previously mentioned was designed specifically as a screen for depression in primary care settings, and has been used with a wide and inclusive age-range (e.g., Almeida et al. 2012), but would not be as good as the GDS in general clinical practice based on existing research. The Hospital Anxiety and Depression Scale (HADS; Bjelland et al. 2002; Flint and Rifat 1996b), originally developed for the assessment of hospitalized individuals, is similar to the GDS in that it largely avoids somatic items. However, the HADS has also not been shown to be as robust as the GDS, at least in hospital settings (Dennis et al. 2012). Finally, the Hamilton Rating Scale for Depression (HAM-D; Hamilton 1960) has been shown to be relatively weak psychometrically (e.g., Bagby et al. 2004), and not well-validated in geriatric populations (Lichtenberg et al. 1992). In general, more comparative work on general psychiatric populations of older adults with respect to instrument sensitivity and specificity across screening tools is required, although such work with specific geriatric populations (e.g., patients with Parkinson's disease) appears to be progressing (Mondolo et al. 2006).

A promising tool, the Hopkins Symptom Checklist-25 (HSCL-25; Fröjdh et al. 2004), while not specifically developed for older adults, assesses for major, minor, and subsyndromal depression, but to date has only been validated with older patients in primary care settings. The relatively high sensitivity and specificity (both 94%) reported by Fröjdh and colleagues make this a tool to consider if subsyndromal depression is suspected. Measures that include a component of general distress, such as the Depression Anxiety Stress Scale (DASS; Lovibond and Lovibond 1995) have been validated in older populations (e.g., Gloster et al. 2008) and may be useful when a single parsimonious measure of multiple domains, including stress, is desired.

Psychotic symptoms in depression

Psychotic symptoms may occur in depression in later life. Meyers and Greenberg (1986) reported delusions occurring in 45% of older depressed inpatients; in such patients the delusions may include guilt, suspiciousness, and persecutory thoughts. Hallucinations may include directives to self-harm (Thorp 1997), and so assessment and proper treatment is important. However, the greatest assessment challenge in an older adult with a psychotic presentation may be the ability to gather any information at all from the patient. In such a situation, depending on the setting and context, either picking a different time for the assessment or relying on (multiple) informants may assist in the short term with a diagnostic question and the formulation of short-term treatment strategies.

Assessing specific suicidal ideation

Mohlman and colleagues (2012), in their suggestions for successful interviewing of older adults, mentioned suicidality as a key content area to cover, including probing for risk factors for suicide and following-up on suicidal ideation with an inventory or protocol in order to ascertain risk. Risks as well as putative protective factors such as social support networks and adaptive coping styles (e.g., Heisel and Duberstein 2005), should be assessed in an interview. Older White and Asian men have the highest suicide rates of any age and gender demographic group. The ratio of completed suicides to suicide attempts is higher in late life and so suicide risk needs particular attention in older clients. Older adults who commit suicide are more likely to be depressed, use a firearm, experience social isolation, and to have physical illness or functional impairment than younger adults. They are less likely to have substance abuse problems or to have previous suicide attempts than younger adults who die by suicide (Conwell and Thompson 2008).

As with younger adults, standard professional practice is to interview for suicidal ideation, a specific method, available means, and the intent to carry out the plan. One distinction that can be quite important in assessment with older adults is the distinction between frequent thoughts of death, normative in advanced age at least with current and recent cohorts of older adults, and thoughts of taking one's own life. In our experience, most older adults readily make the distinction between thinking about death—perhaps even wishing that life would end soon on its own—and actually taking one's own life.

Because of the potential for lethal outcomes if suicidal risk is missed, it is important for assessment and response to a risk of suicide in an older patient to be effective; use of a standardized protocol (such as the Suicidal Older Adult Protocol (SOAP) by Fremouw et al. 2009) is cited by Mohlman and colleagues (2012) as good practice if suicidal intentions are suspected. Several assessment tools are available to assess suicidality, but few instruments are specifically developed for older adults. A scale designed specifically to measure suicidal ideation in older adults is the Reasons for Living Scale-Older Adults version (RFL-OA; Edelstein et al. 2009), which assesses beliefs associated with an orientation toward living and away from ending one's life. This scale has demonstrated good psychometric properties in inpatient, community, and nursing home settings. The Geriatric Suicide Ideation Scale (GSIS; Heisel and Flett 2006) is a self-report measure, tapping into a wider set of constructs including depression, hopelessness, suicidal ideation and behavior, and lack of life satisfaction. An instrument to assess suicidal ideation specifically in nursing home patients was developed by Draper and colleagues

(2002); this Harmful Behaviors Scale (HBS) has good psychometric properties and requires direct behavioral observations to be made.

Once depression is identified in the assessment and suicide risk is known, psychological therapy begins. In the next sections, we discuss the implications of the CALTAP model for therapy with older adults.

Psychotherapy with depressed older clients

The essence of a book focused on a particular population is to emphasize what makes that group of clients different from other clients. That said, working with older clients who are depressed can be very much like working with younger clients. It is worth noting for the mental health practitioner embarking on working with older adults for the first time that often there is very little difference once the assessment has been completed and the work in therapy begins. The therapist works to help the client understand the nature of their depression and what experiences in their lives are due to being depressed. The psychological techniques and interventions are generally the same and involve increased behavioral activation with a focus on increasing the number of pleasant activities, changing negative thoughts into non-negative ones, improving coping skills, encouraging a realistic hopeful outlook, suicide prevention, and other psychological methods. Therefore, it is possible to work with an older client and see the depression resolve without needing to attend to any of the special issues described in this chapter. On the other hand, it is unlikely that one can work with many older clients without attending to some or all of those specific issues and adaptations.

Several evidence-based psychological treatments for depression in older adults exist, including behavioral, cognitive behavioral, cognitive bibliotherapy, problem-solving therapy, brief psychodynamic therapy, and reminiscence therapy (Shah et al. 2012). There are also several antidepressant medications with a strong evidence base, with little evidence of difference in effects of medications and psychological interventions (e.g., Pinquart et al. 2006). Despite conventional wisdom to the contrary, older adults in general are open to psychological interventions for depression once they identify depression as the problem. For example, Robb et al. (2003) reported similar attitudes between old and young toward mental health service use, with older adults being open to referrals from a wider range of sources (including physicians, clergy, friends, and family). Rokke and Scogin (1995) found that older adults prefer psychological interventions to medical ones. In a study by Walker and Clarke (2001), younger adults showed higher rates of non-attendance and higher dropout rates than older adults participating in a cognitive therapy intervention for depression; otherwise in this study younger and older adults had similar treatment outcomes.

Developmental issues and the older client

Late onset versus lifelong depression

A key issue in working with older adults with depression is whether the depression is a late-onset first occurrence, or another episode of a lifelong struggle with depression. Detailing an older adult's long history with recurring depression can be quite helpful in treatment planning, since there are likely to have been several previous treatments, some helpful and some not. Understanding this history, and the reasons for the successes and failures, provides a valuable guide to treatment planning. The vulnerability to depression is an issue in itself and part of the therapy should focus on how to lessen the likelihood of future relapses in the face of the challenges of later life.

However, older adults with a lifelong history of depression can come to think of themselves as a "depressed person." We have seen clients who continue to think of themselves as depressed after their mood has apparently improved a great deal and they are pursuing active social lives with many activities that they enjoy. A common observation, in fact, is that they were having more fun than we the therapists were, in part because they have more free time in the post-retirement lifestyle. A lasting intervention then depends on working on changing this self-schema and helping the client define a concept of self that does not include being a depressed person. This work typically includes both challenging the evidence for being depressed as a personality trait and working out a new self-definition that the client feels comfortable accepting (see Case Example 3.2).

> ### Case Example 3.2 A depressed self-schema
> For example, one male client near 70 years old had shown considerable improvement in mood after years of therapy for chronic depression and after working through his feelings about the death of his wife. He was starting to date again, had resumed a couple of pleasurable hobbies, and was going out to social events or concerts two or three times per week. He had, however, thought of himself as depressed for decades and identified with a cartoon character who had a black cloud following him all the time. The final weeks of therapy were spent contrasting his continuing identification of himself as a depressed person with his actual level of activity and mood and finding substitute self-descriptions that he could accept. He felt it was dangerous to see himself as a happy person and that this would invite disaster, so we worked on calling himself a competent guy, an active man, and a reasonably likeable person.

Overly general attributions to aging

Perhaps the most pervasive use of lifespan developmental thinking in therapy with older adults is its use in educating older adults to rethink their implicit assumptions about the nature of aging (see Case Example 3.3A). Older clients often attribute many of the changes in their lives to the aging process and so assume that the problems they are facing are irreversible ("I'll never be young again..."), generalized across their bodies and their lives, either in the present or in the near future ("My eyesight is failing, so my hearing, my ability to walk and my mind will all go soon..."), and are such that everything can only grow worse ("I'm getting older every day...").

> ### Case Example 3.3A Eleanor: specificity of functional disability in late life
>
> Eleanor was in her early 80s when referred by her family physician for therapy for her depression. She had moved recently from the East, where she had lived in her own home for many decades, to an assisted living facility in Southern California to be near her daughter who was concerned about her increasing disability and depression. Eleanor had two diseases of the eyes that were well on the way to effectively eliminating her vision and she was also very hard of hearing. She was able to walk without difficulty. She hated the assisted living facility she was in and disliked all of their activities, complaining about the lack of services that she wanted, and the rules and restrictions. She attributed all of her problems to aging, and assumed that she would soon be completely blind and deaf.
>
> At this point, a key element was attributing her problems to disease rather than aging, which helped her to see that the course of her blindness was severe and there was little likelihood of meaningful change, but that she still had hearing and there was no current reason to see hearing loss becoming much more severe in the near future. Reviewing the history of how the decision was made to move into the assisted living environment and opening the question of what options she might have, decoupled the living situation from her age and the progressive disabilities, and gave her a greater sense of control over her life. In effect, she came to see the move as a bad decision that she had made and regretted, but still one that she had made rather than one forced on her by aging.

Life expectancy as cognitive intervention

Another common aspect of helping older clients understand the nature of aging is educating clients about the likely amount of time left in their lives. Clients frequently see no point in thinking about the future, starting new activities, or even overcoming depression, because they assume that death is quite near. In the absence of life-shortening diagnosed illnesses, most older clients have several years, quite possibly a decade or two ahead of them. Helping clients understand this can be an important component of engaging them in planning for the future in ways that can help with the current depression and also provide inoculation against future relapses. When the client is feeling depressed and overwhelmed by current circumstances, the notion of many more years of life may not always be completely positive in emotional impact, but it is usually strategically useful in getting the client to take the future seriously and to begin making forward-looking plans.

The downs and ups of developmental aging

Acknowledgement of some of the negative components of normal aging can be quite useful in rapport building and in helping clients cope with depression. As noted in Chapter 1, in general, normal developmental aging brings a slowing in cognitive processing, greater difficulty in focusing attention with distractions around, and a somewhat smaller working memory capacity. This tends to mean that the world appears to be moving faster, that it can take longer to learn new information, and that thinking may take more effort than in the past. Normalizing these changes, distinguishing them from early dementia, and discussing what they do and do not mean in terms of taking on new activities and new learning can be quite important in understanding aging and in increasing behavioral activation. Clients often have given up early on activities they would like to take on because of these difficulties (whether perceived or real). There is also often an additional layer of thinking that young people are learning new things easily and well, and also overestimating how well they used to learn new things when they were younger.

Positive aspects of aging can be a help to the therapeutic process and can also make therapy with older adults *feel* different from work with younger adults. Older adults have many years of adult life experience, and a drive to reminisce and make sense of life (Butler 1963). Out of this life experience, they almost always have previous experience of responding to problems similar to the ones that have brought them to therapy (see Case Example 3.3B). Maintaining a purely present-oriented focus with older clients in therapy is seldom possible and, in most instances, doing some exploring of similar problems in the past can lead to the discovery of client strengths, coping styles, and problem solutions that may not have occurred to the therapist.

> ### Case Example 3.3B Eleanor: discovering past successful coping
> In the midst of a therapy session focused on her current problems, Eleanor remarked that she did not understand why these were so difficult for her when she felt she had dealt with equally difficult problems in the past. We shifted into reviewing these past successes and what she thought the key strengths were that enabled her to overcome them. She took considerable pride in finding solutions and sticking to them, even when they were hard to put into action and took a long time to show results. She rather quickly introduced these traits into her current situation, with marked improvement in mood.

This wealth of experience can also mean that the focus of therapy may embrace multiple examples of problems separated in time and that the target of change may be at a more abstract level than concrete, present time, automatic thinking. The sheer amount of experience involved may be challenging for the therapist to take in and process and the shift to a different level of abstraction may be novel for therapists used to working with very specific automatic thoughts.

Using the client's history to change depressive thoughts

A trainee working with a depressed older man of about 70 was focusing on negative self-talk related to low self-esteem. For the client this quickly led to a lifetime of examples of people telling him he was not as bright as others, not as successful, and so on. Drawing on what was known about his life history, the change strategy focused on how much he had accomplished in his life with several advanced degrees and successful work histories in more than one line of work. Therefore, it was more schema-focused than on current depressive thoughts.

Social context and the older client

A frequent theme related to social context for older clients is the depressing aspect of living in an age-segregated environment of any type due to the frequency with which other residents are taken to the hospital or die. The presence of other residents who are losing cognitive ability to dementias is also a common concern. In general, it is more strategic therapeutically to validate this reaction, and sympathize with it, rather than to try and change it. Others around them—family and other supportive younger adults—are probably already trying to cheer them up. The simple reality is that it is both distressing because of concerns about the friends who are sick or who have died, and because of the constant reminders of one's vulnerability and mortality.

It can also be useful to explore how the decision was made to move into the age-segregated environment and whether it is possible to move out again into a different living arrangement. This review reminds the client of why they are where they are and what the current viable options are. Occasionally this discussion may lead to a move and to living in a more desirable environment. More commonly, the review leads to a sense of deciding to remain in the facility given the range of choices available based on the client's health and level of functioning (see Case Example 3.3C). This acceptance often leads to a more positive appraisal of where they currently live, or at least a decision to make the best of it.

Another common social context that affects older clients is the health care environment, including hospitals, physician offices, pharmacies, insurance companies, and so forth. As a health care professional who is likely to know some of the players in this environment personally, the therapist may have a tendency to see the health care world from the provider's perspective. However,

Case Example 3.3C Eleanor: rethinking the move to assisted living

Returning to Eleanor, helping her to see the move into assisted living as a decision she had made, albeit a bad one, was helpful in lowering her depression. As the therapy went on, she considered other options, and recalled having looked at other assisted living in the area and liking the other places even less. She thought briefly about living on her own, but rapidly decided that her limited sight and hearing ruled that possibility out. She then discussed having other family members who were moving to the area, and that it might be possible to move out and live close to them once they settled in. However, The recognition of depression in the context of residential care for the elderly can also be difficult, especially if there are hints of psychotic symptoms. Case Example 3.4 example illustrates this problem. Of interest, once she went through this decision process, her attitude toward the assisted living place improved, and she started going to some activities that she had avoided up to that point. She was not especially impressed with the activities and the ability of the staff to include her with her disabilities, but felt that "it's better than sitting in my room alone, even when I can't tell what's going on."

Case Example 3.4 Molly: depression with some dementia in age care facility

Molly was a 78-year-old resident of an aged care facility in a rural area. She had lived almost her entire life in a small town about 150 miles from the nearest large city, and with her husband Dave had run a successful store selling saddles and equestrian equipment. In her youth she competed successfully at the national level in dressage, before marrying and having three children. After her husband's death, her children placed her in a nursing home close to her place of birth and early childhood, perhaps with a romanticized vision of their mother finding being in this setting peaceful. Yet in reality none of Molly's friends from her adult life made the three-hour trip to this relatively isolated small town and, indeed, her children rarely visited.

Molly was an only child and had been doted upon by her parents. She was somewhat of a local celebrity in her youth; Dave also idolized his wife, and her children described her as "always knowing how to get her way." In recent times it had appeared to her children that Molly had become "eccentric," and Dave had appeared to tolerate his wife's odd impulsive purchases and increasing reluctance to socialize.

When Dave died suddenly of a heart attack, two years previously, Molly was devastated and took it very badly. Her children had by that point moved to a nearby city, and in recent years had only been occasional visitors to their parents' home. Molly began to act strangely after her husband's death. She claimed that she spoke regularly to Dave, but these conversations began to have a flavor of paranoia, with Dave warning Molly that people were after her money. She began withdrawing from her friends, and accusing her children of wanting to take her home and possessions from her. Eventually this extended to the government wanting to take her house from her. (It was notable that at one stage Dave had been faced with foreclosure on his home due to bad business debts.) Molly began to show signs of hoarding food and household items. On one visit her son Mark claimed he could not even enter several rooms of his parents' home because of the crowding.

One day, Molly had left a pot on the stove and a small fire in the kitchen was the result. A neighbor noticed the smoke and knocked on the back door; when there was no answer, he forced open the back door and attempted to extinguish the flames. Molly came through to the kitchen and began throwing objects at him, shouting abuse; the neighbor was injured and was taken to the hospital for stitches to his head. At this point Molly's children moved her to the rural nursing facility, stating that they felt "the quiet will do her good."

However, the move away from familiar surroundings seemed only to amplify Molly's agitation. She believed that the government had succeeded in taking her home and that now she was in "prison." When the consultation was received by the community mental health outreach team to evaluate Molly, she was indeed on a locked ward, following several attempts to abscond.

The psychologist began her visit by chatting to the nursing staff. One nurse in particular was very forthcoming about Molly's behavior, stating that she was sure that she had a personality disorder "because she is so manipulative." The staff cited her aggression and extreme paranoia as reasons for giving relatively high doses of atypical antipsychotic medications. Conversations with Mark, who had made the trip out to the nursing home due to concerns for his mother's deteriorating mental state, revealed that Molly was well-known to some staff members from her earlier life in the small town, and that some had confided to him that they believed Molly resented being back in her home town; they felt she was deliberately being difficult to show her displeasure. Molly in turn insisted that people were stealing her things and "talking behind my back." Mark stated that he now felt that perhaps placing their mother there had not been a wise decision.

Molly had no previous psychiatric history. Other than non-insulin dependent diabetes, Molly was in relatively good health. She was very non-compliant in her diet, however, and ate other residents' desserts when the opportunity presented itself. She would often sleep in the afternoon, but then be quite restless at night, often staying up all night and going into other residents' rooms looking for sweets, but sometimes looking for Dave or other people known to her from her childhood and early adult years in this small town. If residents awoke and tried to stop her, she would often strike out at them. The afternoon shift was reluctant to keep her awake as sleeping through the afternoon ensured a calmer environment, but the night staff were adamant that she was unmanageable, and hence her prn medications had been increased.

Prior cognitive assessments had revealed that Molly had a moderate level of dementia; staff questioned whether her symptoms of paranoia reflected her dementia or were a late onset psychotic presentation. The NPI revealed the presence of delusional thinking, but this was not as significant as her depressive symptoms. This was echoed in results on the Cornell Scale for Depression in Dementia.

Many things in Molly's environment served to reinforce what were largely thought to be misperceptions, rather than frank hallucinations. It was, in fact, true that several staff were known to Molly from her childhood. She had experienced a prolonged period of time in mid-adulthood where there was real fear her home would be taken from her. She sometimes received boxes of chocolate from well-meaning friends, and these were always first given to Molly so she could open them, but then removed "for her own good." The psychologist, in conducting the assessment, had noticed that Molly often gave strange responses to questions, but it became apparent that this was due to Molly not understanding the questions because of poor hearing; a subsequent evaluation revealed markedly deteriorated hearing bilaterally. Molly had often claimed that people were "talking behind her back"; paranoia may develop in older adults with significant hearing loss.

In the absence of a psychiatric history, it was felt most likely that Molly's symptoms were more reflective of a combination of a psychotic depression, as well as what, with hindsight, was a progressive deterioration in cognitive functioning predating Dave's death. Although it was impossible to rule out the role of dementia (and, thus, Behavioral and Psychological Symptoms in Dementia (BPSD)) in some aspects of her current functioning, it appeared clear that Molly had not received any treatment for her depression following Dave's death.

In consultation with the psychiatrist, Molly was started on an antidepressant and her atypical antipsychotics were titrated down. She was encouraged to not sleep through the afternoon, and this attention to sleep hygiene routines led to decreased nocturnal disturbance. Four weeks after the introduction of the antidepressant, staff were pleased with the changes in Molly's behavior, and Molly herself appeared more settled and engaged, especially now that she could better understand those around her with her new hearing aid. Mark and his siblings had informed Molly's friends that sending cards and notes were more appreciated than chocolates. One or two of Molly's oldest friends made the journey out to visit and took her out to lunch in town, delighted to hear about the earlier equestrian exploits of her youth. Molly herself still had unsettled periods and periodically still lashed out at others, but staff had come up with a few strategies for redirection, which for the most part worked well.

it is important to be able to enter that world from the perspective of the older client, who is often engaged with the system on a regular basis due to chronic illnesses and frequently finds it quite frustrating. Following the client's viewpoint, it is almost always therapeutic to validate the feelings. Occasionally it may be possible to do some problem solving that will help the client move through the health care world more effectively. More often, the path to reducing frustration is lowering expectations about what is likely to happen (see Case Example 3.5).

Case Example 3.5 Sally: depression with chronic physical illness and health care system issues

Sally was a woman in her 60s with several chronic physical conditions. She was deeply depressed and a common trigger for deepening of her depressed mood were the vicissitudes of interacting with the health care providers in her life—doctors who did not return calls, doctors who were behind schedule when she came for an appointment, delays in getting prescriptions filled at the pharmacy, and unpleasant interactions with insurance claims agents regarding coverage of the bills for her care. On the whole, these are the normal frustrations of dealing with getting health care in the USA at this point in time. However, for Sally these were unacceptable and overwhelming failures of these health care providers to care for her.

> The trainee therapist spent a lot of time supportively listening to the emotional outbursts and reflecting them sympathetically to Sally. There was little work on problem solving, both because many of these problems are common and essentially unsolvable and because Sally was actually rather good at getting her needs met, but suffered a great deal emotionally in the process. Over a period of months, she gradually came to accept her ability to handle these situations most of the time and so reduced the level of distress felt somewhat. With yet more time, the problem came to be redefined in terms of her depression over having chronic illnesses, and the dual frustration of being told there was nothing more that could be done to help her and the failure of the attempts made by those who acceded to her constant requests for help.

Cohort effects and therapy

Another source of confusion concerning aging is the confusion of cohort effects with developmental aging effects. In general, older people tend to attribute differences between themselves and younger people around them to age. Cohort effects suggest that many such differences are due to when we are born and the resulting differences in sociohistorical experiences. From clinical experience, it appears that the period from childhood to young adulthood may be of particular importance in shaping values and self-perceptions, but this can vary by individual, of course (see Case Example 3.6, for example). In the popular media, these distinctions are roughly captured by discussions of differences among the World War II generation, the Baby Boomers, Generation X, the Millennials, etc.

> **Case Example 3.6 Sam: cohort differences shaping an older gay man's self-perception**
>
> Sam turned 70 while being seen in a university training clinic for depression. There were several factors influencing his depression, which he had for a number of years. One consistent element was that he was gay and unable to accept his sexuality. He perceived a need to keep it secret and in doing so was quite isolated in his life. While he was intermittently sexually active, in a casual way, he neither formed lasting relationships nor was he at all interested in integrating into the gay community in the city. His opinion of gays as a community was quite similar to the negative views he perceived society as having toward himself as a person. Understanding Sam and his attitudes, and the resulting isolation, depended in a large part in placing him in the context of his cohort, in which being gay was seen in highly negative terms, and spending a lifetime closeted and isolated was not as atypical as it was in the life experience of most of the trainees who worked with him in therapy. It also led, in his case, to setting the goals as working on his self-acceptance and not on greater social contact in the gay community, although the latter did seem like a sensible solution to many of his problems before we understood the depth of his homonegativity. He did eventually accept his own sexuality, and his mood and self-esteem improved.

In general, understanding such differences in terms of different histories tends to decrease the negative tone often associated with the perception that "I am different because I'm old." For most of us, the shift in perception suggests the possibility of change in behavior, which can be emotionally helpful, whether or not the change is acted on. As an everyday example, if I (BK) perceives myself as too old to use computer-based social media, it can contribute to negative mood and I am not likely to learn to use it. If I think instead that this is something that the Millennial generation takes to very easily and that, as a Baby Boomer, it's not a natural part of my experience in the same way, I feel better about myself, and am more likely to learn to use it. I also feel better about myself, however, even if I choose not to use it, in part because it is now a choice that I have made.

On the therapist side of the room, understanding cohort effects and breaking out of one's own cohort's frame of reference are important elements in establishing a rapport with older clients and in understanding them accurately. Showing some knowledge of World War II, and the music, values, and common social experiences of that era can go a long way in developing a good relationship with someone of that cohort. Being able to anticipate, or at least understand and accept, differences in world views between a Korean War era parent and a Baby Boomer child greatly facilitates the work of therapy. In all cases, what is important is understanding the individual client's experience of growing up when and where she or he did.

To some extent, many older adults live with a remembered past that shadows the present world. Southern California, for example, has grown a great deal since the end of World War II and has seen the immigration of a number of different cultural groups and the relocation within the city of others. For the older clients that we see here, all remember a smaller city that many prefer to the current larger and more crowded one. Many have seen the neighborhoods in which they grew up changed, torn down, or taken over by a different cultural group, often with a different language. Most older adults remember a time when current poor health behaviors were seen as acceptable (eating lots of meat and potatoes) or even healthy (drinking sodas, smoking tobacco). They have also seen many fads of all kinds come and go, and predictions about the future that came true or faded away unrealized, while other unexpected changes occurred. These experiences can lead to a skepticism about "new" discoveries and predictions that often strike younger people as stubbornness or as a failure to be modern.

Cultural differences and therapy with older clients

Cultural competency is important in working with any client, of course. Much of cultural competency is being aware of the possibility of differences and following the individual client's lead on what the cultural effects mean in his or her own life (cf. American Psychological Association 2002). An additional complication in working with older clients is that the cultural differences intersect with cohort effects and can be quite distinct from differences one has learned from interaction with friends of the same age. Older adults may have had the experience of being discriminated against or being insulted for being Italian or Irish, for example. Certainly, any older African American adult who lived in the segregated South will have a different experience of being African American in the USA than those raised after integration and civil rights (see Case Example 3.7).

> ### Case Example 3.7 Cultural differences between therapist and client
> One middle-aged white trainee worked with a young-old African American client. Both had been born and raised in Los Angeles, but had very different experiences. The African American client had devoted her life to her community, and to preserving its history and culture. When she was younger, she had been active in the civil rights struggles and for a while affiliated to some degree with the Black Panthers. She was frequently challenging to the therapist, who openly and undefensively acknowledged that she had no real idea what the client's life had been like, but proved herself open to learn from the client. They developed a warm therapeutic relationship, and were able to effectively pursue therapeutic goals and resolve much of the client's depression. Along the way, the client acknowledged having worked through some of her own stereotypes about Whites.

Often, cultural value conflicts are played out within the client, rather than between client and therapist. One middle-aged Mexican American woman described it as "I'm American enough that I can't imagine living with my aging mother all the time and Mexican enough to feel very guilty about it." Another young-old client with an Afro-Caribbean heritage struggled with being the primary caregiver to both parents and two disabled brothers. As the only daughter, the work was clearly her responsibility culturally, but she also longed for independence, the ability to focus on her career, and a desire for her own social and romantic life. Much of her depression stemmed from being unable to decide to move in either direction.

When these internal conflicts are not present, the cultural differences can support and sustain positive mood and self-image. The African American client mentioned earlier was quite proud of her history and of her role in the community. Older clients dealing with family caregiving issues often take pride in doing things differently and in feeling better about the caregiving role than they perceive Whites do.

Older adults themselves often have a more positive self-image based on the cultural perception of age as a time when one is wise and has earned respect. This positive self-concept may or may not be actively supported by younger family members, often depending on some mix of acculturation to Western values and the history of family relationships with the older adult. In the absence of support from younger family members, contact with other older adults from the same culture or with younger people from that culture who actively respect older adults can be helpful in alleviating depression.

Complications in therapy for depression with older adults

As noted, therapy for depression with older adults often goes fairly smoothly. Older adults often have a lot of unstructured time and have ample opportunity to practice therapeutic interventions. The motivation to change often seems to be higher than in younger adults, perhaps driven in part by what Nemiroff and Colarusso (1985) called "the race against time." Knowing that life is limited can be a stimulus for change.

Change does not always go quickly or smoothly, however. One of the most common differences in working with older adults is that the stressors are often chronic, and either progressive or recurring. Common classes of challenges in later life are chronic illness and disability, and family caregiving (see Chapter 1). Many chronic illnesses of later life (although not all) are progressive, and so the stressor changes for the worse over time. This is in contrast to the usually one-time, short-duration stressors that confront younger clients. In working with younger adults with depression, one is often dealing with an issue that has already happened, is over, and is not likely to recur soon. With older adults, the stressors are ongoing, and likely to continue and worsen. Thus, as progress is made on one aspect of the stressor, it is likely that the situation will change and another aspect will need to be dealt with. Older clients often have new stressors that appear during therapy as well—another diagnosis, a spouse who falls ill, a close loved one who dies.

The reality of late life problems

On the therapist's side of the consultation room, working with older clients tends to confront the therapist very frequently with an array of problems, many of which are clearly real and often quite sad. The reality of the client's problems is especially an issue if the therapist assumes (implicitly or explicitly) that psychological interventions mainly work by modifying unrealistic negative thoughts or emotional reactions. Eleanor's situation provides an apt example of a time when anyone might well say, "Of course she's depressed, she going blind and deaf!" In fact, part of the ongoing therapeutic process with older clients is being clear with the client about what is changeable and what is not. For Eleanor (Case Example 3.3), the impact of her progressive vision loss had been substantial and unchangeable. Acknowledging this with sympathy and showing an understanding of how difficult adjustments to lost vision will be is a key part of developing the therapeutic relationship and showing appropriate warmth and empathy. Steps toward increasing pleasure in her life to alleviate depression depended on helping her discover ways to maximize the use of the hearing she had left to continue to enjoy books, music, sports, etc., by using headphones with adjustable volume on the various playback devices that she had.

Bereavement and grief work

Psychologists often seem to have difficulty focusing on grief as a key presenting problem in therapy with older adults. BK has frequently noted that trainees and peers seeking consultation are often focusing on other issues when a client's presenting problem included grief for a loved one. The complications in general appear to be mainly in the therapist's comfort in talking about and encouraging the client to talk about the loss, and to express feelings openly (see Case Example 3.8). Much of the work is active listening and reflection and is not technically difficult at all. But it can be quite uncomfortable to listen to stories about death and the feelings of loss, which inevitably confront the therapist with the likelihood that they too will lose loved ones. The work of grief is generally divided between expression of feelings and working through the loss on one hand and adjusting to a new life without the deceased and to the social role of widowhood on the other (Stroebe and Schut 1999). See also Worden (2008) for a further explication of therapy for clients experiencing grief as a primary symptom.

Case Example 3.8 Trudy: depression during bereavement

Trudy was 80 when she started therapy at the suggestion of her daughter and her physician for severe depression following the death of her husband of nearly 60 years. She was very positive about the marriage and her husband as a person, and saw no future for herself as a single person.

Therapy focused in the early sessions mainly on talking about her husband, the way he died, how much she missed him, and just letting her cry. As is often the case for the bereaved after a brief period of time following the loss, no one else in her life was willing to listen without telling her she needed to move on, get busy, and so forth.

As time went on, this focus on grief expression was punctuated occasionally, then more frequently, with discussion of things she used to enjoy, but did not now feel like doing. The therapist would discuss the pros and cons of resuming these activities to increase enjoyment in life versus the quite real possibility that they would lead to more intense grief reactions. Over a period of several weeks, some activities became more acceptable to her, and she resumed going to arts events in her community and volunteer work that she had done for years.

As a few months went by, it became apparent that a couple of men she knew were interested in a relationship with her. At first this was unthinkable to her. The therapist empathized with how hard it was to think of dating at this point in her life and being with anyone other than her husband. As these discussions went on, he also noted that she seemed to show some signs of interest and some pleasure in being found attractive. Without urging her to take any particular action, he also shared some stories of widows who found new relationships of different sorts, always emphasizing that what she did was totally up to her. Eventually she decided on some lunch and coffee meetings, and one of these developed into a more serious relationship. Among other things, she enjoyed the fact that she was getting more male attention than her single daughter who was in her 50s.

Summary

Depression is a common focus in therapy with older adults and a good introduction to issues that arise in working with older adults. It provides some good examples of ways that the CALTAP model is useful in therapy by providing the older client with different ways of thinking about aging and about problems occurring in late life. It is also valuable in illustrating some of the common reactions of therapists to working with older adults. Depression is not the most common psychological disorder in late life, however.

The linkages between depression and anxiety have been a matter for research and debate for years. Clinically, we have noted that there are times when the alleviation of depressed mood reveals anxiety disorders. For example, one client in her late 80s was referred for depression, which seemed to be occasioned by the strain of caregiving for her husband, his controlling and sometimes insulting interaction style, and other changes in her life that threatened her sense of independence and control. After a couple of months of therapy focusing on different approaches to caregiving (hiring a caregiver from a home care company), on being more assertive with her husband, and thinking about the possibility of leaving him, her depression improved considerably. Then she became highly anxious, with chronic worrying and difficulty making decisions. Depending on the client's preferences, some clients may well avoid letting go of depression in order to not feel the anxiety. In the Chapter 4, we discuss assessment and treatment of anxiety disorders in late life.

Chapter 4

Anxiety in later life

Introduction to anxiety in later life

Anxiety, and not depression, is the most common psychiatric disorder in later life (Beekman et al. 1998; Kessler et al. 2005a), yet it remains relatively under-researched in older populations compared with depressive disorders (Byrne and Pachana 2010). Late life anxiety prevalence estimates range from 3.2% to 14.2%, depending on age and specific diagnoses (e.g., generalized anxiety disorder (GAD), simple phobias; Wolitzky-Taylor et al. 2010). According to a recent systematic review (Baxter et al. 2013), the current prevalence of anxiety disorders is 7.3% worldwide, but significantly higher (10.4%) among developed (i.e., Anglo/European) compared with developing (i.e., African) nations (5.3%). Using the National Comorbidity Survey Replication (NCS-R), Byers et al. (2010) found 12-month prevalence rates in community-dwelling persons aged 55 years or older of 5% for mood and 12% for anxiety disorders, with women at increased risk for anxiety disorders compared with men. The prevalence of anxiety symptoms (as opposed to disorders) is much higher, ranging from 15% to 52.3% in older community samples, and 15% to 56% in older clinical samples (Bryant et al. 2008).

The most common anxiety disorders reported in older adults are phobias and GAD (Beekman et al. 2000; LeRoux et al. 2005). Panic disorder is a relatively less common anxiety disorder in later life, as are obsessive compulsive and post-traumatic stress disorders (Wolitzky-Taylor et al. 2010), these latter two disorders being classified as separate from anxiety disorders in the Diagnostic and Statistical Manual of Mental Disorders, 5th edition (DSM-5; American Psychiatric Association 2013). Anxiety disorders, although common in older adults, are less prevalent than in younger age groups (Kessler et al. 2005b). Subsyndromal presentations of anxiety are also common among older adults (e.g., Lenze et al. 2005).

Anxiety disorders in later life have been shown to:

- increase morbidity and health care costs, including primary care visits;
- be associated with several medical conditions, including coronary artery disease, mobility and functional limitations, and sleep disturbance;

- increase distress, impair social functioning, and lower quality of life and life satisfaction;
- predict institutionalization in those with dementia (e.g., Gellis 2006; Lenze et al. 2000; Scogin et al. 2000; Wetherell et al. 2003).

In short, anxiety disorders significantly impact the length, the quality, and the manner in which life is lived for older adults. Unfortunately, as with depression, both health professionals and older adults themselves often believe that increases in anxiety are part of normal aging. Furthermore, compared with younger adults, older adults tend to minimize and under-report anxiety symptoms (Levy et al. 2003), which has implications for epidemiological data, as well as assessing and treating these disorders clinically.

There are several identified protective factors and risk factors for anxiety in later life. Protective factors include high levels of perceived social support, regular exercise, and higher levels of education (Vink et al. 2008). Risk factors include female gender, lower levels of education, poor self-rated general health, current anxiolytic use (which is a risk factor, as well as a common form of treatment of anxiety), physical or sexual abuse in childhood, current smoking and excessive alcohol use, stressful life events, and neuroticism (Beekman et al. 1998; Vink et al. 2009). Depression is also a risk factor for anxiety (Wetherell et al. 2001). Not enough research has been conducted to date to comment on culture and ethnicity with respect either to risk or protective factors, or symptom presentation differences (e.g., Wolitzky-Taylor et al. 2010).

Comorbidity between anxiety and depression in later life is high; in one study 47.5% of those with major depressive disorder also met criteria for anxiety disorders, and 26.1% of those with anxiety disorders also met criteria for major depressive disorder (Beekman et al. 2000). These rates are similar to co-occurrence rates in younger adults (Cassidy et al. 2005). In older adults, comorbid anxiety in depression is associated with poor treatment response and increased likelihood of treatment dropout (Lenze et al. 2003); older depressed patients with higher levels of comorbid anxiety at pretreatment have also been shown to take longer to respond to treatments and also be at greater risk for recurrence of depression (Andreescu et al. 2007). Older people with anxious depression are also at greater risk for suicidal ideation and attempts, as well as reduced psychosocial supports (Jeste et al. 2006; Lenze et al. 2000). Comorbid anxiety and depression in later life can be conceived of as a type of double jeopardy: subjecting already vulnerable older clients to additional emotional distress, compounding burden, and diminishing quality of life (Beattie and Pachana 2010). In one study, primary care physicians noted the high number of their patients with symptoms of both anxiety and depression, who nevertheless failed to meet diagnostic criteria for either disorder (Sartorius et al. 1996). Distinguishing between anxiety and depression, particularly subthreshold presentations of the two conditions that are comorbid, poses a difficult diagnostic challenge in clinical settings (Cassidy et al. 2005).

Assessment of anxiety in later life

In a similar way to assessment approaches with depressed clients, tools and approaches used with older adults with anxiety must consider issues such as sociodemographic characteristics, cognitive status, and possible comorbid medical and psychiatric conditions. Assessment strategies, goals, and procedures should be clear in the mind of the therapist and clearly articulated to the older adult undergoing assessment. This is particularly important with anxious clients, who may feel heightened anxiety in the face of assessment and may need more reassurance as part of the assessment process. A client's excessive anxiety may serve to inhibit the assessment process, as well as affect assessment data. The anxiety of the client, if not addressed in the assessment process, could color the data collected, making interpretation difficult; this issue is discussed further in the following sections.

Clinical interview

Much of discussion of clinical interview techniques (e.g., the advantages of structured or semi-structured interviews over unstructured interview formats) remains the same for anxiety as for depression (refer to Chapter 2 for detailed discussion of structured vs. unstructured interviews). It is important for clinicians to gather detailed data on the nature and circumstances surrounding instances of anxiety symptoms, and hence structured interviews help insure pertinent areas of interest are covered.

Clinicians who have not seen a lot of older clients may underestimate the presence of anxiety symptoms of concern by attributing their appearance to "normal aging." For example, they may feel that it is "normal" for older adults to be more socially isolated or to see people less often. This represents an age-biased view of behavior in later life. An older adult's current patterns of behavior needs to be compared with past behaviors and not evaluated in light of the clinician's impressions of what is "normal" for an older person.

An interesting point in using diagnostic interviews with older clients is that whatever the interview structure chosen, particularly for anxiety disorders, one must be cognizant of the ways that the current diagnostic criteria (both DSM-IV and DSM-5, as well as ICD-10) are not well-tailored to the common presentations of anxiety in older adults. As part of the Advisory Committee to the DSM-5 Lifespan Disorders Work Group, Mohlman and colleagues (2012) discuss a variety of specific presentations of anxiety in later life, which make diagnosis difficult if not taken into account by clinicians. For example, excessive anxiety and avoidance are basic features of all anxiety disorders. Accurate recognition and diagnosis requires that age-specific presentations are recognized and behaviors that could signal the presence of an anxiety disorder are not misattributed to normal aging. Thus, the older adult who rarely ventures out of the home should not be viewed as typical, as their behavior is not normal for, nor explained by, their age. There is also the broader issue of heterogeneity in older adults with respect to behaviors, descriptions of symptoms, medical conditions and treatments, unique life circumstances, and so forth, which makes discussion of potential anxiety symptoms challenging (Bryant 2010).

Mohlman and colleagues (2012) suggest asking probing questions of anxious patients with medical comorbidities to determine whether "excessive" worry is present; some examples include "Do your health care providers say you worry too much?" and "Do you think you check things like your blood pressure more often than you need to?" Such questions can help determine not only the presence of excessive worry related to health concerns, but will provide useful information for treatment. They also describe many age-specific presentations that can be useful in diagnosing anxiety in later life. For example, they detail age-specific examples of maladaptive avoidance, such as avoiding exercise or public transportation due to excessive fear of falling, excessive checking on the health of self or loved ones (e.g., multiple calls to adult children per day), and refusal to use any type of aid to enhance functioning (e.g., cane, walker, hearing aid) for fear of appearing "old."

This group also underscores the fact that older adults may not endorse particular clinical criteria, particularly of "excessive" anxiety, either because they are unsure themselves about whether or not it is excessive, or because they lack insight into whether or not it may be excessive. The criteria of "excessive" can be difficult to pin down at any point in the lifespan; in later life some issues to consider in making (or assisting the older adult to make) this judgment may include considering past patterns of behavior, whether others have commented on or worried about the amount or frequency of behaviors, or whether the older adult themselves has seen such behaviors interfere with activities or functioning. Mohlman et al. (2012) also suggest using the patient's own descriptive words in place of the term "excessive" during a standardized interview, as in older adults a denial of "excessive" worry may be accompanied by descriptions of cognitive and emotional processes that clearly are "excessive" in relation to peers of a similar age.

As in depression, physical illnesses and medication side effects may mimic symptoms of anxiety. Older clients are more likely to be on medications, which may make accurate diagnosis of an anxiety disorder challenging; medications may also have side effects such as fatigue and cognitive confusion, which not only mimic the symptoms of anxiety disorders, but also may impact treatment. For example, shortness of breath may be a symptom of a physical illness, such as chronic obstructive pulmonary disease (COPD), a symptom of an anxiety disorder, or may, in some cases, be related to comorbid anxiety and COPD. Similarly, tachycardia may be the result of stress and anxiety, may reflect a symptom of an illness or a medication side effect, or again may be partly attributable to multiple causes. The clinician working with older adults would be remiss if he/she did not have a full understanding of the potential etiologies of such symptoms in later life.

Older adults with anxiety may also have other comorbid medical conditions that could impact on assessment, diagnosis, and treatment (see, for example, Case Example 4.1A). Research shows that between 80% and 86% of older adults over age 65 years have at least one chronic medical condition (e.g., Haley 1996). Gastrointestinal illnesses (Kane et al. 1993), hyperthyroidism (Kathol et al. 1986), cancer (Deimling et al. 2006), and diabetes (Blazer 2003b) have all been associated with anxiety disorders in later life. Respiratory (Yohannes et al. 2000) and cardiac conditions (Todaro et al. 2007) and symptoms, such as shortness of breath, are also associated with anxiety in this age group, and are of particular note in anxiety disorders because their symptoms are reciprocal. Thus, symptoms such as shortness of breath from asthma can exacerbate anxiety, and tachycardia from increased anxiety can exacerbate cardiac conditions. Older adults can also develop anxiety about specific symptoms associated with illnesses common in later life, such as chest pain in the case of cardiac illness (Goldberg et al. 1990). Further complicating accurate diagnosis is the fact that older adults tend to somaticize psychiatric conditions, including anxiety (Lenze et al. 2005).

Case Example 4.1A Marlene: history of anxiety with recent macular degeneration

Marlene, aged 66, was referred to Jennifer from her primary health care physician. She had recently received a diagnosis of macular degeneration, which was in its early stages. Unfortunately, after receiving the news about her sight, she asked her ophthalmologist what she could do now and was told "Better see the things you want to see in this world in the next 5–10 years." When Marlene and her husband Michael came to a follow-up visit at the health care clinic, he was livid about how his wife had been treated. "What sort of a thing is that to tell a person? Now all she does is worry about how much time she has left to see things."

By her own admission, Marlene had always been a nervous person. In her twenties she had been to see a psychologist, and received treatment for panic attacks and mild agoraphobia. The treatment had been successful, and she had resumed her activities and work as a librarian. When her first husband was killed in an auto accident, she again sought treatment for recurrent panic attacks brought on by the sudden loss. Again, her symptoms resolved and she was able to resume work. Marlene's current presenting symptoms included headaches, nausea, shortness of breath, heart palpitations, and poor sleep, which had increased since she was told of her prognosis with respect to her vision loss.

Marlene and Michael, whom she married approximately 10 years ago, had no children, and she had no children from her first marriage. Michael was a computer programming consultant, and they lived in a small house on the outskirts of town. Marlene's passion was her garden and particularly creating "a little bit of wild nature at our doorstep." She and Michael were avid birdwatchers, and she hung various feeders around her garden so she could photograph the birds that visited them.

Many of Marlene's hobbies and activities involved sight—photography, bird watching, and reading. She had become obsessed with the eventual loss of her vision. This seemed exacerbated by the ophthalmologist's instructions to monitor all changes in her vision closely. This was to determine whether she had the so-called wet or dry type of macular degeneration, as this would be important for both prognosis and possible treatments. However, in either case, her sight would continue to decline over the next 5–10 years.

Marlene documented all observed changes in her vision in a small diary. She would often work on it in the middle of the night, also recording her thoughts about her vision changing. "It is all futile—don't know why I am continuing to record any changes—nothing can be done." Despite the sleeping pills prescribed by her physician, Marlene was often up most of the night.

Her husband Michael reported she had stopped filling her bird feeders, and had not picked up her camera since the chat with the ophthalmologist.

In addition, the medications prescribed to older adults to combat anxiety bring with them age-specific potential side effects in this population. In particular, sedative-hypnotics have many negative side effects in older adults, including increasing drowsiness and exacerbating cognitive impairment. Gray and colleagues (2006) reported that older adults using benzodiazepines were more likely to develop mobility problems and have issues with activities of daily living. The use of benzodiazepines in older adults is also related to an increase in risk of falls (Ray et al. 2000). In the USA, one in three adults aged 65 and over will have a fall each year (Hausdorff et al. 2001). Falls result in morbidity and hospitalization due to injuries and fractures, as well as other less apparent consequences, such as the post-fall syndrome of immobility, anxiety, and depression (Zeimer 2008). The consequences of falls for older adults go beyond the physical injuries sustained—those aged 75 and above who fall are four to five times more likely than those aged 65 to 74 to be admitted to a nursing home for at least a calendar year (Stevens and Dellinger 2002). Fear of falling itself is an important issue, with about 3% of older adults in the community avoiding leaving their homes and yards due to fear of falling (Arfken et al. 1994), with some acquiring an agoraphobia-like syndrome as a consequence of fear of falling, rather than an actual fall (van Haastregt et al. 2008).

It is important for the clinician working with older adults with comorbid medical conditions to bear in mind that some level of anxiety may be expected and, in some cases, useful for the client. Anxiety serves a biologically useful purpose in alerting us to potential danger and to heightening awareness so that appropriate action can be taken. It is unrealistic and possibly counterproductive to attempt to alleviate all anxiety. Moreover, both anxiety and depression may be natural and appropriate reactions to diagnoses of serious medical conditions. For the older adult now having to closely monitor diet in the face of a diagnosis of Type 2 diabetes, some amount of worry about their health may actually enhance treatment compliance, although more research in this area is warranted. However, the inability of clinicians to distinguish between adaptive and pathological anxiety in older adults is a barrier to correct diagnosis and, by extension, treatment (Lenze and Wetherell 2009).

Finally, similar to depression, cognitive screens to ascertain level of current cognitive functioning may be useful, especially if there is a suspicion that cognitive difficulties may be a sign of an incipient dementia. Brief cognitive screens such as the Montreal Cognitive Assessment (MoCA; Nasreddine et al. 2005), Modified Mini-Mental State Exam (3MS; Teng and Chui 1987), and the Rowland Universal Dementia Assessment Scale (RUDAS; Storey et al. 2004) are appropriate for older adults. It is important to note that moderately low scores on any of these screening measures could be ascribed to either anxiety, impaired cognitive functioning due to MCI or incipient dementia, or any combination of these. Teasing apart the degree to which anxiety might contribute to cognitive impairment is tricky, but retesting with such a screen following successful treatment of the anxiety may offer some insights.

A challenging and stimulating aspect of working with older adults is this ongoing interaction of physical, cognitive, and emotional symptoms that span the mind–body interface. As a practical matter, assessments are often tentative and result in hypotheses tested by treatments rather than in firm conclusions. This is especially true in anxiety where many of the emotional symptoms involve physiological arousal. It is, of course, very useful to be able to get as much information as possible from the client and their physician about potential physical causes of the symptoms. It is also important to recognize that the physician is also dealing with the same mind–body interface and may not be absolutely certain or correct in medical diagnosis. Tracking the time course of symptoms and their relationship to various illness onsets, as well as medication start and stop points can be helpful in making such distinctions. Comparisons to other older adults with similar disorders may be helpful for the clinician, and consultation with a clinician more experienced in late-life anxiety disorders may be helpful for therapists new to this population. In many cases, treatment and retesting and reassessment will be an expected and valued part of the process.

Assessing symptoms of anxiety

Research on the assessment of anxiety in geriatric populations, and on the development of targeted instruments measuring anxiety in this age group, lags behind similar research on depression. This has been written about by many authors (e.g., Pachana and Byrne 2012) and, in part, may spring from the fact that anxiety consists of several subclasses of disorders, rather than being a more unitary condition, such as depression, and also from the stereotypical thinking that older adults are very likely to be depressed or anxious simply due to aging. Nevertheless, in the last decade a number of instruments designed specifically for use with older anxious patients have been developed. As with depression, instruments developed for younger age groups are also in use with older adults. Similarly, specific instruments for assessing anxiety in those with cognitive decline or dementia have also been developed.

There are three instruments that have been designed specifically for use with older adults with anxiety disorders. The Short Anxiety Screening Test (SAST; Sinoff et al. 1999) was designed specifically to detect anxiety symptoms in older adults (specifically age 70+), particularly in individuals with comorbid depression. The original validation article by Sinoff and colleagues describes the SAST as an interviewer-assisted instrument taking 10–15 minutes to administer. The scale has ten items rated on a 4-point severity scale, and a score of 24 or greater suggests a diagnosis of anxiety. A time frame for responses to the instrument is not given in the original article. In individuals with anxiety, but without depression, the SAST showed a sensitivity of 75.4% and specificity of 78.7%; in the presence of comorbid depression, sensitivity and specificity were 83.3% and 70.5%, respectively.

The Geriatric Anxiety Inventory (GAI; Pachana et al. 2007) was developed to measure dimensional anxiety symptoms in older adults over the age of 65, although its use on populations younger than 65 has been reported (Poulsen and Pachana 2012). The items of the GAI were specifically crafted to exclude somatic symptoms of anxiety that overlap with medical conditions common in later life (Pachana et al. 2007). In contrast to the SAST, the GAI has a simplified agree–disagree response set modeled on that of the GDS (Yesavage et al. 1982). There is a 20-item and a shorter 5-item version (Byrne and Pachana 2011) of the GAI; both have a 1-week response framework. The 20-item version has a cut-off of 9 and above, and the short form a cut-off of 3 and above, to indicate clinically significant anxiety. The sensitivity and specificity of the 20- and 5-item versions are 73% and 80%, and 75% and 87%, respectively. The GAI has been translated into over two dozen languages (Pachana and Byrne 2012) and has gained acceptance as a reliable measure of anxiety in later life (e.g., Diefenbach et al. 2009; Edelstein et al. 2007).

The Geriatric Anxiety Scale (GAS; Segal et al. 2010) was developed to measure cognitive, somatic, and affective symptoms of anxiety in adults over the age of 65; its three subscales reflect these three domains of content. The items for the GAS are reflective of the full range of anxiety disorder symptoms as described in the anxiety disorders section of the Diagnostic and Statistical Manual of Mental Disorders (DSM-IV-TR; American Psychiatric Association 2000). The scale has 30 items rated on a 4-point severity scale; each item is rated in relation to the respondent's last episode of significant anxiety. The GAS total score is based on the first 25 items; potential scores range from 0 to 75 with higher scores indicting higher anxiety levels. An additional five content items assess areas of anxiety often reported to be of concern for older adults and are designed to be used clinically (e.g., "I was concerned about my children."). A 1-week response time frame is given.

In 2012, Therrien and Hunsley reviewed the extant literature to assess which anxiety assessment tools had the strongest empirical support for use with older populations. The majority of commonly used published measures of anxiety lacked sufficient evidence to warrant their use with older adults. Based on the psychometric evidence at that point in time, the authors suggested that three measures, the Beck Anxiety Inventory (BAI; Beck et al. 1988), Penn State Worry Questionnaire (PSWQ; Meyer et al. 1990), and the Geriatric Mental Status Examination (Copeland et al. 1976), had sufficient evidence to justify their clinical use in older adults, with two scales developed specifically for older adults, namely the Worry Scale (Wisocki et al. 1986) and the Geriatric Anxiety Inventory (Pachana et al. 2007) also found to be appropriate for use with older adults, although each had a less developed empirical base.

As with the depression screens discussed in Chapter 3, a few words may be appropriate here with respect to other anxiety screens that may be used with older clients. The HADS (Bjelland et al. 2002; Flint and Rifat 1996b), as noted in the chapter on depression, has some limitations in its use with older adults (Spinhoven et al. 1997). The Adult Manifest Anxiety Scale-Elderly Version (AMAS-E; Reynolds et al. 2003) is adapted from a measure originally designed for younger populations. Its three subscales derived from factor analysis-worry/stress, fear of aging, and physiological symptoms of anxiety are broad, and may suit some patients with respect to presenting concerns. Unfortunately, the research base for this instrument is rather limited.

The BAI (Beck et al. 1988) has been shown in a number of studies to have sound psychometric properties when used with older adults (e.g., Wetherall and Arean 1997), but some researchers have reported limitations with respect to certain cognitive features of anxiety, such as anxious apprehension (Wetherall and Gatz 2005). The PSWQ (Meyer et al. 1990) mentioned above is a measure of trait pathological worry with good psychometric properties in older adults with GAD (e.g., Stanley et al. 2001), but a caution is offered about the difficulty some older adults may experience with the sometimes tricky wording of the reverse-scored items (Hopko et al. 2003). For both the BAI and the PSWQ, the clinician may wish to restrict their use to more well-educated and cognitively intact older adults, and for situations in which either a more nuanced reporting of symptom severity, or more detail about worry as opposed to pure anxious symptomatology, respectively, is desired.

Assessment instruments themselves can demonstrate such age biases. Dennis and colleagues (2007) found that while self-rated screening tools, such as the HADS, were adequate as screens in older anxious adults, they were less reliable at picking up the magnitude of change in anxiety symptoms over time in this population. Interestingly, in their study, 57.5% of older adults with clinical anxiety symptoms recruited in an outpatient mental health clinic required assistance in completing the State Trait Anxiety Inventory (STAI; Spielberger 1983) and 30% required some assistance in completing the BAI (Beck et al. 1988). Dennis and colleague's participants also had difficulties on the STAI with reverse-scored items being endorsed in the wrong direction. For the over 50% of subjects requiring assistance with the instrument, the assistance took the form of rephrasing and repeating the scoring instructions for items, as well as pointing out missing items. Previously McDonald and Spielberger (1981) had noted that the format of the STAI is easy to misinterpret. The ease with which older adults can complete self-report measures, including understanding the response options and the wording of items, is therefore important to consider.

In the case of Marlene, the news about her condition and prognosis was delivered in a way that caused an exacerbation of a pre-existing anxiety disorder. So an important aim of clinical intervention, even at the stage of assessment, is for reassurance about understanding the nature of her concerns (See Case 4.1B). In reality, anyone receiving such a diagnosis would have cause to worry, and so it is important here that the goal is not to deny or extinguish what is a normal human reaction to such news, but to work with the client to insure that she is able to work toward goals, including quality of life, and the regaining of equilibrium in her daily functioning. Here, the relationship with the spouse is also important to consider moving forward.

> ### Case Example 4.1B Marlene: anxiety with depression and memory impairment
>
> Marlene was very pessimistic about visiting a psychologist. "I am not crazy—I am going blind!" Michael also was focused on the loss of sight in his wife. They had taken a trip to Alaska—something they had always talked about doing—including a visit to Attu, the westernmost island in the Aleutians. Attu is a birdwatcher's paradise but with extremely primitive conditions, and Marlene had not coped well with this trip. Despite some stunning photographs from the trip and many interesting places and animals seen, Marlene had not enjoyed the trip. "I just keep thinking this is the last time I will see any of these things."
>
> Jennifer gave Marlene the MINI, which revealed major depression along with GAD. Marlene's scores on the GAI and the GDS (15 item version) were 18 and 13, respectively, indicating clinically significant anxiety and depression. On the MMSE, Marlene's score of 25 was due primarily to poor memory, with most points lost on recall of the three items, as well as poorly drawn intersecting pentagons and one point lost on serial sevens. A risk assessment revealed no suicidal ideation, and there was no history of suicide in Marlene's family.
>
> In giving feedback about her assessment results to Marlene and Michael, Jennifer pointed out that Marlene had moved successfully past prior episodes of anxiety, and that even though the current stressors were significant, that she had confidence that therapy could assist them both with coping with Marlene's diagnosis. She noted that in their reports of changes in their lifestyle since the diagnosis of macular degeneration, their social contact with friends and family had declined precipitously. Jennifer also noted that anxiety and depression often occur together, and that this "double-whammy" can significantly impact coping strategies. She also reassured Marlene that some amount of concern over her vision was normal, but that perhaps having to document and in essence pay such close attention to changes in her vision served to fuel her anxiety, to the point where it was seriously interfering with her daily life. Both Marlene and Michael agreed with this assessment, and Marlene expressed relief at being "heard" in the sense of the loss she was feeling at the prospect of losing her vision. Recommendations for on-going therapy as well as the benefits of joining a support group for adults with macular degeneration were explored. By the end of the session, Jennifer had gotten both Marlene and Michael to agree to try the support group and to come in for some counseling sessions, both as a couple and separately.

Psychotherapy for anxiety disorders in older adults

As is true of the other psychological disorders discussed in this book, therapy for anxiety in later life is often quite similar to the work one would do with younger clients. Various combinations of teaching relaxation methods, changing anxiety arousing thoughts, changing attitudes toward the physiological symptoms of arousal, and learning early cues for impending anxiety attacks are common treatment methods. Comorbid presentations of depression and anxiety in older adults are a particular therapeutic challenge, especially in the face of the presence of one or more medical illnesses (Lecrubier 2001). In general, however, psychotherapy techniques are used with little or no modification with anxious older clients. However, similar to the discussion in Chapter 2 on depression, the assessment tools and approaches used with younger populations are sometimes different to those used with older adults. Therefore, making good choices about which tools to use to measure anxiety in this population is important.

The evidence base for effectiveness of psychological interventions with anxiety is also strong. Cuijpers et al. (2014) in a meta-analytic review found strong effects of cognitive behavior therapy (CBT) for anxiety with older adults, with similar effect sizes for alleviation of depressive symptoms in these anxious older adults. Pinquart and Duberstein (2007), in their meta-analysis, reported similar effect sizes for CBT for anxiety with older adults. They also compared CBT outcomes with pharmacological outcomes. The effects of medications for anxiety compared with placebo were stronger than effects of CBT compared with wait list controls. However, if the placebo effect is subtracted, the specific effects of medication and CBT were similar.

Developmental aging and therapy for anxiety

The aging body is more prone to disease, and many chronic illnesses occur in midlife or later, and generally worsen over time. When the chronic illness or disability is a major focus of the therapy, it is more useful to consider it as one of the challenges of late life (see Chapter 1) and as a topical focus of therapy (see Chapter 6). When the presenting problem is the anxiety itself and the physical problems are context, it can be useful to think of the physical changes as part of the aging process. These changes affect anxiety in later life in two main ways: the content of worry in later life tends to be focused on health issues, rather than on social anxiety and achievement concerns as in earlier adulthood (Lindesay et al. 2012), and pain and other symptoms associated with medical illness may complicate relaxation methods.

The physiological profiles of emotions in later life appear to be similar to those of younger adults, but lower in amplitude (Levenson et al. 1991). In general, self-reported arousal also seems to be lower, probably due to the positivity effect and to enhanced self-regulation with aging (see Chapter 1). However, there is also evidence that, once aroused, older adults take longer for fear and anxiety responses to return to baseline. Therapists may need to keep in mind that a more muted presentation of anxiety may be due to these developmental aging changes and still reflect important changes from the client's older adult baseline. The symptoms from any one stress reaction are also likely to be longer lasting than in younger clients. In tracking responses to therapeutic interventions, using the client's own ratings and expecting possibly longer periods of adjustment can be useful in monitoring treatment effectiveness and progress.

While the focus of anxiety in earlier adulthood is often unrealistic, and the construction of future-oriented scenarios occurs largely in an information vacuum (see Miloyan et al. 2014, for an interesting discussion of the clinical implications of future orientation for mental health), health-related anxiety in later life can be rooted in real illness or at least be related to the exaggeration of real illness concerns. Getting a sense of the realistic component of the anxiety is important, but can also be quite difficult. Asking the client for information about what their physician has actually said about diagnosis and prognosis is an essential step. If these responses are unclear, talking with the treating physician and getting copies of medical reports can be useful. It is important to recognize what is medically caused, and to be appropriately sympathetic and supportive about the impact of those symptoms on the client's life. At the same time, the therapist helps the client to carry out a reality test and to substitute realistic thoughts for anxiety-driven thinking that exaggerates the impact of the illness. Adjusting to heart disease, for example, is a difficult process, but being chronically worried about an impending heart attack adds additional distress, can lead to panic symptoms that mimic cardiac symptoms, and in some instances can trigger arrhythmias. Working with anxiety around health issues constantly confronts the therapist with mind–body issues, and is quite professionally challenging and stimulating. Recognizing a rapid heartbeat as a sign of high anxiety, for example, can be anxiety reducing in itself, if it was formerly being interpreted as a sign of an impending heart attack (see Case Example 4.2). This recognition can then trigger additional steps to recognize what the cue for the anxiety was and the use of anxiety reduction strategies, such as calming breathing or stress-reducing thoughts.

Case Example 4.2 Anxiety with cardiac symptoms

For example, an older client in her mid-70s came in for therapy for panic attacks and other anxiety-related symptoms. She felt that she needed psychotherapy in any case, due to a history of generalized anxiety disorder going back a bit more than 10 years. A recent panic attack with tachycardia had resulted in a visit to the ER and referral to a cardiologist. The ER doctor told her it was panic and not heart disease. The cardiologist then told her, before testing, that it was not anxiety, but something was really wrong with her heart. After a couple of weeks of testing, the cardiologist told her she had some mild problems with her heart, but did not need ongoing treatment for it. Fortunately, her primary care physician was more supportive and more oriented to patient education, and explained the heart condition; that it was quite mild and of no concern, and that it was probably not responsible for her panic attacks with tachycardia, but that the panic could trigger worse cardiac symptoms. Part of the therapist's role in these early weeks of treatment was being empathetic and supportive about the additional anxiety aroused by the conflicting reports and helping her decide how best to get a clearer explanation of what was happening to her body. The therapist also proceeded with an intervention to reduce anxiety.

Anxiety about illness onset can also be triggered by aspects of normal aging. The slowing in thinking and in retrieving memories, changes in the span of working memory, and normal changes in word- and name-finding abilities (cf. Salthouse 2010) can easily trigger concerns about the onset of Alzheimer's disease and other dementias. In some instances, cognitive assessment and educating clients about the differences between normal aging and dementia can settle these concerns fairly quickly. In others, it may take a more prolonged period of tracking when normal memory failures occur and substituting realistic, stress neutral thoughts, such as (if true): "I've always had trouble finding my keys around the house." Or "This is normal forgetting, I don't need to worry about Alzheimer's yet."

Social context and anxiety in older adults

As a close corollary of the role of physical illness as a major source of worry for older adults, the medical system and the long-term care system are key social contexts for worry in later life. In general, there is much more interaction with physicians, and more time spent in clinics, medical laboratories, medical imaging facilities, and hospitals in older adulthood than in the younger years. People of all ages can have anxieties about one or more of these settings (e.g., hospital anxiety, panic related to needle sticks or the sight of blood, claustrophobia cued by being in MRI tubes), and the likelihood of exposure to the feared stimulus is higher in older adulthood. In addition to these physical cues for anxiety, the social ecology of the settings often increases anxiety as well: the inherent uncertainty of diagnosis and treatment, combined with organizational structures that do not always communicate well, or clearly, what is known and what is going to happen to the patient next.

Some degree of concern about being placed in a nursing home is part of the background of the lives of most older adults (see Case Example 4.3). Especially for the anxious older adult, it may well be a perceived threat associated with any medical procedure, any decline in physical health, and also in any family argument. Keeping one's "third ear" attuned to these concerns and encouraging the client to discuss them with you as the therapist, and then to explore how realistic they are, can be essential parts of therapy. It is also important to be clear in one's own mind, and then with the client, about whether there is any likelihood that topics discussed in therapy could be used by others to decide that placement is appropriate. In most instances, this is unlikely since the therapy is confidential and the client controls how any information shared in therapy will be used. When there are exceptions, they should be clearly discussed with the older client (e.g., an appointed conservator, a child who sits in on therapy sessions, written consents to share information with family).

> **Case Example 4.3 Anxiety about husband's functional decline**
>
> One client in her late 80s with a mixed diagnosis of depression and anxiety became progressively more worried about loss of independence after her husband returned home following a rehabilitation stay in a nursing home after briefly being admitted to hospital. Both of them were moved to the first floor of their home for safety reasons and paid in-home caregivers were hired to help them. Some aspects of this she appreciated, such as not having to cook for her husband. On the other hand, she felt that the caregivers watched over her too much, and that between the caregivers and her husband, she had less independence than before. She had mixed emotions about the current situation, but worried about what would happen in the future, feeling that this was quite likely the beginning of a sequence of events that would lead to admission to a nursing home for both of them. Reviewing what her health condition was and her recollection of family discussions was reassuring that it was neither highly likely nor likely to happen soon. In fact, family reassured her often that she and her husband should be able to stay in the current arrangement indefinitely.

Cohort differences and anxiety in late life

One general effect of cohort differences is that we all eventually become old-fashioned, in the sense that our identity and our original sense of what the world is like were fashioned in an earlier era, which we, of course, experienced as the modern era in our youth. Relatively new inventions and new changes in society can be sources of anxiety for persons raised in earlier cohorts. Later born therapists need to be able to break out of their own cohort perspective in order to understand that older clients' anxieties may be triggered by things therapists born later take for granted as a natural part of life. The pervasiveness of computer-based technologies and social media can be disquieting for some older adults. Social shifts, like the rise of the religious right in American politics for older adults who came of age in the liberal to radical 1960s, may be harder to understand and accept. The influx of newer immigrant groups with different customs and languages may well cause anxiety, even to people who were entirely comfortable with the range of cultural diversity present in their youth. Recent events, like the global financial crisis, can also trigger memories of earlier lived experiences such as the Great Depression in older clients, which might be at odds with a therapist's own views of the current situation.

In our experience, these cohort differences are seldom the explicit and main cause of anxiety in older clients. However, they often arise as part of the background of why the client is feeling uneasy. Being able to recognize these effects and to sympathize appropriately with the experience of living in a world much different than the one the client grew up in, and was comfortable with in young adulthood and middle age, can be an essential part of building rapport. It is important to be able to do this even for perceptions with which the therapist may disagree. Helping the client put this experience into the framework of changes in society that are somewhat stressful for everyone, rather than seeing them as something wrong with themselves as individuals, can be helpful in reducing overall levels of stress.

Parents never stop being concerned about their children, even when the children are in late middle age or the young-old years. In people with a propensity toward anxiety, these concerns easily become worry and other symptoms of anxiety (see Case Example 4.4). Cohort changes can exacerbate these worries to the extent that cohorts differ in the nature of jobs and careers, attitudes toward borrowing and credit, attitudes toward divorce, and child raising practices. Reinterpreting these worries in terms of cohort differences can help to allay chronic worrying (see Case Example 4.5).

> **Case Example 4.4 Anxiety about family members flying**
>
> For example, a highly anxious client in her mid-70s was often extremely worried about family members traveling, especially if they were flying somewhere without her. Her children and grandchildren were scattered around the USA and Europe, so her fear over their flying was a frequent trigger for anxiety. Part of her anxiety was driven by her sense that people used to stay closer to home, and traveled by car and train when she was younger. She saw "this constant flying all over the place" as a new trend that she felt was entirely unnecessary. Implicitly (not overtly) she felt that family were doing this to her. One part of her therapy was talking about social change over her lifetime and how her children, and especially grandchildren, had grown up taking flying for granted, seeing the world as smaller and more unified than she had. This discussion of their cohort perspective took place within a context of recognizing and expressing empathy for her perception of the situation, and the difficulty for her of living through this change in the perceived size of the world.

> **Case Example 4.5 Anxiety about granddaughter's lifestyle**
>
> For example, a woman in her early 90s worried frequently about her granddaughter's lifestyle. She felt that her granddaughter was not managing money well, and took too many vacations and other trips out of town. Her trainee therapist helped her think about these behaviors both in terms of what the client would have done when she was that age and in terms of changes that the client saw as being typical of people in her granddaughter's generation. While she continued to disapprove, she worried less.

Cultural influences on anxiety in late life

One of the most salient influences of cultural issues on anxiety in late life occurs when the older adult emigrates in later life, typically to follow children or grandchildren who have emigrated. When this occurs, the older adult is usually relatively unacculturated to the new country, and can find the language differences and much of the newness to be triggers for anxiety. These anxieties and chronic worrying can easily extend to younger family members who are becoming acculturated faster and to a greater degree, and often in ways that the older person is unhappy with.

For example, for many older immigrants, including those who arrived in their younger years and grew older in the USA, there is a perception that White non-Hispanic culture does not show proper respect to older adults, and that older family members are placed into institutional care quickly and easily. While this is not factually accurate, the perception can be quite influential. As older adults see their children becoming acculturated, they may begin to worry that their Americanized children will be quick to place them into nursing home care.

In general, the therapist can work with these cultural differences by exploring why the children decided to emigrate, why the older adult decided to follow them, what the pros and cons of living in the USA are, and how these differ for the older person and younger family members. Part of this process is likely to be greater communication with younger family members about these concerns. Encouraging the older adults to gather information and check the reality of their worries is often useful. It may also be helpful to encourage the older adult to find non-family-related activities and support when it is available. Being able to visit and talk with other older adults from the same nation of origin, or (language abilities permitting) older adults from other nations who are in similar places with regard to acculturation, can be very helpful. For example, one Latina in her 70s who had married outside of her culture found a great deal of support in a multicultural singing group, some from finding that others loved to hear her explanations of what songs from her country meant within that culture, and also from meeting another Latina woman, albeit from a different nation of origin.

The influences of culture in understanding and treating anxiety can be quite varied, but this does not necessarily complicate treatment. In working with Latino elderly, experience suggests that anxiety is often identified mainly in terms of physical symptoms. On the other hand, there is often much less belief in the separation of mind and body than is common in Anglo culture, and so the idea that changing thoughts or changing relationships with family members will have a curative effect on these physical symptoms is more easily accepted. There appears to be less of the resistance to psychological solutions to physical symptoms than often appears with White non-Hispanic clients, who tend to perceive the psychological treatment to imply the problem is imagined.

Less is written about anxiety in the Asian cultural context in general, although it is a population of increasing interest and concern (Sue et al. 2012). Underreporting of affective disorders in Asian cultural groups has been noted in the literature (Woodward et al. 2012), and this has implications for diagnosis, assessment, and treatment in this population. Prevalence rates for psychiatric disorders among all racial groups may vary to some extent by whether they are first- or second-generation migrants (Jimenez et al. 2010). The authors' experience with Asian caregivers suggests that stances toward mental health in general may influence the seeking out of psychological assistance for mental health issues.

Generally speaking, it is always safest to rely on the client for information about what the cultural values and beliefs are for their group. There is not a great deal of reliable information available about cultural differences in general and especially not with regard to old age. Much of what we think we know, and unfortunately a fair amount of what is written in the clinical literature, is based on stereotypes. There is always a lot of variation within cultural groups, and immigrants can be anywhere on the various dimensions of change between their culture of origin and the one to which they are adjusting. In any case, it is the client's perception of their culture that is shaping the client's cognitions and behaviors.

Problems that arise in therapy with older adults with anxiety

While progressive muscle relaxation and other relaxation methods often work quite well and easily with older adults, problems can arise (see Case Example 4.6). When introducing progressive muscle relaxation with older clients, checking first about parts of the body where there is chronic pain or where muscle tightening is likely to trigger pain or distress is an important first step. Clients can then be encouraged to skip that part or to imagine tensing those muscles if this type of covert tensing makes sense to them. Similarly, breathing exercises for relaxation should be tailored around any illnesses that affect breathing or previous abdominal surgeries that may make deep breathing distressing.

> ### Case Example 4.6 Obsessive practice of progressive relaxation
> A client in her late 80s was so pleased with the fairly quick effect that relaxation had on her ability to sleep that she started doing it obsessively throughout the day (two or three times an hour by her report). She then reported getting cramps in one of her legs. This was an unusual occurrence in our experience, and the first hint of obsessive compulsive tendencies on her part. She was encouraged to do the exercise less frequently and, of course, to skip doing the leg that cramped until the cramping was over for a few weeks.

It is quite common for older adults to do the muscle tightening in areas of the body susceptible to pain, even though instructed in the session to skip those areas. There is also a frequent tendency to rush through the exercise. Generally speaking, it is a good idea to have the client demonstrate in session how they do the exercise at home, especially if they report doing it regularly and getting no result. Commonly they go through the entire exercise in less than five minutes. One older client did it so quickly that it looked somewhat like a seizure that started at the feet and went quickly to her head. In general, the response to these problems is to first try and correct issues with the procedure and then to explore whether other alternative methods of relaxation might work better for the individual client. Various forms of breathing exercises can be helpful, as can aerobic physical exercise consistent with the client's health and abilities. It is also useful to explore what kinds of relaxation techniques the client knows from past experience, which ones work the best, and any preferences the client might have. Many older clients will have had some positive experience with progressive relaxation, breathing techniques of different types, meditation, or using aerobic exercise to relax. At times all that is needed is to ask the client to resume doing whatever worked well in the past on a regular basis.

On the other hand, some clients will have only had experience with one or two methods, and will not have liked the experience. Talking through what was unpleasant about the ones they have tried before and discussing possible changes in one of those, or reviewing alternatives that would avoid those pitfalls is good therapeutic strategy (see Case Example 4.7). In general, clients who find passive relaxation methods boring or even somewhat anxiety arousing tend to do well with aerobic exercise and vice versa.

> ### Case Example 4.7 Changing relaxation methods
> One client in her mid-70s was unsuccessful with progressive relaxation because she worried constantly if she was doing it correctly. We decided to switch to a focus on breathing, which she reported worked better. We also explored possible relaxing activities to add to her day. In between sessions, she independently decided to leave her arts and crafts materials set up all the time so that she could work with them whenever time permitted. She reported this was one of very few activities that fully occupied her mind and nullified her chronic worrying.

As with depression, a difference in working with older adults about their anxiety arousing cognitions is that many of the topics of concern will be reality based. It is a good strategy to anticipate this in all discussions about changing thoughts to reduce worry and anxiety. Showing an understanding that there are real medical problems to worry about, that a spouse's physical decline realistically raises the possibility of their death and the client's widowhood, or that ongoing progressive decline may in the future raise the need for 24-hour nursing care is an important first step before suggesting that the degree of distress may be higher than it needs to be, or that it could be reduced to improve the client's overall health and well-being.

Then, the suggested changes in thinking need to be appropriately realistic and are generally aimed at the reduction of excess anxiety, rather than relaxation. For clients with very serious problems, it may be a better strategy to aim at replacing stress-enhancing thoughts with stress-neutral, rather than stress-reducing, thoughts. The latter may be seen as unrealistic, overly positive, and not showing an understanding of the client's problems. Examples of potential stress-neutral thoughts include: "I have serious medical problems and I'm doing everything I can to take care of myself." "I've handled major changes in my life before and I can handle this one." The stress-reducing or stress-neutral thoughts must, of course, be tailored to the individual client. Their past history of coping with stress, typically quite rich by the time one reaches old age, can be a very helpful resource for these cognitions. The artistic client in Case 4.7 did very well with telling herself that she could not control what happened by worrying; in large part, this worked because she had the underlying belief that worry prevented bad things from happening. Clearly, some other individuals would have found saying to themselves that the situation was not under their control anxiety arousing, rather than calming.

Finally, negotiating introducing psychological strategies in dealing with anxiety while the older adult is simultaneously taking anti-anxiety medications can be problematic. For an older woman without dementia who was on multiple anxiolytics, the client's progress with relaxation and other coping strategies was undermined by her psychiatrist saying "you have to be on those drugs for the rest of your life." The client was confused about the effect that increased coping with her anxiety would have on her continuing to take the anxiolytics; here, consultation between the physician and the psychologist can be very important to maintain progress in treatment. Many commonly prescribed anxiolytics offer almost instant relief from the experience of anxiety symptoms, and simultaneously may make the ability to use the experience of such emotions in the course of treatment more problematic (e.g., when working through a fear hierarchy). Zinbarg et al. (2006) comment on this in their discussion of efficacious treatment for anxiety disorders, such as phobias.

Summary

Anxiety in later life is generally underdiagnosed and undertreated, despite it being relatively common, as well as highly comorbid with depression and a range of medical conditions. Similar to depression, assessment approaches to anxiety must take account of the potential overlap in depressive symptoms with medical disorders. Treatment considerations in late-life anxiety include sensitivity to how different cultures and cohorts may experience and talk about anxiety symptoms in the therapeutic context. More research is warranted in how anxiety symptoms are expressed in very old age.

This chapter and Chapter 3 have often mentioned progressive dementias of late life (neurocognitive disorders in DSM-5) as alternative diagnoses. In the following chapter, we turn to the question of how to recognize these disorders and then implement psychological interventions for people with dementia.

Chapter 5

Dementia

Introduction to dementia

Dementia is an umbrella term for a suite of disorders related to degenerative brain impairment typically associated with later life and characterized by changes in cognition, behavior, and personality, to the extent that the ability to carry out everyday activities of living is compromised. Approximately 7% of people over the age of 65 years, and approximately 40% of people over the age of 85 years, have some form of dementia (Alzheimer's Association 2012). Prince et al. (2013) estimated that globally, 35.6 million people lived with dementia in 2010, with numbers expected to nearly double every 20 years, to 65.7 million in 2030 and 115.4 million in 2050.

Dementia in the DSM-5

Mild NCD (neurocognitive disorder), a newly introduced term, recognizes a level of cognitive decline that goes beyond declines associated with normal aging changes, but is not yet at the level of a major NCD. Mild NCD is similar to the levels of functioning previously captured by terms such as mild cognitive impairment (MCI; Petersen 2004), and like MCI represents a level of cognitive decline that may progress to a form of major neurocognitive decline, or may remain stable (or in some cases even improve, depending on the etiology of the initial decline). In most studies, conversion rates between MCI and some form of dementia (usually Alzheimer's disease) have been reported as ranging between 20% and 40%. Generally, those who continue to decline experience impairment in other cognitive domains in addition to memory, with the presence of depression and a relatively high degree of functional impairment at baseline testing, also having an increasing risk of conversion (Farias et al. 2009; Gabryelewicz et al. 2007; Mitchell and Shiri-Feshki 2009).

Mild NCD can be defined cognitively as a decline of between 1 and 2 SDs below average. Major NCD includes performance below 2 SDs below the mean. The diagnosis of a mild NCD requires that the patient experiences cognitive changes that negatively affect functioning, which are observable by the individual, others, or on objective cognitive testing, and that the changes in cognition require some compensatory strategies to help maintain independence and perform activities of daily living. Critics have pointed out that while being able to identify a person with such a decline early may improve access to assistance and potential early interventions, it may not be straightforward to ascertain such changes accurately across settings with varying expertise with measurement of cognitive decline (Morris 2012). It is important to recognize that mild and major NCDs exist on a continuum and that in many cases a variety of factors, including the sensitivity of cognitive tests used, the presence of comorbid psychiatric or medical conditions, and prior levels of education, may affect judgments about whether a person meets criteria for mild or major neurocognitive impairment.

In the most recent revision of the *Diagnostic and Statistical Manual of Mental Disorders* (*DSM-5*; American Psychiatric Association 2013), the terms major or mild NCD serve as a first-order diagnostic differentiation. Major NCDs include diagnoses such as dementia from the previous edition of the DSM (*DSM-IV-TR*; American Psychiatric Association 2000), and disorders that constitute a substantial level of cognitive decline (two or more SDs) from previous functioning and interfere with the person's independence (Siberski 2012). However, the DSM-5 expands the category of major NCDs to include diagnoses that encompass other etiologies and age groups, such as traumatic brain injury.

Since this change with respect to terminology is relatively recent, most of the existing literature still refers to dementia as the umbrella entity. The DSM-5 also recognizes the term dementia as continuing usage for NCDs affecting older adults, although it notes that NCD is a broader term and includes disorders not subsumed under dementia in earlier DSMs. In this chapter, we use the term dementia in large part because reference is being made to research and conceptualization of the disorder of dementia prior to DSM-5. For example, the recent US National Institutes of Health-Alzheimer's Association (NIA-AA) research criteria and guidelines for diagnosing dementia due to Alzheimer's disease (McKhann et al. 2011) refer to dementia, because they both predate DSM-5 and are referring to dementia disorders specifically.

An important concept underpinning these changes, however, namely the idea that impaired memory *might not* be the first sign or symptom of neurocognitive decline indicating possible dementia, as well as it being important to try to identify cognitive changes that adversely affect the individual as early as possible (i.e., even while still of a mild nature), is welcome. In a variety of settings a diagnosis of dementia was either put off or deemed less important, due to reluctance on the part of family (and sometimes health professionals) to recognize the disorder early. Often family and health care professionals state that the person with suspected dementia would not want to know if they had the disorder, and families often fight to keep the diagnosis from their relative. Elson (2006) eloquently answered these statements with the empirical finding that 86% of persons with dementia wanted to know the cause of their altered cognitive state, while 69% wanted to know if they were diagnosed with Alzheimer's disease.

This paralleled earlier debates about telling people with cancer and other terminal illnesses about their diagnoses. In general, the reluctance is more on the side of the family and health professionals who do not wish to impart bad news, rather than on the part of the affected person who often wants to know what is happening and to participate as much as possible in future planning. We often find that knowing the diagnosis is reassuring to persons with dementia who otherwise are facing changes in their thinking and abilities that are unexplained and therefore frightening. On the flip side, if there is an insistence on secrecy and keeping the diagnosis from the person, this can then complicate the situation when concrete plans such as a move to residential care need to be executed.

Subtypes of dementia

After a clinician determines whether the NCD is major or minor, a subtype is listed (e.g., "major NCD due to Alzheimer's disease"). The four primary forms of dementia included under major NCDs are Alzheimer's disease, vascular dementia, dementia with Lewy bodies, and fronto-temporal dementia, which are diagnosed following the preliminary determination of the presence of major NCD. For the four major types of dementia, the estimated prevalences are as follows: Alzheimer's disease, 60–80%; vascular dementia, 20–40%; dementia with Lewy bodies, 5–20%; fronto-temporal dementia, 5–20% (Fratiglioni and Rocca 2001; Lee 2011; Ratnavelli et al. 2002; Wakisaka et al. 2003).

Alzheimer's disease is the most common form of dementia. It is the sixth leading cause of all deaths in the USA and is the fifth leading cause of death in Americans over the age of 65 years (Alzheimer's Association et al. 2011). Alzheimer's disease most commonly affects individuals over age 65, but early onset dementia can affect individuals in their 40s and 50s.

Vascular dementia includes, in addition to the presence of cognitive decline, cerebrovascular disease (CVD) defined by the presence of focal signs on neurologic examination consistent with stroke (with or without history of stroke); and evidence of relevant CVD by brain imaging (usually computed tomography (CT) or magnetic resonance imaging (MRI)). More recent reviews suggest that vascular dementia is relatively rare on its own and, importantly, can magnify the impact of comorbid disorders such as Alzheimer's disease (Series and Esiri 2012). There is also the suggestion that Alzheimer's disease on its own is more uncommon than was previously thought (Holmes et al. 1999).

The core symptom components required for fronto-temporal dementia include an insidious onset and gradual progression of symptoms over time, early observed declines in social or interpersonal interactions, early impairment in the self-regulation of behavior, and early emotional blunting and loss of insight. Similar to Alzheimer's disease, neuropathological, neuropsychological, and neuroimaging work has focused on revealing more precisely the relationships between outward signs of change and impairment, and the underlying neuropathological mechanisms (Schroeter 2012; Schroeter et al. 2012). This increased neuropsychological and behavioral inquiry into fronto-temporal dementia has resulted in a recent explication of the behavioral variant of fronto-temporal dementia (bvFTD), now believed to be a common cause of early onset dementia, roughly equal in prevalence to Alzheimer's disease in individuals aged 65 and under (Knopman and Roberts 2011; Ratnavalli et al. 2002).

Dementia with Lewy bodies is characterized by a progressive decline in cognitive functioning accompanied by at least two of the following symptoms:

- fluctuating cognition with pronounced variations in attention and alertness;
- recurrent visual hallucinations that are typically well-formed and detailed; or
- spontaneous motor features of Parkinsonism (Leverenz and McKeith 2002).

Key differential diagnoses here include psychotic disorders and delirium. Since Lewy bodies tend to be comorbid with Alzheimer's disease pathological changes, it may be difficult in some cases to distinguish the two dementia subsyndromes, particularly earlier in the disease process.

Psychiatric comorbidities

A number of psychiatric conditions may coexist with dementia. In the early stages of the disease, or around the time of diagnosis, depression may occur. Depression has been both proposed to be a risk factor for dementia as well as an early symptom of some forms of dementia. In addition, approximately half of older patients with late-onset depression have some degree of apparent cognitive impairment (Butters et al. 2004; Köhler et al. 2010). Symptoms of anxiety frequently co-occur with both MCI and Alzheimer's disease, and have been reported to range in prevalence from 47% to 50% in the former and 48% to 70% in the latter (e.g., Ferretti et al. 2001; Gallagher et al. 2011). Similarly, comorbid late-life anxiety has been found to contribute to greater declines in cognitive functioning, as well as poorer outcomes in persons with dementia, including early institutionalization (Beaudreau and O'Hara 2008; Butters et al. 2011; Spector et al. 2012).

There is evidence that the presence of mood or anxiety symptoms or disorders increases the risk of developing dementia. For example, in a prospective study of conversion to Alzheimer's disease, 185 persons with no cognitive impairment and 47 persons with MCI (mean age 84 years, range 75–95) were followed for 3 years (Palmer et al. 2007). Psychiatric symptoms occurred more frequently in persons with MCI (36.2% mood and 46.8% anxiety symptoms) than in cognitively intact individuals (18.4% mood and 24.9% anxiety symptoms). Moreover, of persons with both MCI and anxiety symptoms, 83.3% developed Alzheimer's disease over a 3-year follow-up as opposed to 40.9% of persons with MCI without anxiety; only 6.1% of the cognitively intact participants developed Alzheimer's over the 3 years. Among persons with MCI, the 3-year risk of progressing to Alzheimer's in this sample almost doubled with each anxiety symptom reported (relative risk (RR) = 1.8 (1.2–2.7) per symptom). Conversely, among cognitively intact subjects, only symptoms of depressive mood were related to development of Alzheimer's disease (RR = 1.9 (1.0–3.6) per symptom); in persons with MCI presence of depression did not increase risk of progression. Anxiety and, to a lesser extent, depression increase the likelihood of progression to dementia, particularly Alzheimer's disease, although the mechanisms for this are still being explored (Palmer et al. 2007).

Assessment of persons with dementia

A wide range of dementia-specific assessment tools for both persons with dementia and caregivers have been developed, spanning behavioral, affective, and cognitive domains, and including numerous screening instruments. Many of these assessment tools involve informant ratings of prior or current functioning. These tools include observational scales, as well as self-report inventories. Tools for assessing dementia exist both in print (e.g. Burns et al. 2004), as well as on line (e.g. <www.nia.nih.gov/research/cognitive-instrument>). Another example of the latter is the Dementia Outcomes Management Suite (DOMS), an initiative of the Australian Dementia Collaborative Research Centres and the Australian Commonwealth Government to assist health professionals to select appropriate tools with which to evaluate persons suspected of having dementia. The suite is aimed at appropriately qualified health professionals and may be accessed at: <http://www.dementia-assessment.com.au/>.

Clinical interview

The clinical interview should not be neglected in persons with dementia. For clinicians seeing such patients in a private practice or outpatient setting, this is natural and expected. However, in consultation and liaison work with persons with dementia in inpatient and nursing home settings, often contradictory information is provided by various referral sources, particularly those unfamiliar with various presentations of dementia. In such cases, scheduling an interview with the patient, without family members or caregivers present, is essential. Often this may be tricky, as there may be a belief either that the person with dementia cannot speak for him- or herself, or will be distressed. Again, a clinician's primary assessment strategy is the initial clinical interview, which can assist in building up a picture of this patient and their circumstances, as seen through their eyes. Interviewing other significant parties is important for a variety of reasons, but the clinician should hold firm in seeking to speak to the person with dementia directly and in private.

There are several tools that may assist in the clinical interview; one is the Clinical Dementia Rating Scale (CDR) developed at the Alzheimer's Disease Research Center (ADRC) at Washington University, St Louis (Morris 1997). It is designed to assist the clinician in staging the severity of dementia across a variety of domains, including memory, orientation, judgment and problem-solving, community affairs, home and hobbies, and personal care. Ratings on the CDR range from no impairment through to severe impairment. Although originally developed for use with individuals with Alzheimer's disease, the instrument is appropriate for use in other forms of dementia. The utility of the scale for the psychologist using it in the interview is not so much to ascertain stage of illness (though such a global rating may be useful), but to gauge performance across these domains. If individuals have areas of severe deficit along with islands of preserved functioning, this is very important for both feedback to the person with dementia and their caregiver, but also may help in formulating a treatment plan. The CDR collects information in a standard way from both the patient and an informant, and the tool provides useful examples and guides to assist the clinician. Videotapes to aid in scoring the CDR also are available from the ADRC at Washington University in St Louis, Missouri.

The Camberwell Assessment of Needs in the Elderly (CANE; Reynolds et al. 2000) is another useful tool to incorporate into a clinical interview. The CANE is a semi-structured interview consisting of 24 domains that cover physical, social, psychological, and environmental needs of the person with dementia. The CANE provides perspectives on the needs of the person with dementia from the patient's perspective, as well as family and professional caregivers. The interview starts with an open question about each domain, followed by questions regarding help, and any formal or informal support the patient receives, as well as any unmet needs in that area. Items are scored on a three-point scale ranging from little (1) to a lot of help (3). Satisfaction with the amount and quality of support received is also noted. A study by Walters and colleagues (2000) found "psychological distress" among the most frequently identified unmet needs in a primary care setting for persons with dementia based on CANE interviews.

Cognitive screening

Basic cognitive screening approaches for use with both depressed and anxious older individuals were discussed in the chapters on depression and anxiety. Here, this material is reviewed for use in a dementia population, with additional useful tests cited. Changes in cognition in later life may arise from a number of factors, including medical illnesses and medication side effects, and comorbid psychiatric presentations such as depression or anxiety. Screening of cognitive functioning is often useful for clinicians working with older clients, but is particularly important if dementia is suspected or diagnosed, and recent cognitive data (e.g., neuropsychological testing within 3 months) is not available. Even if neuropsychological testing has been carried out in the recent past, screening may be useful to document current level of cognitive functioning. Such screening may also pick up previously undocumented cognitive declines or changes, and may serve as a useful basis for a referral for neuropsychological testing.

Older adults with depression and particularly late-onset depression often cite memory problems as a significant symptom, more so than younger populations (Blazer 2003b). As such, a common referral question (in the minds of either the referral source and/or the clinician) may be whether the client is experiencing depression or the onset of a dementia. Thus, use of a cognitive screen in such circumstances can help the clinician to see how the client is faring with respect to cognition in the present moment, as well as offering data to compare with other administrations of cognitive screens. As a rule, it is wise for the clinician to administer a cognitive screen him- or herself if cognitive functioning is an important question, rather than simply accepting results that may have been administered earlier. Cognitive screens are susceptible to when and where they were administered (e.g., hospital-based test results may be lower than results obtained in the community setting due to health status, as well as the often disconcerting nature of the acute medical environment). Cognition also may change in response to a variety of circumstances, including medication and health changes. So an up-to-the-minute picture of cognition is useful on multiple counts.

The individual's cultural background, presenting issues, comorbid conditions, and level of education, as well as awareness of deficits may all influence selection of cognitive screens. A complete review of all potential screening instruments for cognition is beyond the scope of this chapter, but the interested reader is referred to recent reviews by Edelstein (2007), Pachana and colleagues (2010a), and Cullen et al. (2007).

The Mini-Mental State Exam (MMSE; Folstein et al. 1975) is still the most widely used instrument for cognitive screening across a range of disciplines and circumstances, and is simple and easy to administer in clinical practice. Although limited in terms of the scope of information it provides to the clinician, it is a useful way to communicate results to other professionals in a lingua franca. MMSE scores should always be interpreted in light of age and education (Crum et al. 1993), rather than simple cut-off scores (as unfortunately is widely practiced).

Brief cognitive screens, such as the Montreal Cognitive Assessment (MoCA; Nasreddine et al. 2005), Modified Mini-Mental State Exam (3MS; Teng and Chui 1987), and the Rowland Universal Dementia Assessment Scale (RUDAS; Storey et al. 2004), are all in relatively wide use, have good psychometric properties, have some advantages over the MMSE with respect to overcoming educational and cultural biases (e.g., relatively less reliance on orientation, prior learning, and language facility), and are appropriate for older populations (Ismail et al. 2010). The MoCA has the advantages that it is in the public domain, is easily administered and scored, and provides good data on the evidence of cognitive impairment and particularly MCI. Domains assessed include visuospatial and executive functioning, confrontational naming, memory encoding, attention, language, abstraction, delayed recall, and orientation. The MoCA has been used with a wide range of clinical conditions, including various types of dementia, Parkinson's disease, HIV, multiple sclerosis, stroke rehabilitation, and substance use disorders.

The 3MS offers a much more comprehensive survey of cognitive functioning, including executive functioning, while still only 27 items. It has the added advantages of a more standardized administration than the MMSE, while also yielding the original Folstein MMSE score as an option. The domains sampled include those of the MMSE (orientation, registration, mental reversal, recall, naming, repetition, reading, 3-stage command, and copying pentagons) with the addition of cueing prompts and multiple choice options to gauge cognitive limits, and additional items such as similarities and language generativity (animal naming). The 3MS is useful in situations where a finer-grained picture of cognitive functioning is required. It has been used in a variety of clinical settings.

The RUDAS is a brief screen particularly designed to minimize the effects of culture and language diversity on assessment of current cognitive functioning. The domains assessed in the RUDAS include registration, body orientation, praxis, drawing, judgment, recall, and animal naming. Designed in Australia to be applicable to a broad range of individuals, the items on the RUDAS were developed in consultation with a wide variety of health care professionals, as well as representatives from a diverse range of cultural and linguistic backgrounds. The test provides a range of response formats (verbal, non-verbal, written, and praxic) to ease test-taking. A comprehensive manual describes details to insure smooth test administration, down to a diagram of how the test taker, test administrator, and a translator should be seated with respect to each other. Despite the attractions of culture and language bias minimization, the RUDAS is most appropriate for those already displaying some evident cognitive decline; in those with more intact cognition or higher socioeconomic levels a ceiling effect is a distinct possibility.

An Australian tool, the Informant Questionnaire on Cognitive Decline in the Elderly (IQCODE, Jorm and Jacomb 1989) is an informant rating scale to assess cognitive impairment in older persons. The IQCODE, when combined with another cognitive screening tool such as the MMSE, can improve sensitivity and specificity (Mackinnon and Mulligan 1998). There is also a 16-item short form of the IQCODE (Jorm 1994), which is very useful in busy clinical settings.

If the results on a basic cognitive screening test are suggestive of more profound cognitive impairment, referral to a neuropsychologist for a more complete work-up is usually warranted, especially if diagnosis of a progressive neurological condition is queried (see American Psychological Association Taskforce on Dementia Assessment (2012) for further explications of best practice in detection of dementia, the most common of progressive neurological conditions affecting older adults). A general medical work-up to rule out other potential causes of cognitive decline (usually by a geriatrician or a neurologist) also may be warranted.

It may be useful to screen for depression and anxiety during the interview (see Case Example 5.1A). As has been alluded to previously, late-onset depression in particular is characterized by significant complaints of cognitive impairment and the differential diagnosis between depression and dementia, particularly in frail or very old persons, can be difficult. Also, treatment of persons with dementia who have comorbid depression or anxiety is important, as left untreated these psychological disorders increase burden unnecessarily. Brief age-appropriate screening tests such as the Geriatric Depression Scale (GDS; Yesavage et al. 1982) and the Geriatric Anxiety Inventory (GAI; Pachana et al. 2007) are appropriate for persons who can still manage self-report inventories. The Cornell Scale for Depression in Dementia (Alexopoulos et al. 1988) and the Rating Anxiety in Dementia scale (Shankar et al. 1999) are used if informant reports on mood and anxiety are necessary.

> ### Case Example 5.1A Sandy: assessment of dementia referral
>
> Sandy was referred to John by her primary care physician for what she stated was "to check why my brain isn't working anymore." A neuropsychologist with a mixed assessment and limited psychotherapy practice, primarily with traumatic brain injury patients, John approached Sandy's referral with both his neuropsychological and clinician's hats on, so to speak. The interview started out awkwardly, however, as John was in possession of the referral letter, which pithily stated "depression; query dementia," whereas the patient informed the psychologist that her primary care physician had assured her that her memory problems were "definitely not dementia."
>
> Sandy presented as a well-groomed 64-year-old woman who looked about a decade younger than her age. She worked in a local high-end clothing boutique and was divorced. She appeared nervous and fidgety, and during the clinical interview she often needed prompting and was extremely tangential. She appeared distracted and at one point excused herself for what turned into a 10-minute trip to the women's bathroom.
>
> On a screening test for depression (GDS-15) Sandy scored in the mildly depressed range. On the MoCA she scored in the moderately impaired range. At this point John was becoming convinced that despite the physician's assurances as reported by the patient, Sandy was indeed perhaps faced with a possible diagnosis of dementia.
>
> John decided to proceed with a few neuropsychological tests with a plan for completing a neuropsychological assessment of Sandy's cognitive functioning at a second session. After an unremarkable completion of a basic trail-making test, John administered a list-learning test. During the second recitation of the list, Sandy broke down completely. "I cannot do this. My brain is not working right!" It took 30 minutes and several cups of tea to stem the flood of tears and a near panic attack from Sandy.

Talking with patients about cognitive symptoms

One of the most frequent questions we receive when lecturing about cognitive assessment in persons with dementia is whether and how to share news of a diagnosis of dementia with a patient. As discussed, persons with suspected dementia would usually value knowing the source of their cognitive decline. How to discuss the positive findings of a dementia assessment is a matter best tailored to the individual patient, their family context, and the circumstances. Often the person is diagnosed within the context of a memory assessment clinic; here, the members of the team may have established protocols for discussing findings with clients. In our clinical work we find that families and health care professionals who strive to keep a diagnosis from a person with dementia inevitably face elaborate maneuvering to keep the secret safe.

Did Sandy have cognitive decline in addition to her high levels of anxiety (see Case Example 5.1B)? In this case, John's decision to cease cognitive assessments beyond screening measures until her high levels of anxiety could be addressed was mostly driven by the fact that any declines on cognitive testing could, at

> **Case Example 5.1B Sandy: addressing anxiety first**
>
> Given Sandy's distress, John decided against continuing with cognitive tests, instead exploring Sandy's reaction to the memory testing. At one point, when he mentioned the word anxiety, Sandy spontaneously volunteered that she had a long history of anxiety and specifically panic attacks. She had not experienced these for over a decade. However, she had recently relocated across the country to be near her daughter and her first grandchild. She had found work quickly when she moved, but she found the traffic congestion and loss of her friends disorienting after many years of living in a relatively small community. She had had difficulty settling on a primary care physician, and she noted that she had felt very flustered when she visited the referring physician, after arriving 30 minutes late due to traffic.
>
> Sandy appeared relieved to be talking about her distress and John scheduled another session for later in the week. He obtained permission to have her records from her previous therapist sent to him. They arrived promptly, and revealed a long history of anxiety in the face of stress, with some panic attacks, but which had responded well to a CBT approach.
>
> Sandy appeared much less flustered at this second interview; the appointment had been scheduled for a day she did not work, in the middle of the day to minimize traffic hassles. John administered the GAI to Sandy on this second interview, and her score of 15 out of 20 revealed significant anxiety symptomatology. John decided to forego further memory testing in favor of addressing Sandy's high levels of current anxiety. Sandy was keen to start therapy to address her anxiety symptoms, as she was keen to enjoy her time with her grandchild and her daughter.

least in part, be attributed to anxiety, thereby clouding the picture of whether true cognitive decline was present. In cases where high current levels of anxiety and/or depression are present, it may be wise to forego testing until the affective/anxiety symptoms resolve or at least current distress is alleviated.

Depression in dementia

Depression, as a differential diagnostic question, is one of the most common queries encountered by a psychologist who regularly sees older clients. There are many symptoms of these two disorders that overlap, with memory complaints, apathy, agitation, and decreases in activities of particular note. Particularly in prodromal phases of dementia, these symptoms may in fact represent the co-occurrence of both a mood disorder, together with incipient cognitive decline.

Particularly in the early stages of dementia or in the case of MCI, a wide variety of depression screens may be useful to augment data gathered during the clinical interview. Choosing between the use of, for example, the Beck Depression Inventory or the Geriatric Depression Scale may, in this case, depend more on the clinician's preferences and usual practice, or the presence of data from earlier clinical testing, which might then warrant a repeat administration of the same instrument for the sake of comparison with previous scores. However, assessment tools specifically designed for use with patients with suspected depression in the presence of dementia have been developed. The most widely used, the Cornell Scale for Depression in Dementia (Alexopoulos et al. 1988), uses information from the patient, as well as a caregiver or other knowledgable informant. Information is elicited through separate semi-structured interviews with both parties separately; these two interviews together take approximately 20–30 minutes. Each of the 19 domains assessed with the Cornell (e.g. lack of energy, pessimism, suicide) is rated on a scale of 0, 1, or 2 (absent, mild, severe); scores above 10 indicate probable major depression; scores above 18 indicate a definite major depression. The final ratings of each item are based on the rater's overall clinical impression, having resolved any discrepancies between informant data and observed behaviours and (if possible) the patient's own self-report.

As mentioned in Chapter 3, informants may under-report depressed mood in persons with dementia (Towsley et al. 2012). Here a strategy of gaining multiple perspectives from those who know the patient well both in their current and recent past contexts is useful, and direct observation of the person with dementia is critical, preferably across several instances, at different times of the day and in different contexts. Other pertinent assessment data include medications or medical conditions that may be mimicking depressive symptoms (e.g. decreased appetite, disturbed sleep). Finally, it is worth reflecting on whether behaviours exhibited by the person with dementia that might be interpreted as reflecting depression may actually have other drivers. For example, a person with dementia may be withdrawn and reluctant to participate in activities due to conflicts with other residents in a nursing home facility.

Anxiety in dementia

Anxiety presents a specific diagnostic challenge in the face of dementia. The agitation typical of dementia may be difficult to separate from anxiety. Similarly, impaired memory may be interpreted as a sign of anxiety, depression, or dementia.

The Rating Anxiety in Dementia (RAID; Shankar et al. 1999) scale was designed for the measurement of anxiety in persons with dementia and is currently the most used instrument for this purpose. The scale has 18 items that are rated on a three-point scale using a combination of direct observation and interview, and the report of a person who knows the older person well. A score of 11 has good sensitivity (77–90%) and specificity (79–82%), with excellent internal consistency reliability (0.83) and adequate inter-rater reliability (kappas from 0.51 to 1.00). Snow and colleagues (2012) have recently published a structured interview guide for this instrument, developed to standardize administration and scoring, which improves reliability and validity. This is an important consideration, given that interviewing persons with profound cognitive impairment can make administering screening tools challenging.

Anxiety and agitation both describe a complex set of behaviors with some overlap. Agitation is used to describe behaviors associated with anxiety, dementia, and delirium. In a large factor analysis study of persons with untreated Alzheimer's disease, Spalletta et al. (2010) found that anxiety and agitation loaded on separate factors—anxiety loading with depression, and agitation loading with irritability and aberrant motor behavior.

Agitation in dementia

The Cohen Mansfield Agitation Inventory (CMAI; Cohen-Mansfield et al. 1989) is a caregivers' rating questionnaire consisting of 29 agitated behaviors, each rated on a seven-point scale of frequency. Ratings are for the two weeks preceding the administration. The purpose of the CMAI is to assess the frequency of manifestations of agitated behaviors in older persons. It was originally developed for use in the nursing home and is one of the most widely used specific rating scales of agitation in dementia. An on-line manual is available for the CMAI, providing instruction in its administration (<http://www.dementia-assessment.com.au/symptoms/cmai_manual.pdf>). It is important not to influence the caregiver, but rather let them tell you what they know about the behaviors of the person with dementia they are caring for. It is best to leave at least 20 minutes for the interview. A short version of the CMAI is also available (Werner et al. 1994).

Delirium and dementia

An important differential diagnosis for dementia is delirium. The prevalence of delirium in older hospital patients has been reported as ranging from 11% to 24%, with higher rates found in post-surgical patients (Fann 2000). Many older adults with delirium go undetected; in a survey of patients in a Veteran's Administration (VA) hospital in the USA being evaluated for depression, 40% actually had delirium (Farrell and Ganzini 1995). Delirium may have many etiologies, but underlying medical illnesses, such as infections or drug toxicity, are common causes in older people. In order to treat the delirium it is important to ascertain its cause. Common disorders with this risk in older persons include thyroid disease, diabetes, sodium–potassium imbalance, sleep deprivation, and dehydration (Levkoff et al. 1992), the latter being a common concern in older adults with dementia who are in care.

The Confusional Assessment Method (CAM; Inouye 2003) is the preferred tool for ascertaining the presence of delirium. The CAM can be administered in about 5 minutes, and has good sensitivity and specificity (94–100% and 90–95%, respectively; Inouye 2003). The CAM has two parts—part one is an assessment screen for overall cognitive impairment, while part two includes only those four items found to have the greatest ability to distinguish delirium from other disorders. The CAM simply assesses the presence or absence of delirium, rather than severity, so it is not really useful for detecting improvement; here, a brief cognitive screen such as the MMSE (Folstein et al. 1975) or the MoCA (Nasreddine et al. 2005) may be more useful. The CAM has been particularly designed to help improve rates of detection of delirium in a wide variety of settings (Inouye et al. 1990). Unfortunately, in clinical practice, delirium often goes undetected. A wrong diagnosis of dementia when delirium is present:

- may exacerbate the delirium;
- results in inappropriate medication and perhaps restraint;
- as there is a risk of self-harm due to the confusional state of delirium, untreated delirium carries significant risk of negative outcomes for patients, including older adults.

Pain and dementia

The assessment of pain in persons with dementia is important. Swafford and colleagues (2009) conducted a review of systemic pain management assessment and intervention strategies used in nursing homes, and found that pain management practices can greatly improve with the adoption of systematic assessment and/or management practices. The systematic assessment and management of pain benefits patients in all settings, including home-based care. Systematic assessment includes having caregivers regularly monitor whether the person in dementia is in pain, either due to a new acute cause that may provoke new behaviors such as agitation, or chronic conditions such as arthritis, which can severely decrease quality of life if pain management approaches are erratic.

Assessment of pain is challenging in those with impaired cognition or communication abilities. Pictorial or visual analog rating scales may be quite useful here (Hadjistavropoulos et al. 2007; Scherder and Bouma 2000). Unidimensional verbal descriptor scales (e.g., "no pain," "mild pain," "moderate pain," "severe pain") may be more suitable for those with more intact verbal skills. Scales that use drawings of faces (from smiling to distressed) are more suited to those with higher levels of cognitive impairment. Finally, the Abbey Pain Scale (Abbey et al. 2004) is a clinical observational pain assessment tool, highly suited to assessing pain in those with limited communication skills. Items include six questions about physical or observable signs of pain (e.g., vocalization and facial grimacing). In their study, Abbey and colleagues demonstrated that the pain scale ratings in older adults fell by half on average following a pain-relief intervention (Abbey et al. 2004).

Systematic management of pain includes combining psychosocial and pharmacological intervention strategies to keep pain in check. Again, haphazard and erratic pain management can increase agitation and other behaviors, and lead to decreased quality of life. For a detailed discussion of pain management strategies in persons with dementia the reader is referred to Snow and Jacobs (2014).

Psychotic symptoms and dementia

Up to 50% of patients with Alzheimer's disease have been reported to experience psychotic symptoms (Lacro and Jeste 1997), and 19% of patients with dementia with Lewy Bodies (McKeith et al. 1996). In assessing psychotic symptoms in the presence of dementia, it is important to distinguish true psychotic symptoms from misperceptions that may result from either sensory impairment, an impaired ability to interpret the environment, or some combination of the two. This may be most acutely difficult in older persons in residential aged-care settings, where often the environment is noisy and confusing, patients often have sensory impairments, and severity of dementia makes misperceptions probable and communication difficult. Because psychotic symptoms are a relatively common presentation in dementia, use of a rating scale for Behavioral and Psychological Symptoms in Dementia (BPSD), such as the Neuropsychiatric Inventory (NPI: Cummings et al. 1994) with its psychosis item, is useful both for assessing for psychotic symptoms, as well as putting these in context with other BPSD. The NPI (Cummings et al. 1994) is useful for tracking changes and improvements in BPSD. For those unfamiliar with the scoring procedures of the NPI, Connor et al. (2008) provided a useful summary. If the query is couched in a more general disquiet over the patient's level of agitation and aggression, use of the Cohen Mansfield Agitation Inventory (CMAI) in its full (Cohen-Mansfield et al. 1989) or short (Werner et al. 1994) form may be useful both for exploring the level and type of agitation, as well as serving as a baseline measure from which to ascertain any improvement, whether from pharmacological and/or behavioral and environmental interventions.

Psychotic symptoms may also co-present with a number of progressive neurological conditions, including Huntington's disease, Parkinson's disease, multiple sclerosis, and amyotrophic lateral sclerosis (Masand 2000). Psychotic symptoms occur in approximately 40% of Parkinson's patients, being a function of the disease process, medication side effects, and/or incipient dementia (Cummings 1992). Anti-parkinsonian drugs are perhaps among the most prominent medications associated with psychotic symptoms, but others commonly used in older populations, such as sedative-hypnotics, some analgesics, both tricyclic antidepressants and selective serotonin reuptake inhibitors, anticonvulsants (such as carbamazepine), and antidysrhythmics (such as digoxin) may also produce psychotic symptoms (Targum 2001). In a psychotic presentation in the face of comorbid medical and/or neurologic illness, careful history taking with respect to the course of the illness and medication schedules is invaluable.

In summary, assessment of persons with dementia and those with suspected difficulties with cognitive functioning presents unique challenges to the clinician. It is useful for the clinician to keep an open mind about the direction that the referral may take—gathering data from an interview and with objective measures is key here. Often therapy directions can be informed by measures of domains beyond cognitive and affective functioning. Likewise, the success of interventions is best demonstrated by changes in such measures.

Therapy with people with dementia and their caregivers

Over the past 30 years, the idea of psychological interventions for persons with dementia has been gaining in acceptance. The wider acceptance is based in part on more accurate and earlier identification of people with dementia, so that now the diagnosis may be made while the person with dementia is sufficiently cognitively intact to benefit from therapy. It has also been rooted in increasing understanding of dementia, and a decline in all or none thinking about the cognitive abilities of persons with dementia. As such, it is now more widely understood that while memory and learning may be more difficult, they are not altogether absent until very late in the process of dementia. Finally, there has been additional research (including the rediscovery of older research, e.g., reviewed by Gatz et al. 1998) on the use of behavioral methods, and the training of family and other caregivers in behavioral methods (Logsdon et al. 2007). This means that there is more understanding of the ways in which the person with dementia can be helped later in the dementia process by getting caregivers to use behavioral methods to improve the care receiver's mood and behavior.

Interventions for persons with dementia

Psychological work with persons with dementia, particularly those with more moderate or severe dementia, differs from that discussed in Chapter 3 and

Chapter 4. Here, both assessment and treatment approaches are tailored relative to the individual with dementia. By this, we mean that in such cases, the combination of the behaviors of concern, and the psychological impact of those on the people in the immediate environment, often require a set of interventions that include not only more standard behavioral management techniques, but also involve very specific reference to aspects of the person with dementia's earlier life, prior to the onset of disease. The pairing of very familiar activities, personally meaningful stimuli, and so forth can increase the efficacy of the suggested interventions. At all times and at all stages of the disease process, including the prodromal phase or diagnoses such as MCI that may progress to dementia, the person with dementia remains a person whose unique personality and preferences often hold the key to effecting positive change.

Psychologists working with individuals with dementia and their families often need to work in a multidisciplinary environment, with good liaising with the family and other health and mental health professionals vital to positive intervention outcomes (Pusey and Richards 2001). Psychotherapeutic interventions with persons with dementia include cognitive and behavioral approaches (Spector et al. 2012). Evidence-based interventions with caregivers include cognitive behavioral therapy (CBT; Pinquart and Sorensen 2006), interpersonal therapy (IPT; James et al. 2003), and family therapy approaches (Qualls and Noecker 2009). A variety of psychosocial strategies to assist persons with dementia, professional carers, and families in residential aged-care settings have also received good empirical support for improving quality of life and well-being in these settings (e.g., Konnert et al. 2009).

Attitudes toward dementia

In our experience, both trainees and health professionals find that encountering dementia brings up fears and negative feelings about aging, decline, and profound cognitive and behavioral changes. Sometimes there is a tendency to think that little can be done psychologically, that options are limited, so that an almost nihilistic stance is adopted. Others approach this population with the feeling that they do not know enough about dementia or persons with dementia, and so avoid providing services fearing they will make a mistake.

This negativity in attitude and language is often understood by, and can have negative consequences for, persons with dementia (Hubbard et al. 2002). Persons with dementia at all points in the severity range of the illness can benefit from psychological interventions. Psychological assessment can help ascertain which treatment approaches may work best, can chart positive changes in response to treatment, and can assist in how the intervention proceeds (e.g., in choice of therapy materials or the frequency of scheduled sessions).

Even family members may become paralyzed, unable to decide the best way forward in dealing with a loved one who appears so changed. In many ways the person with dementia is the most robust person in the scenario who, once engaged in a meaningful way, can often show remarkable adaptivity and even humor in the face of their circumstances. After gaining the support of both family and care staff, trying out a variety of approaches with the person with dementia, and certainly shifting approaches in the face of increasing cognitive decline or behavior changes, is often required to arrive at an intervention that is effective.

Developmental influences on work with clients with dementia

In working with persons with dementia, development can refer both to the process of aging itself and also to the developmental process of a progressive dementia. Changes in cognition with normal aging raise concerns about dementia in many older adult clients. As noted earlier in this chapter, it can be unclear for months to years whether relatively minor changes in cognition are normal aging, represent a change that will not progress, or are the beginning of a progressive dementia. Dementia is a common concern in therapy with many older clients and the therapist needs to be prepared to provide realistic feedback about the current impact of the reported cognitive changes. They also need to be prepared to help allay unrealistic anxiety, while not being overly dismissive of the possibility that dementia may be formally diagnosed in a year or two.

Advancing age also affects the ways in which dementia presents, especially if aging has brought on additional health problems or declines in sensory abilities. The physical diseases or impairments result in higher levels of overall functional decline. The dementia also complicates attempts at treatment, rehabilitation, or compensation for the physical disorders. A frail 90-year-old with dementia is a very different person compared with an otherwise healthy 70-year-old with dementia. The person with dementia may also use the physical frailty to cover for cognitive deficits. For example, several clients with dementia have covered visuospatial orientation problems and difficulties finding their way around familiar environments by blaming their decreased range of walking on physical pain or weakness in their legs. This misdirection away from the cognitive losses on the part of the person with dementia may be intentional or may simply reflect the person's decreasing insight and increased discomfort as a result of the progression of the dementia.

The developmental progression of dementias

In general, the more striking developmental influence will be the progression of the dementia itself. As noted earlier, most of the dementias of later life are progressive. Most unfold over a number of years and move somewhat slowly from normal aging to very severe cognitive impairment with most memory (including personal autobiography) gone, and language very limited and eventually absent. In the early phase of a dementia, the person with dementia can benefit from therapy focused on emotional reactions to learning the diagnosis and acceptance of changes in lifestyle and behavior that may be necessary in these early phases. Since the dementia is progressive, the therapist must be mindful of the client's ability to recall what is discussed from session to session, and monitor positive change even more carefully than is done with other clients. Working with a person with dementia who is able to benefit from therapy can be very helpful in alleviating depression and anxiety, and so improving overall functioning. Working with a person with dementia whose cognition is so poor as to be unable to recall prior sessions or to benefit from the therapy is unethical and can lead to charges of fraud.

There are many approaches to thinking about stages of progressive dementias. While all have some value, it is also important to keep in mind that the course is often quite variable in terms of speed of progression, and in terms of what abilities and behaviors are affected. This variability can be influenced by:

- premorbid personality factors;
- by the size, timing, and location of the brain pathology;
- by environmental characteristics;
- by comorbid physical and mental health disorders.

Different treatment and dementia services settings often serve people in particular phases of the dementias and may have different, sometimes non-overlapping, notions of the stages of dementia. Professionals who mainly work with early-stage dementias may think of what others would call middle stages as late and those working with late-stage dementias may think of middle stages as early. Obviously, this can lead to miscommunication and confusion when talking across these settings about a particular patient and so being aware of this as a potential issue can help to insure accurate information is shared.

Examples 5.1–5.3 give a sampling of issues that arise in therapy with persons at the early to middle stages of dementia, at differing ages, and with differing health profiles.

Example 5.1 Recognizing dementia in client with high premorbid education and intelligence

One man in his late 60s in the early stages of dementia was feeling depressed with a sense of loss that was mainly focused on realizing that he was no longer able to play bridge well and that the group that he played with on a regular basis was "carrying" him in the game. He also missed doing the kind of complex thinking and problem solving he had done in his career as an engineer. He was still doing quite well in the less complex activities of life. His wife was very reassuring regarding her affection for him and her commitment to staying with him and caring for him as the dementia got worse, and so he was not at this point very concerned about the future. Much of the therapeutic work around these issues consisted of letting him talk about and grieve for the abilities he no longer had and then refocusing his attention on what he could still do that he enjoyed. It is worth noting that it is not uncommon that persons with dementia are much less distressed about the illness than might be expected and also less distressed than their family members often are. An important lesson from this example is that the therapist was inclined at first to see the client as depressed, and not cognitively impaired, and so worked at minimizing the client's concerns about his cognitive losses. When a review of neuropsychological test reports done over a period of a few years convinced the therapist that there was, in fact, cognitive decline, the therapy moved more quickly toward resolution of the depressed mood as the therapist accepted the reality of the cognitive losses. The client was facing the same lack of acceptance of his cognitive decline from many family members and friends as well, so the therapist's acceptance was a welcome relief.

Example 5.2 Dementia emerging in therapy as emotional distress declines

A woman in her late 80s began therapy with clear indications of depressed mood and cognitive screening scores that could be attributed to advanced age, MCI, or the impact of depression on executive functioning items. The therapy focused on her emotional distress in caring for her husband who was quite physically impaired, and had a very negative, dominating, and angry style of interacting with her. The therapy had a positive impact on her depressed mood and increased her assertiveness with her husband. At about the same time her depression was improving, she gave up driving, attributing the decision to a hand tremor that, in fact, only lasted a few days. Her conversation in sessions became more repetitive and there was a notable increase in word-finding difficulties as she talked. A second cognitive screen at this point showed a steep drop in the total score and also a new failure in delayed recall ability. Although she still remembered session content week to week, gradually she withdrew from the therapy.

Example 5.3 Middle to late-middle phase dementia

A woman about 90 years old was brought into therapy by her daughter. She had multiple physical problems including severe visual and hearing impairments, needing a wheelchair for mobility, and moderate cognitive impairment. She was depressed about her current situation, and the focus of the depression was on her relationship with family members,

> rather than her physical problems, which she mostly accepted as part of being 90. While much of the therapeutic work focused on improving communication between the client and her daughter, one theme was helping the client to recognize that some of the things she did not know about her living situation and her finances were due to her memory impairment and her difficulty in doing arithmetic, rather than to family plots to keep the knowledge from her.

Working with the patient

In thinking about the likely role of the therapist, it can be useful to distinguish between stages. In earlier stages, adjusting to the diagnosis and thinking about the future are key issues, and memory is still clearly intact enough for verbal therapy. In middle, moderate stages, memory is declining more markedly, and the therapist needs to assess frequently whether progress is being made and the client is remembering the content of past sessions. Note that failing to remember the therapist's name is not a reason in itself to stop therapy, but failing to remember the therapist altogether or remember past sessions is. The focus at this stage is generally on adjustment to functional losses and finding ways to manage life that do not rely on lost cognitive functions. As the moderate stage progresses, the intervention will need to involve caregivers more than the person with dementia, and will rely on teaching them how to manage their own emotions and to use behavioral strategies to bolster functioning as much as possible.

Working with the caregiver

As the dementia progresses into moderate levels of impairment and memory declines to the point where direct work with the person with dementia is no longer feasible, the focus shifts to working with caregivers to improve the mood or enhance the behavioral functioning of the person with dementia. One initial hurdle in this work is often helping caregivers understand why they need to change when the person with dementia is the one with the diagnosis. The simple answer, of course, is that the person with dementia is not capable of change on his/her own at this point. Frequently, there will need to be some allowance for working through the caregiver's perception that this is unfair, or simply very new and therefore odd. In part, this can also stem from the difficulty that many caregivers (both family members and paid caregivers) have working out the implications of dementia in an everyday applied way. What the therapist often hears is some variation on "Yes, I know she has dementia, but why can't she do X?" A similar issue is the caregiver's perception that the person with dementia's behavioral problems or dependent behaviors are interpersonally motivated, rather than a result of the dementia. Changing these perceptions can take some time and require a combination of psychoeducation about dementia and therapeutic work.

Once the caregiver truly accepts the idea that their behavior can change the person with dementia's behavior, the work to be done is largely behavioral analysis of the targets for change in the person with dementia: What are the antecedent stimuli? ("What was happening before she did X?"), and what are the reinforcers? ("What happens after he does X?"). Along the way, the caregiver learns to think in terms of increasing or decreasing the frequency of behaviors, rather than in strict all or none terms. There is also often some reassessment of how important the behavior initially targeted is. While any behavior is changeable in principle, behavior change requires work and time. It is fairly common that the caregiver decides that behavior change is not worth the effort and accepting the behavior problem is preferable. A fairly common solution may be, for example, to accept the person with dementia's desire to wear two shirts, rather than one, or to bathe less frequently rather than to engage in the behavior change process. If the target is improving depression, increasing pleasant activities, and decreasing stress are common techniques.

Environmental modifications follow the same principles. Many concerns about the person with dementia's behavior center on safety. Providing a safe environment for the person with dementia to walk in can be more strategic than trying to reduce or prevent wandering. Dementia proofing the home by making certain dangerous items inaccessible is likely to be less stressful than constantly monitoring where the person with dementia is at and what they are doing. Learning how much environmental stimulation is beneficial, and how much is overwhelming and stressful is important in reducing problem behavior. This threshold will keep moving as the dementia progresses, of course.

Helping caregivers understand the impact of their own emotional state on the person with dementia's behavior can also be very helpful in reducing behavior problems and general strain in caregiving. Persons with dementia tend to have at least normal and often enhanced responses to the emotions of those around them, even when they do not understand what is going on in the environment. Becoming frustrated and even angry with the person with dementia is not uncommon, nor is feeling depressed or anxious in their presence. Caregivers should be encouraged to have outlets and support for these emotions outside the person with dementia's presence and to find ways to stay calm while with them. Relaxation approaches can be helpful with staying calm, as can cognitive change strategies such as reminding oneself that the dementia is the cause of the frustrating behavior, not the person they once knew.

Improving the caregiver's emotional state

In general, therapeutic work with caregivers should be a blend of the approaches described in this chapter to help the caregiver manage the care receiver's dementia related behaviors and changes in the relationship, as described in this chapter, and therapy aimed at treating depression or anxiety disorders as covered in Chapter 3 and Chapter 4. The psychologist should be prepared to discuss available supportive services, both information and support groups, for family caregivers, as well as possible respite options for the care of the person with dementia. While the nature of the stress of caregiving is very long term (typically years and sometimes decades) and the progressive nature of the dementia means that the stressor is constantly changing, the change processes for treating depression and anxiety in caregivers do not differ from those used with other people with those diagnoses.

End-stage dementia and the psychologist

In the end stages, the person with dementia will be non-verbal and have difficulty with basic functioning. The psychologist's role is likely to be mainly helping carers with their emotional adjustment and thinking through behavioral issues in patient care activities. Problem solving skills and applied behavior analysis interventions may continue to be helpful in solving care problems that arise. The psychologist's skill in using non-verbal behavioral cues to detect emotions and pain may also be helpful in assessing the person with dementia's state at this point. The role of psychology in end-stage dementia care is similar to the role in hospice care for persons with cancer and other terminal illnesses who are in the final stages before death.

Social context influences on working with persons with dementia

A major social context factor in work with persons with dementia is whether they are still in the home setting with family or in a 24-hour care setting. The work with persons with dementia (and older adults with serious physical frailty) in 24-hour care settings requires expertise in the social ecology of the setting, as well as expertise in working with older adults.

Working in the residential care environment

There are several approaches that the psychologist can take toward improving quality of life, functionality, as well as psychological functioning for persons with moderate to severe dementia in the nursing home. The first key point is to recognize that the care facility is a system, and approaches to individual patients must acknowledge that informal interactions, as well as formal care proceed within this system. Institutional systems, as with all systems, may function with greater or lesser efficacy, and so the therapist should be cognizant of how functional this particular system is, as this may impact interventions.

Behavioral and psychological symptoms of dementia (BPSD; Finkel 2000) include disturbed perception, thought content, mood, or behaviors in persons with dementia, which frequently cause distress to themselves and their carers (International Psychogeriatric Association (IPA) 2002). A large number of persons with dementia exhibit such symptoms over time, but often these behaviors reflect the person with dementia trying to communicate or react to their environment or internal states. Too often, these symptoms are labeled as undesirable and medications are prescribed to decrease agitation and aggression in particular. While these symptoms are distressing and potentially dangerous in the clinical setting, an attempt to uncover the potential cause or trigger for the symptoms is essential to working out an effective management strategy.

One system that NP has found useful in employing as a basic strategy in nursing homes is to teach staff how to recognize that particular behaviors of the person with dementia may signal an unmet need (McAiney et al. 2007; P.I.E.C.E.S. Canada 2008). This system is as useful for care staff as it is for the consulting psychologist and concerned family members. It offers a checklist of potential underlying causes of behaviors that should be explored before either pharmacological or psychosocial interventions are put in place. If the person with dementia is in pain and this is not recognized, or if the person is responding to distressing elements in their environment (and this includes other persons in the environment who may be causing distress) then interventions that do not first address this are at best misguided, and at worse may seriously compromise health and quality of life (see Box 5.1 for the PIECES framework).

Box 5.1 PIECES framework for understanding BPSD

- Physical problem or discomfort.
- Intellectual/cognitive changes.
- Emotional.
- Capacities (including sensory impairments).
- Environment.
- Social/cultural.

Common *physical* causes of behaviors in a person with dementia could include undiagnosed delirium or pain. *Intellectual/cognitive changes* can result in the person with dementia misperceiving information from staff, or being unable to clearly express their wishes or concerns. *Emotional* changes in the person with dementia (such as increased anxiety) can result, in part, from the decreased ability to process what is going on in the environment due to their impaired cognition. The prior *capabilities* of the person can spur behaviors, as well as being a means of redirecting energies (e.g., in the case of a former nurse in a facility who is intent on helping others; recognizing this capability and employing it, rather than attempting to block it would be an effective strategy). The *environment* is often a trigger for behaviors (e.g., long confusing hallways triggering wandering and agitation). *Social/cultural* factors must be recognized for effective dementia care (and fit nicely within the CALTAP model that we have been using). For example, a woman with dementia who has experienced trauma, particularly physical or sexual abuse, may feel uncomfortable having personal cares delivered by a male nurse attendant.

A second strategy, useful both for institutional carers as well as caregivers in the home, is to maximize the efficacy of communication with the person with dementia. The FOCUSED strategy (see Box 5.2) is useful here (Ripich et al. 1995). This mnemonic reminds the person communicating with the patient with dementia to speak directly at the person, so their lip movements and facial expressions are clearly visible, to stay short and sharp with respect to the information to be conveyed, and to as much as possible use a normal conversational tone of voice. If the person with dementia is unable to think of a word and the conversation stops, suggesting a word may help "unstick" the conversation and get good communication flowing again. NP has found this technique useful for students encountering their first experience in residential care, especially if they have not had much direct contact with patients with dementia.

Box 5.2 FOCUSED strategy

- Face-to-face communication.
- Orientation (repeat key words).
- Continuity of topic.
- Unsticking (suggest candidate words).
- Structuring questions (provide one/two options).
- Exchanging normal conversation.
- Direct, short, simple sentences (but not delivered too slowly!).

Working in the home environment

In the home as well, the environmental context is a major influence on the emotions and behavior of the person with dementia. As discussed in the section on developmental progression of dementias ("Developmental influences on work with clients with dementia"), helping the caregiver and other family members understand the dementia, and the changes it is causing in their loved one, and then helping them handle their own emotions and change their own behavior to reach as harmonious a balance as is possible in the home, is an ongoing challenge for the family with which therapy can be helpful. The balance point itself keeps changing over the years of the progression of the disorder.

Another theme in adjusting the home environment is finding the balance between too little and too much stimulation. From the early stages of the illness onward, the person with dementia will tend to try and simplify life in order to avoid overly demanding situations that place demands on them that they can no longer meet. This can involve complex activities, but also commonly includes being in large groups of any kind. In group settings, the complexity of keeping up with the conversation and the challenge of remembering who the people are typically too demanding as dementia progresses. Given that Western culture tends to emphasize activity and socialization, and sees stimulation as being good for cognitive and emotional health, family members often push the person with dementia to do more than they are able to do. This can lead to stress, frustration, and outbursts of anger or other behavioral problems. Too little stimulation can also be a problem and lead to boredom, depression, and agitated behavior, as a way of increasing activity and discharging energy. As with other chronic illnesses that impair functioning in later life, sorting out the balance between too much and too little activity is an ongoing issue that requires trial and error learning. In progressive conditions like most dementias in later life, the condition itself is changing over time, and so the trial and error process has to be repeated periodically as the person with dementia's abilities change.

Sometimes it is the client's children who can bring pressure to act on the latest bit of health advice promulgated in the mass media. For example, adult children of a parent with moderately advanced Alzheimer's disease insisted to care staff at a nursing facility that they make their mother complete Sudoku puzzles every day "to stop her mental decline." This was seen as very distressing for the patient, but the children were quite adversarial in their stance: "It is for her own good."

There is a general tendency to withdraw socially from the person with dementia and their family. Dementia is rather scary to a lot of people, and they may prefer not to witness the effects on a friend. It is also simply not easy to know what to do or what to talk about. Part of the social context for the person with dementia and the family is this loss of old friends and social contacts, and perhaps an adjustment to new contacts as they enter the world of dementia services and supports.

Cohort influences on working with persons with dementia

The common influence of cohort in understanding dementia is that earlier born cohorts are likely to use diagnostic categories and have ideas about the etiology of dementias that were common earlier in their lives. These differences can arise in understanding the current dementia and also in understanding family history of dementia. Understanding and being able to explain in jargon-free language, how terms like senility, senile dementia, Alzheimer's disease, hardening of the arteries, and so forth, have changed over the years is helpful in orienting the person with dementia and the caregiver to the current illness, and to understanding family risk. An important aspect of this psychoeducation is distinguishing normal aging from the neurological disorders causing the dementia. It is usually also important to take the initiative in explaining the difference between somewhat increased familial risk associated with family history of most dementia disorders, and the high level of risk associated with a single gene dominant inheritance pattern. Many people from earlier born cohorts have dated understanding of genetic influences in terms of classic genetics, rather than changes in probable risk.

Cultural influences on working with persons with dementia

In cultures where respect for older adults is a highly valued cultural tradition, a diagnosis of dementia may be seen as disrespectful. This may keep the family from taking steps to understand the problem or prevent them from using the diagnosis to guide future decision making. In therapy with family members, it can be helpful to explore whether other illnesses (e.g., cancer, heart disease, diabetes, etc.) would be seen as disrespectful of the older adult, then exploring what it is about the neurological disorder underlying the dementia that makes dementia a violation of respect. When this step is successful, then the therapist can move to problem solving about ways to handle the changes that are brought about by the dementia, while still maintaining a respectful stance toward the person with dementia. This is usually a collaborative process with the clients acting as experts on their culture and what is likely to work in their particular family, and the therapist guiding the discussion with questions and supportive problem solving.

This sense of possible disrespect can be complicated further when the cultural understanding of dementia is rooted in traditional views of dementia as resulting from moral failures or from evil spirits, and so involving shame for the individual and probably also the family (Sayegh and Knight 2013). These differences in comprehension of the nature of dementia need to be addressed tactfully and respectfully, but it is likely that the difference between the Western scientific understanding and the family understanding will need to be explored. It is generally a good strategy for the therapist to take the stance that "Well, here is what Western science has to say about this, what do you think?" This position takes the therapist out of direct confrontation with the family's views, and engages them instead in a conversation about why there are different views. This approach is more useful to the family in terms of how to handle the problems confronting them, whichever viewpoint is taken.

In cultures in which a parent maintains a very strong authoritative role in the children's lives, the parent's dementia can result in a very dysfunctional situation, in which the person with dementia is still making decisions for middle-aged and young-old children, even though the decisions no longer work or make sense. Working through this dilemma with the family can be very difficult and requires considerable cultural sensitivity. One potential way toward resolution is exploring gently whether the children have actually always obeyed the parent and how they have handled it in the past when they made other decisions. These past methods may or may not be appropriate to the handling of the person with dementia in the present, but the acknowledgement that the family has ways to make their own decisions is a useful start toward changes that make sense for the whole family.

Issues in working with people with dementia

An advantage that professionals generally have over family members in recognizing and working with persons with dementia is that we usually meet them after the dementia is under way and so do not have the history of knowing them as a cognitively intact individual. The great majority of persons with dementia are pleasant, socially charming people. Discussing the changes in their mental abilities and their attempts to cope with those changes is intrinsically professionally interesting. It is often inspiring to hear their attitudes about decline and their insights into how others in the family are reacting.

This advantage is absent when a client that we meet as a cognitively intact person develops dementia. This can happen either because the initial assessment missed the dementia or, by coincidence, a client whom we have seen for depression or anxiety develops dementia. When this happens, the therapist experiences more of the depression, anxiety, and sense of loss that family feels as the person's level of cognitive function diminishes. It is also fairly common that the therapist first reacts with denial of the dementia.

Summary

Opportunities for psychologists to participate in the assessment and treatment of persons with dementia are growing as the numbers of individuals identified with possible neurocognitive decline increase. This is due to both increased public awareness of the signs and symptoms of dementia, as well as better identification of individuals at an earlier stage in the disease process. However, many myths and stereotypes of people with dementia persist; an important role for the psychologist is in helping all of the individuals involved in the client's care to have a good understanding of the context of the disease, and its attendant issues and concerns, so that good forward planning can occur. In the dementia area, more work on how culture and context influence dementia symptoms and behaviors is warranted.

As noted herein, dementia is just one of the chronic illnesses that affect older clients. It is the one most common disorders and clearly associated with old age, and one often addressed in the literature on psychological assessment and therapy in late life. In the Chapter 6, we discuss issues related to chronic illnesses of late life whose impact is on physical functioning, rather than on cognitive abilities.

Chapter 6

Psychological issues affecting medical conditions

Introduction to psychological issues affecting medical conditions

Chronic medical conditions in later life are largely caused by non-communicable diseases such as cardiovascular diseases, cancers, diabetes, and chronic lung diseases. Three quarters of deaths from non-communicable diseases are in those aged over 60 (World Health Organization 2010). Psychological issues intersect with such conditions in three ways: first, these conditions are related to lifestyle behaviors such as tobacco use, an unhealthy diet, insufficient physical activity, and the excessive use of alcohol; secondly, they are negatively impacted by psychological disorders such as depression; thirdly, they increase the risk of psychological disorders. Thus, psychologists are well-placed to both advise about lifestyle options, as well as offer direct psychological interventions to older adults affected by such non-communicable illnesses. The increasing proportions of older adults affected by such illnesses means that we will see burden of disease and associated costs rising globally in the coming decades (World Health Organization 2004).

The great majority of older adults have at least one chronic physical condition, which impacts upon functioning and usually requires some intervention, not uncommonly, some form of medication. As noted in the World Health Organization (WHO) reports cited above, the impact of chronic medical conditions on social and economic well-being is a global phenomenon. In 1999, individuals in the USA aged 65 years and older with three or more chronic medical conditions represented 48% of Medicare beneficiaries and accounted for 89% of Medicare's annual budget (Anderson and Horvath 2002). In Australia, chronic diseases are the leading cause of illness and disability in those aged 65 years and over (Australian Bureau of Statistics 2006) and accounted for nearly 70% of all health system expenditure in Australia (over $AU35 billion) in the years 2000–2001 (Dowrick 2006). The 2004–2005 Australian National Health Survey (NHS) reported almost all Australians aged 65 years or older have at least one chronic condition, with 80% having three or more chronic conditions (Australian Bureau of Statistics 2006). In Europe, chronic diseases are linked to premature retirement (Jimenez-Martin et al. 1999).

Medical comorbidity itself is associated with poor QOL, multiple medications, and increased risk of side effects and other adverse drug interactions, morbidity, and mortality (Gijsen et al. 2001). Polypharmacy in particular has been an increasing topic of research in geriatric patient populations, and researchers have called for rethinking approaches to patient care (Nobili et al. 2011). The roles that chronic illness and functional disabilities play in later life can be significant, and include triggering psychological distress. For example, when the onset of a medical condition leads to new functional decrements in older adults, there is a high risk of the development of depression (Ormel et al. 2002). Thus, the interaction of medical problems with psychological distress is a common topic in therapy in later life.

Psychological illness and distress can also impact the development and course of chronic illnesses. For example, a recent meta-analysis of 11 studies by Rugulies (2002) demonstrated that major depression is a predictor for development of coronary artery disease. The overall relative risk for development of heart disease in depressed subjects was 1.64 (95% CI, 1.29–2.08). A history of major depression has been linked to increased risk of developing Type 2 diabetes by a factor of two over one's lifetime (Eaton et al. 1996; Kawakami et al. 1999). In fact, diabetes is a classic case of reciprocal impacts of psychological health on disease onset—depression has been shown to contribute to the onset of diabetes (Mezuk et al. 2008), and diabetes has been shown to contribute to the onset of depression (Anderson et al. 2001).

Moreover, psychological factors can directly influence adherence to treatment recommendations, and can often influence the degree of physical pain and distress related to the medical condition. Depression and anxiety can add additional disability to the impact of the physical condition on the client's life and can thus be thought of as a source of "excess disability."

When seeing older adults, it is always possible that an undiagnosed medical condition is contributing to presenting symptoms. There are non-specific physical complaints, which could point to any one of a number of medical conditions, including confusion, self-neglect, falling, incontinence, apathy, shortness of breath, anorexia, and fatigue (Ham et al. 2002). If these symptoms are part of an initial presentation, a referral to a primary care physician to rule out a physical cause is warranted. Often the identification and treatment of medical illness in older adults is delayed due to misinterpretation or dismissal of early and vague symptoms presented by the older person, resulting in increased morbidity and decreased QOL. Older adults themselves, as well as their families and carers, may underplay the significance of such symptoms, attributing changes in health and functionality to "old age," rather than to a potentially treatable physical condition (Williamson and Fried 1996). Although acute symptoms may garner attention, the onset of illness in older adults can be insidious.

A range of medical conditions can present as psychiatric illness. Both hypo- and hyper-thyroid disease may manifest with diminished energy and apathy, and thus may be misdiagnosed as depression in an older adult. Vitamin B_{12} deficiency can present with depression and irritability, along with memory loss. Similarly, memory loss and agitation are often features of depression, anxiety disorders, and dementia syndromes. Importantly, if such presenting symptoms are mistakenly believed to be a part of normal aging, then appropriate treatment may be delayed. In some cases, such as with Vitamin B_{12} deficiency, lack of timely treatment may result in symptoms becoming permanent.

Familiarity with psychiatric symptoms arising from or co-occurring with common medical conditions (Box 6.1) and medications (Box 6.2) is useful for the clinical psychologist. It may be relatively easy to separate psychiatric symptoms from symptoms of physical illness, but more often it is not. In a careful clinical interview, the timing of onset of symptoms, especially with respect to

---

Box 6.1 Major medical illnesses associated with anxiety or depression.

- Asthma.
- Cancers (e.g., pancreatic cancer).
- Chronic obstructive pulmonary disease.
- Cardiac disease and vascular disorders.
- Drug withdrawal.
- Epilepsy.
- Gastrointestinal disorders.
- Genitourinary conditions.
- Endocrine conditions (e.g., thyroid disease).
- Musculoskeletal conditions (e.g., chronic back pain).

Data from Culpepper, L. (2004) Effective recognition and treatment of generalized anxiety disorder in primary care. The Primary Care Companion to the Journal of Clinical Psychiatry, **6**(1), 35–41.

Gagnon, L.M. and Patten, S.B. (2002) Major depression and its association with long-term medical conditions. Canadian Journal of Psychiatry, **47**, 149–152.

> **Box 6.2 Major classes of medication that may cause depression and/or anxiety**
>
> - Analgesics.
> - Antibiotics.
> - Antihistamines.
> - Antihypertensives.
> - Antipsychotics.
> - Anxiolytics.
> - Cancer drugs.
> - Corticosteroids.
> - Digitalis.
> - Estrogen.
> - Insulin.
> - Non-steroidal anti-inflammatory drugs.
>
> Data from Culpepper, L. (2004) Effective recognition and treatment of generalized anxiety disorder in primary care. The Primary Care Companion to the Journal of Clinical Psychiatry, 6(1), 35–41.
>
> Gagnon, L.M. and Patten, S.B. (2002) Major depression and its association with long-term medical conditions. Canadian Journal of Psychiatry, 47, 149–152.

external events, may offer a clue. Similarly, if medical symptoms are successfully treated, psychological symptoms may abate. Often the presenting symptoms, for example, sad or anxious mood, may spring from either a primarily psychological or medical origin, and this may also change over time. In the end, careful assessment of psychological as well as medical symptoms serves as an important base for the primary task, which is constructing an intervention strategy that acknowledges both medical and psychological influences. Then, these same assessments can demonstrate the efficacy of the intervention strategies and guide refinement of same.

Medical conditions can exacerbate presentations of psychiatric illness and vice-versa. There are extensive data about the negative reciprocal relationship between depression and medical illnesses in later life (Katon 2003) and a growing body of research about the similar reciprocal effects of comorbid anxiety and medical illnesses (Culpepper 2004). Often these relationships are complex. For example, there is a large literature about the difficulties in disentangling symptoms of depression from the symptoms of cancers and their treatments, but this literature is much more sparse for older patients (Weinberger et al. 2009). Depressive symptoms may not easily be distinguished from such issues as pain, anxiety, and adjustment issues related to cancer diagnosis and treatment (Massie 2004). The presence of depression in older cancer patients is as high as 25% (Massie 2004), yet often depression is even more likely to remain unrecognized for older as compared with younger adults (Extermann and Hurria 2007). Older adults with cancer are also less likely to receive treatment for depression and psychological distress (Morley 2004).

When the older medically ill patient presents to the psychologist, both assessment and intervention issues may be complex. Assessment of psychiatric symptoms in the presence of medical conditions, particularly multiple comorbid medical conditions, may be difficult: one cannot be sure exactly which underlies the symptom, and quite possibly both could contribute to the symptom presentation. Long-standing medical conditions may have resulted in a significant period of time where maladaptive coping strategies and behaviors have been in play, which can be challenging to confront and manage in therapy. Psychiatric conditions may be exacerbated by external events (e.g., bereavement) that in turn can negatively impact or exacerbate the medical illness. Finally, patients with chronic illnesses may have difficulty adhering to a regular schedule of psychotherapy sessions, they may fatigue easily within session, and require a level of health care coordination that may fall to the psychologist in some cases. These patients are increasing in both age and number, a result of changing demographics and morbidity patterns. They are certainly an increasing proportion of the geropsychologist's caseload.

Assessment in persons with psychological issues affecting medical conditions

Assessment approaches with older adults with comorbid medical conditions, suspected or confirmed, requires careful gathering of data about symptoms and timelines. Older adults may describe symptoms of distress with respect to physical complaints, or alternatively they may fail to mention physical ailments and symptoms, believing them to be consistent with normal aging and, therefore, not worth mentioning. It may be useful for the clinician to directly assess aspects of physical functioning that may be impaired due to comorbid medical conditions. There are also some assessments of physical and emotional functioning specifically designed for use with patients with specific physical disorders.

In assessments of emotional and cognitive functioning in older adults with comorbid medical conditions, it is important for the clinician to insure that the medical conditions themselves do not contaminate the testing process or data in unexpected ways. For example, if patients need frequent breaks for testing, to take medication or ingest food, the testing sessions should be constructed with this in mind so that timed tests can proceed as intended.

Functional assessment

It is useful for clinicians to be aware of the World Health Organization's (WHO) Classification of Functioning, Disability and Health (ICF). Disability (now referred to in WHO guidelines as activity limitation) refers to restrictions in performing everyday tasks. WHO's ICF guidelines recognize two other levels of functioning: physical impairment and handicap; all of these various levels of functioning are interconnected.

Assessment of activities and functionality can assist in determining areas of preserved functioning, as well as areas to target for rehabilitation or compensation, particularly in a multidisciplinary context. Alternatively, the psychotherapist may wish to use this assessment to gauge changes in pre- to post-therapy functioning. For certain patient groups, for example, persons recovering from stroke, there may be conflict between the patient's and family's expectations for recovery and actual recovery, or even the expected time line of recovery. Sometimes, such an assessment can be useful to generate conversations about adaptive equipment that could help increase functionality (or spark discussion of avoidance of using such equipment, i.e., "It makes me feel old"). For example, older persons with sensory or movement disorders may be amazed at the range and price of devices that can add significantly to independence and QOL. There are web-based providers of such devices, and in such instances, referral to a knowledgeable occupational therapist or physical therapist may be wise. Finally, such assessments can alert the clinician if a recommendation to consider a move to an assisted living arrangement might be warranted.

Activities of daily living (ADLs) involve everyday tasks ranging from self-care through to more complex (or instrumental) activities, such as shopping or attending medical appointments. A basic ADL scale in wide use clinically is the Barthel index of basic ADL (Collin et al. 1988). This scale is most appropriate for individuals for whom basic self-care activities are an issue; items include feeding, bathing, dressing, and toileting. Versions of the scale have been developed for specific populations such as patients suffering from a stroke (Quinn et al. 2011). Use of such a scale in regular clinical practice can assist greatly in communicating levels of both ability and disability with other health care providers.

When instrumental activities of daily living (IADLs) are of interest, the Lawton Instrumental Activities of Daily Living Scale (Lawton and Brody 1969; Graf 2008) is a brief rating scale, which covers the ability to:

- carry out shopping;
- prepare food;
- negotiate transport systems;
- use the telephone;
- undertake housekeeping and laundry;
- be responsible for one's own medications;
- handle finances.

However, it may be that some instruments measuring ADLs or IADLs are too basic for some patients; in this case, it may be useful to get information from the patient or an informant about what sorts of activities are of most interest and which have been discontinued due to illness. This information can be paired with some of the QOL (QOL) measures described in the following section, both to plan intervention goals and chart progress in therapy.

Quality of life assessment

The WHO defines QOL as "individuals' perceptions of their position in life in the context of the culture and value systems in which they live in, and in relation to their goals, expectations, standards, and concerns. QOL is a broad ranging concept affected in a complex way by the individual's physical health, psychological state, level of independence, social relationships, personal beliefs, and their relationship to salient features of their environment" (World Health Organization (WHO) QOL Group 1995, p. 1405). Quality of life is an important domain to examine in both the assessment and design of interventions with older adults.

A widely used scale to assess QOL in older adults is the WHOQOL-BREF (Skevington et al. 2004). The WHOQOL-BREF is a 26-item version of the WHOQOL-100 assessment instrument and assesses QOL across four domains—physical, psychological, social, and environment. In a cross-sectional survey of adults carried out in 23 countries ($n = 11{,}830$), including participants from a wide range of socioeconomic strata, as well as from hospital, rehabilitation, and primary care settings, the WHOQOL-BREF was found to have good to excellent psychometric properties. The strengths of this measure are its brevity and its application across a wide range of settings as a cross-culturally valid assessment of QOL.

Although enhancing QOL is usually an intended goal of therapy, it is not often measured directly in clinical practice. Part of the difficulty with QOL instruments is that although most researchers now agree that QOL is a multidimensional, rather than a unitary construct, there is little agreement regarding the number or scope of such dimensions (Bowling 2005; Haywood et al. 2004). There have been attempts to match instruments with specific illnesses (e.g., Diabetes Quality of Life Brief Clinical Inventory; Burroughs et al. 2004), or to take the approach that the older adults themselves can best describe what QOL means to them (Bowling et al. 2003). This individualized approach to measuring QOL has gained favor with QOL researchers (e.g., Halvorsrud et al. 2012).

One instrument that appears promising for use in clinical practice is the Schedule for the Evaluation of Individual Quality of Life—Direct Weighting (SEIQOL-DW; Hickey et al. 1996), an abbreviated and more practical form of the original SEIQOL (O'Boyle et al. 1992, 1993). It is an interesting and clinically useful measure, because it builds upon the notion that the older person is the best source of information about what actually constitutes their own QOL. Clients nominate their five most important domains of QOL—whatever they feel best reflects their own preferences. The client then judges the current status of their nominated areas of QOL by rating them on a vertical visual analogue bar anchored at the two extremes by the terms "Best possible" (rated 100) and "Worst possible" (rated 0). Finally, the relative importance of each QOL area is calculated using a sectogram (also called the SEIQOL-DW disk).

This is a cardboard pie chart (see Figure 6.1) calibrated from 0 to 100, containing five independently movable overlapping circles, each representing one

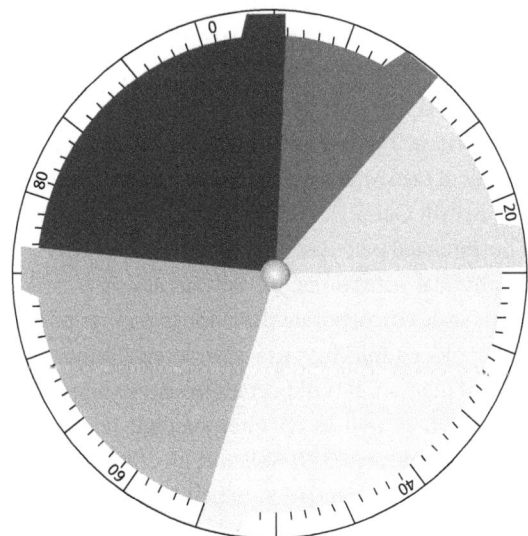

Fig. 6.1 SEIQOL instrument.

QOL area chosen by the individual. Thus, each person can easily visually manipulate the disk to show the relative importance of these areas of QOL.

The overall SEIQOL-DW QOL Index ranges from 0 to 100, with higher scores indicating higher QOL. The semi-structured interview takes approximately 10–20 minutes to complete. Wettergren et al. (2009) reviewed 39 studies using the SEIQOL-DW in order to determine the use, feasibility, and psychometric performance of the instrument. The authors concluded that the SEIQOL-DW was valid, reliable, and of use even among quite disabled patient populations. Construct validity, assessed by means of convergent and discriminant validity, was also shown to be acceptable. The SEIQOL-DW gives the clinician a numerical output, but perhaps its most helpful role to the psychotherapist is the insight it offers into an individual's QOL values and status, as well as their priorities with respect to their individual lives.

NP has used this instrument both in research investigations, as well as in clinical practice; older adults really seem to value the opportunity of describing their own perspective on what gives meaning to their life. Although persons with depressed mood may require more prompting to complete the task, the data collected serves as an important benchmark for how the client sees change in their life as a result of interventions engaged in during the course of therapy.

Assessment of pain

Pain is an important dimension to assess in older adults, particularly those with cognitive or language impairments that make it difficult for them to alert others to their pain. The assessment of pain can be as simple as a 1–10 scale of pain intensity, or can involve more standardized instruments. Pain is under-recognized and under-treated in later life (Brown et al. 2011), particularly among patients in residential aged-care settings (Helme and Gibson 2001), so the careful assessment of pain is important. There are an increasing number of review articles on this issue; Abdulla et al (2013) includes reference to the excellent guide to pain assessment by the British Geriatrics Society, which is useful across settings, but particularly for hospitalized patients.

Pain involves physical sensations, as well as affective and functional responses. Most pain scales incorporate these three aspects of pain. It is important to be aware that older adults may use other words for pain or describe their pain in a roundabout manner. It is important to survey both the impact of pain on functional activities, as well as on interpersonal relationships and social roles. The Brief Pain Inventory (BPI; Keller et al. 2004) is a short instrument with good psychometric characteristics, which is extensively used in clinical settings. The BPI includes a diagram on which patients can indicate the location of their pain, and includes questions regarding pain intensity (current, average, and worst, using a 0–10 rating scale), and includes items that evaluate impairment experienced due to pain. Although not originally designed for cancer pain, it is widely used with this population (e.g., Atkinson et al. 2012).

Psychotherapy with persons with psychological issues affecting medical conditions

Developmental aging and psychological issues with illness

The increase in chronic illness and disability in later life is due in some measure to biological aging and the consequent changes in the body's wear and repair systems (Ricklefs and Finch 1995). Thus, some of the increase in illness and frailty is due to changes in the immune system over time (Efros 2009). Cancers become more common in later life with higher likelihood of the errors in cellular reproduction that lead to cancerous growths. The wear over time on non-renewing cells in heart and brain lead to other common late life disorders. There is ongoing debate in theories of biological aging as to whether these changes associated with age are developmental in the sense of being programmed to unfold as we age or whether they represent accumulated errors with the passage of time (Gonidakis and Longo 2009; Shringarpure and Davies 2009). Certainly, one reason that older adults tend to have more chronic illnesses than younger people is that there has been more time to accumulate them. They can start at any age, but by definition do not go away, and so increasing age makes it more likely that one has one or more. For ones that start earlier and are progressive, they will be further along in the course of the illness as time goes by and age increases.

However, the specific illnesses and functional disabilities acquired, and at what age they occur varies greatly among individuals. A key part of the CALTAP model is this focus on the *specificity* of the challenge and of the attribution of symptoms and dysfunction to disease, rather than the over-generalizations typically associated with attribution to age itself: the Shakespearean "sans teeth, sans eyes, sans taste, sans everything," which is depressogenic thinking, and unhelpful in finding coping strategies and adaptations to illness and functional losses.

In general, in clinical work, more is explained by understanding the illness than by relating it to the aging process. As we have seen in the chapters on depression (Chapter 3) and anxiety (Chapter 4), attributions of symptoms to aging is an important source of the kinds of cognitive distortions that lead to psychological distress in patients, and may underlie potential mismanagement of psychological reactions by inexperienced psychologists and other health professionals.

Communication with health professionals, and accurate understanding of diseases and their treatments can be affected by aging-related changes in sensation and cognition. Even in healthy aging, older adults tend to have reduced visual and auditory abilities, process information more slowly, have more difficulty learning new information, and have some decline in inferential reasoning. All of these factors will make understanding medical information about a disease and complex treatment regimens more difficult. The older the patient, the more influence these changes will have. Obviously, if the changes are further exacerbated by illness, the difficulty with communication will be even more significant. In therapy, showing understanding and empathy for these changes, helping the client understand their impact on communication with doctors and other health professionals, and helping the client problem solve ways to improve communication or find other ways to get the information, are all important skills to bring to this work. Depending on the specifics of the situation, clients should be encouraged to tell the health professionals what their communication issues are, and ask that they speak more loudly or more slowly, ask for printed information, or bring a trusted family member or friend into the consultation room. They may also choose to get some of their information from health organizations, self-help groups, or on-line sources, and may want to ask their physician or clinic staff for recommendations.

In contrast, as seen in Chapter 1, older adults also often bring strengths to coping with chronic illnesses. In general, older adults tend to have better developed coping strategies and rely less on ineffective coping such as avoidance strategies. Active coping strategies may be more easily implemented, particularly in the presence of good social support networks, and a greater sense of self-efficacy with respect to controlling or accepting symptoms or limitations may be achieved. Older adults tend to place a higher priority on emotion regulation and are better skilled at controlling negative emotional reactions to stressors. For many people, age brings with it experience with a variety of medical illnesses, both their own, and those of loved ones and acquaintances. By the time we reach old age, the illnesses of grandparents and parents have been part of our experience.

However, some individuals seem to miss this experiential learning. A common theme across the chapters of this book is the difference between late-onset and recurring problems. For adjustment to physical illness, having the first experience of medical illness later in life appears to make psychological distress more likely and more difficult to deal with (see Case Example 6.1). People who have seen themselves as healthy all of their lives can be quite shocked by the onset of serious illness in late life. This distress is often complicated by the attributions that they have made about their health up to this point. Having the concept that

> **Case Example 6.1 Late life first experience of physical illness**
> One 80-year-old male client was severely depressed after being diagnosed with a progressive lung condition, which would likely eventually lead to his death. He had not only been illness-free until this diagnosis about 5 years earlier, but had been very active, including mountain climbing and ocean swimming, as well as very active socially with former colleagues from his work life. He was severely depressed and refused to use oxygen as prescribed, even though it was quite clear that this refusal led to the weakness and dizziness that severely limited his ability to be active and increased his depression. In his view, using the oxygen simply confirmed how ill and disabled he was. He also had the viewpoint that he did not want to be better unless he could be as good as he had been before the onset of the disease, which was clearly not a realistic medical possibility.

"I am always healthy" as a part of one's self-concept increases the impact of the illness on emotional distress later in life. This impact is even greater if one's health is seen as being due to having been a good person or having had a bargain with God (e.g., "I've been a caregiver to several others and so God has kept me healthy;" or "I suffered a lot as a child and good health is my reward for that").

Social context influences on psychological issues and physical illness

A pervasive social context influence on health care for older adults is the role of ageism, often implicit in behavior, rather than in an explicit dislike of older adults (see Case Example 6.2). Older clients frequently complain of feeling invisible in interactions with health care providers, for example, a physician directing questions to a granddaughter, rather than directly to the client. One 90-year-old woman complained that she frequently has to tell health care providers not to

> **Case Example 6.2 Physician over-attributing symptoms to psychological factors**
> An African American woman in her 70s had multiple medical problems and severe anxiety. Her physician was part of a county health clinic in her neighborhood. Her scheduled appointments were fairly widely spaced and she frequently went to the emergency room of a nearby hospital with medical complications. As the psychological treatment progressed and her anxiety lessened, we became concerned that her medical care at the outpatient clinic was worsened by the physician's perception that most of her symptoms and ER visits were due to anxiety. We conveyed our perceptions (both by phone and in a follow-up letter) that we thought her anxiety had reduced markedly without a change in her symptoms, that the ER visits did not usually coincide with times when she was highly anxious, and that some symptoms (great difficulty in going upstairs to her bedroom) were not likely to be anxiety related.

yell at her, that not all older adults are hard of hearing. It is important that therapists working with older adults not make these same mistakes, and that they express empathy for the client's experience of ageism and be able to suggest appropriate ways for the client to respond to this type of treatment.

For older adults with medical problems, the increased time spent in physicians' offices and other parts of the health care system can greatly increase the salience of the relationship with the physician, and with nurses and other key health care personnel. The necessary dependence on their professional expertise can readily translate into emotional dependency and a greater sensitivity to perceived disapproval, impatience, and judgment. On the provider side, this is complicated by the pressure of time and other demands of their work, such that their global fatigue and stress can easily be misperceived as irritation and other personal reactions by the patient. Older patients with depression, anxiety, or high dependency needs can frustrate physicians who are often not as highly skilled at handling emotional demands from patients and do not have as much time to focus on relationship issues as do psychotherapists. A moderately common reason for referrals from physicians is their experience of the patient as being too emotionally demanding. A ready acceptance of the referral, with an acknowledgement that handling such issues is exactly what psychotherapists do, can help build the relationship with the physician and also clarify the therapist's contribution to the patient's care.

Older adults living in age-segregated environments are surrounded by other older adults with medical problems, and the continual and frequent experience of seeing other residents taken off to the hospital by ambulance, being transferred to higher levels of care, or dying. As noted in earlier chapters, this constant exposure to illness, disability, and death can easily make even relatively healthy older adults sad or anxious, but can also clearly exacerbate the concerns and the distress of anyone with psychological issues centered on their own physical illnesses. The therapist walks the fine line between acknowledging the reality that the situation is genuinely distressing (so as not to be seen as minimizing the client's feelings or their realistic grounding) and helping the client focus on the specific aspects of their own illness, treatment, and prognosis. In the CALTAP model, this focus on the specific challenges of the client's illness is an essential aspect of combating the tendency to over-generalize the course of aging, and so to perceive the worsening condition of neighbors as a sign that one's own decline and death are near.

Cohort effects on psychological distress and physical illness

From the early twentieth century up until cohorts born in the 1970s, successive cohorts have had higher educational levels. Earlier born patients are likely to have, on average, lower levels of formal education and probably less familiarity with medical and psychological terminology. These cohort effects will make learning about an illness and following complex medical treatment plans more difficult for many of these patients. Also, the expression of illness changes over time, as does the health professional's ability to recognize and respond to illness. For example, the specific risks and symptoms of cardiac illness unique to women are being recognized and more effectively treated (van Lennep et al. 2002).

Our knowledge about risk factors for illnesses and the consequences of health related behaviors is constantly changing. Earlier born cohorts can recall when smoking tobacco and drinking sodas were considered healthy. What kinds of foods are considered healthy changes from generation to generation. Whether one should exercise or rest when recovering from illness has changed over the years. One consequence of this is that older patients may feel somewhat guilty for having brought an illness on themselves, whether or not the risk they were taking was understood to be a risk in their young adult years. Another consequence of these changes is that older adults are often skeptical of current health advice, since they can recall when health professionals were giving the opposite advice. Older adults, contrary to popular myths, are also open to the use of complementary and alternative medicines, in part because alternative medical approaches have existed for decades, and are not as new as later born cohorts seem to think, although the earlier born may discuss these in different terms to later born cohorts (Poulsen et al. 2013).

It is common to encounter clients with COPD or heart disease whose depression is worsened by guilt over having done it to themselves by smoking. This perception is often strengthened by comments to that effect from health professionals and younger family members. Exploring how the client really feels about this can be helpful. This exploration can include checking whether the client believes it or is feeling badly about being accused by others, in which case, the true underlying emotion may be anger at others, rather than guilt. It can also include putting their smoking into its historical context, reviewing what they have thought over the years about smoking and its health consequences, and discussing the view that smoking is one risk factor, but not a single cause of the condition that they have. These discussions can also be an exercise for the therapist in putting aside one's own cohort-centered views on the subject and putting the client's emotional health ahead of what the therapist considers to be true.

The concept of patients as active participants in their health care is relatively new. Many older patients have embraced this idea, but others continue to see physicians as authority figures and are less likely to question them, to seek second opinions, or to research alternative explanations and treatments than are their children and grandchildren.

The therapist's response to this style of relating to physicians will depend in large part on how well the client's health care is going. If things are going well, there is no need to intervene. If the client is dissatisfied with treatment, or is confused about the diagnosis and treatment in ways that affect their health, working on ways to communicate clearly with physicians and the exploration of other ways to collect information can be helpful. For example, in many instances it may be easier to talk to the office nurse about questions they have or to contact a local health organization (e.g., heart association, cancer society, etc.) for their brochures and fact sheets. When the focus is on increased communication with the physician directly, anticipating and respecting the client's desire to show respect to the physician can be an important element of making the changes in their approach to asking questions acceptable to the client. The changes tend to be self-reinforcing once started, since increasing a sense of control over one's health care has a positive emotional impact.

The acceptance of psychological and stress-related influences on physical health is also relatively recent, although gaining ground rapidly among earlier born cohorts. Earlier born cohorts are more likely to think of this relationship in terms of psychogenic disorders that are "all in your head." In general, it is good strategy to anticipate this interpretation and explain to the client that psychological or stress-based influences make pain and other symptoms of real physical illnesses worse. In working with clients on pain control, it is wise to educate them on the role that psychological interventions play in pain control in traumatic injuries, cancers, and other clearly physically caused pain. It is also helpful to focus on the physical explanation for the client's pain, and to return to these themes often.

Earlier born cohorts are also more likely to have the belief that the best way to handle physical illness is to ignore the symptoms and continue to be more active than the physical limitations permit (see Case Example 6.3).

Case Example 6.3 Denial of illness and being overly active

One male client in his 70s had COPD and was supposed to be on oxygen 24 hours a day. He used the oxygen less often than directed, but also pushed himself to continue to mow the lawn, do other yard work, paint the house, and over-exerted himself in ways that often led to being debilitated for several days and, at times, to additional visits to the doctor. His wife supported this exertion and, at times, put pressure on him to do things around the house, partly out of this shared cohort belief in the way to handle illness and partly out of denial of his illness.

Cultural influences on psychological factors influencing health in the older client

The most salient cultural issue with regard to the influence of psychological factors on physical health is the strong belief in mind–body dualism that seems to be prevalent among many non-Hispanic Whites. This belief tends to result in a skepticism concerning the role of psychological intervention in helping with physical symptoms and requires therapeutic discussion and explanation of the underlying rationale before treatment can begin (see Case Example 6.4). As noted in the section on "Cohort effects on psychological distress and physical illness," this belief seems less strong in more recently born cohorts of this group, but is still often an influence. In contrast, African American and Hispanic older clients who come to psychotherapy seem to have much less trouble with the interdependent influences of emotional stress and physical illness. In Australia, the traditional Aboriginal model for the causes of illness stresses the importance of social and spiritual dysfunction; these then also provide roadmaps to wellness (Maher 1999).

> **Case Example 6.4 Cultural issues in coping with illness**
>
> In an Afro-Caribbean family with two older parents with dementia, two of the sons were also struggling with medical problems. It seemed clear to the therapists involved (three in the USC training clinic—working with the caregiver (the daughter), the family system, and working on psychological assessments of the parents and the older of the two brothers) that the causes of the problems had not been definitively diagnosed. The reasons for this were a combination of: (a) access issues (no insurance, uncertain and rather low income levels); (b) cultural issues that resulted in distrust of government services. The distrust was rooted in the country of origin, but confirmed by experiences in the USA; (c) a culturally influenced reluctance to explicitly recognize, even within the family, that the older brother was not fully intellectually competent. From our psychological assessment and with the limited history we could gather given this reluctance, we concluded that he either was developmentally disabled, or perhaps had experienced a brain injury in late adolescence or early adulthood.

A salient issue with minority clients will be their experience of racism within the health care network and of other barriers to obtaining quality care, especially for those with lower incomes. While racism still exists in health care, for earlier born cohorts, the expectation and the experience of it tends to be more salient, since the current cohorts of older adults can remember times when legal discrimination was practiced and when overt expression of racism was more commonly accepted socially. Being aware of and acknowledging these realities with clients is important to building a rapport and to reaching an accurate understanding of what the client faces in interactions with health care providers. Moving too quickly to trying to modify thoughts about racism is likely to communicate that the therapist does not understand the client's social reality. It is also important to remember that clients may take some time to build up the trust in the therapist necessary for them to begin to share their social reality, particularly if the therapist is from a different culture to the client.

Issues in psychotherapy with older adults for psychological issues related to physical conditions

In general, experience teaching and consulting with therapists working with older adults suggests that many of the difficult issues in working on psychological issues affecting physical conditions and their treatment, are more on the therapist's side of the room than the client's. Many psychotherapists have little knowledge regarding medical illnesses, and are uncomfortable with discussing physical symptoms and their treatment with patients. Some therapists see a focus on physical problems as avoidance of more important psychological topics. Some are prone to interpreting all physical symptoms in purely psychological terms. Others simply find the topic depressing or overwhelming, and prefer to avoid it. This work can also bring up topics that touch on therapists' own experiences with older parents or family members (e.g., a father who died early of a stroke, a mother who suffered severe dementia for many years). In these circumstances the transference issues need to be recognized.

With an appropriate knowledge base and therapy skills, this work can be exciting and professionally challenging. It is useful to have a good knowledge base concerning the most common types of illnesses that older adults face. The level of knowledge needed by psychotherapists is far less than that needed by physicians, and can be acquired from materials distributed by non-profit health organizations and/or reading the consumer-oriented information brochures put out by government health institutes. National guidelines developed specifically for that country's people, based on epidemiological data, may also be useful. Some working knowledge of common cancers of later life, heart diseases, stroke, diabetes, COPD, and arthritis is a good basis to start. More information about less common disorders can be acquired as clients with those diagnoses appear in one's practice. Building relationships with health associations may be useful for the clinician, through giving informational sessions about the relationship of psychological factors to the illness and, in turn, having access to information from these groups to pass on to clients.

It is of crucial importance to have a clear sense of the psychotherapist's role in working with the psychological issues affecting physical conditions. The role can vary depending on the organizational context in which the therapist works, but the psychotherapist should never veer into practicing medicine or directly intervening in the medical treatment. While this can seem obvious, clients do ask questions about whether they should continue taking certain medications, whether they should pursue a treatment option, etc. Sooner or later, every therapist is faced with situations in which these questions arise and where they do have a strong opinion about what the client should do. The therapist is on firmer ground, however, in helping the client to clarify what they want to do. At times, information on the client's psychological condition or on the range of treatments being pursued may be useful to pass on to the treating physician, with the client's consent, of course.

One general model for thinking about the psychotherapist's role and the likely impact of psychological intervention is to think of the psychological issues as adding excess disability to the level of functioning that is dictated by the medical condition itself. Thus, the client with heart disease and depression can reach a higher level of functioning and a lower level of global distress through psychological intervention for the depression. Acknowledging the reality of the heart disease and the real limitation it places on the client is an important theme for such interventions. The goal of therapy is not likely to be a return to the levels of life satisfaction prior to the onset of the heart disease, but rather an improvement in the mood currently experienced.

Another model for the psychotherapist's role is the removal of the psychological disorder as a barrier to the client's adherence to treatment of the medical condition or the development of a fairly satisfying post-morbidity lifestyle. It is not uncommon for clients experiencing the hopelessness and helplessness associated with depression to decide not to follow through with medical treatment, to fail to take medications as prescribed, or to take the position that if they cannot pursue the demanding activities that they used to pursue, they do not wish to do anything. Helping the client label these thoughts as "the depression talking," spending some time on the emotional work of grieving for lost health and lost activities, and helping the client decide what activities she wants to pursue now are key steps to improving adherence by alleviating depression.

The need to communicate with and coordinate care with physicians does not seem to come naturally to psychotherapists (see Case Example 6.5). Therapists without training in interdisciplinary teamwork or other background for learning how to communicate effectively with physicians may find contacting physicians intimidating and often unproductive. Psychologically oriented professionals in general are used to providing a lot of background information, entertaining hypotheses, and tolerating fairly high levels of ambiguity. Physicians tend to be pressed for time and to prefer concise, definite statements about what is wrong, and a clear recommendation about what needs to be done and who needs to do it. Adapting one's style to the physician's need for brevity and clarity is very helpful to cross-discipline communication. It is also of critical importance not to

> **Case Example 6.5 Coordination of care with physician**
>
> One client in her 80s was being cared for at home by her son, who was also disabled from an accident. In discussing the things in her life that prompted her depressed mood, she put having to depend on her son to change her adult diapers after urinary incontinence high on the list. The therapist asked what her physician had told her about the incontinence, expecting to clarify the cause and prognosis, whether she could expect an end to this stressor or not. The client stated that she had never told the physician. With the client's permission, the therapist called the doctor who, in fact, was completely unaware of the problem, and scheduled diagnostic testing and an office visit. This led to the treatment of a urinary tract infection and some improvement in the incontinence.

appear to be practicing medicine or otherwise crossing into the physician's territory of responsibility for the patient.

It can lower the therapist's anxiety to be aware that physicians are similarly defensive of their territory with other physicians (e.g., primary care versus specialists), and not only with psychotherapists and other non-physician helpers. In NP's nursing home experiences, clinical practice physician colleagues speak of territoriality with respect to patient care, such that advice or suggestions offered by, for example, the geriatrician, are ignored by the primary care physician.

Psychotherapists may also have information and a perspective to contribute to the ongoing assessment of the client's health. While some physicians are prone to discount the importance of psychological factors as an influence on their patient's health, it is also fairly common to find that symptoms without a clear-cut medical diagnosis can be attributed to psychological disorders or to global stress. This may be true, but psychotherapists may also find that a client's symptoms do not fit standard presentations of depression or anxiety; feeding this information tactfully back to the treating physician can initiate further diagnostic work that may lead to a medical diagnosis for the symptoms (see Case Example 6.6).

> **Case Example 6.6 Diagnosing absence of psychological disorder**
>
> A male client in his 70s was referred for psychotherapy by his physician because his symptoms were somewhat non-specific, he had a depressed facial expression, and had become somewhat socially isolated. The therapist's intake assessment failed to find any typical symptoms of depression and, after a few sessions, the therapist was convinced that the client's mood had not really changed in the past couple of years. With the client's permission, the therapist called the physician, with whom he had a good working relationship with several shared patients, and explained why he did not think the client actually was depressed. He expressed concern about potential physical causes for the changes noted by the doctor. The doctor was somewhat annoyed at getting this news, but pursued additional assessment and specialist consultation, and the patient was diagnosed with Parkinson's disease.

More commonly, clients may share side effects of medications or the therapist may note changes in emotionality or behavior subsequent to a change in medication. In general, the first strategy is likely to be encouraging the client to make this known to the treating physician, but some clients may be too cognitively frail, too anxious, or too passive to do so, and the therapist may need to pass the information to the physician, with the client's consent, of course.

In working with the client around issues of adherence to medical treatment, a common issue for older adults is that they receive a lot of advice about what they should do. This advice, even when well-intentioned and presented kindly, taken with the effects of the illness itself can feel like loss of control. Frequently reminding clients that the decisions are up to them, and that they can certainly choose not to take the medication, not to have the surgery, and so forth, is a key element of restoring the client's sense of control. Exploring the pros and cons of pursuing or not pursuing treatment in a pressure-free setting is helpful both in making the decision, and in becoming clearer about one's own feelings and reactions to the options.

Physicians, nurses, and other health care providers rarely have the time or the training to do this, and generally have a strong conviction that their patients should pursue active treatment and want to get better. The psychotherapist has more time, more tolerance for ambivalence, and more commitment to helping clients reach their own decision. Most clients end up choosing adherence to medical treatment, although some find compelling reasons not to continue the treatment. From time to time, clients choose not to have a recommended surgery and then cancel their next appointment because they're in the hospital having the surgery. The complexity of these decisions and the ambivalence that people can feel when confronted with them is often underestimated by health care professionals and by the client's family.

Summary

In thinking about working with older adults with chronic illness, it is clear that many parts of both the assessment and treatment may be impacted by the presence of the condition, and so psychologists need to be mindful of these influences, which may be subtle. There is a need, given the increasing proportion of older clients seen in practice who are both of an advanced age and have multiple medical comorbidities, for research on assessment tools and treatment protocols to be developed that take account of such clients. We will need more of an empirical evidence base if we are to offer the most efficacious interventions for these clients.

In Chapter 7, we move on to discuss substance abuse. Substance abuse is an often unrecognized problem facing older adults, unrecognized in part because professionals do not think to ask the questions that would lead to its recognition. Like working with physical symptoms, substance abuse requires thinking about physical and mental health symptoms together, and often involves a multidisciplinary perspective and interprofessional collaboration.

Chapter 7

Substance misuse and abuse

Introduction to substance misuse and abuse

Substance abuse problems have tended to be overlooked in discussions of mental health and aging until fairly recently. There is to some extent a cultural tendency to underestimate the seriousness of alcohol abuse in later life, perhaps seeing it as a natural antidote to the presumed normative distress of growing old. Alternatively, perhaps it is seen as the "right" of an older person to enjoy what may appear a harmless drink or two. Yet now, we are seeing a rise in physical and psychological problems associated with alcohol use in older adults as this segment of the population increases (Agency for Healthcare Research and Quality 2010). The numbers of older persons engaged in heavy drinking in community surveys ranges from 6% to 16% (Menninger 2002). Similarly, as the Baby Boomer cohort ages, clinicians will be confronted with older patients who have higher rates of alcohol abuse and a wide experience with a variety of substances (Satre 2013; Wu and Blazer 2011), including so-called designer drugs, whose long-term effects are still being researched (Gunderson et al. 2012).

Dependence and abuse of over the counter (OTC) and prescription medications occurs in older adults and clinicians need to be aware of issues pertaining to the context of such use/abuse. Historically in gerontology, there was a tendency to assume that all over-medication of older adults was the fault of the physician, rather than intentional abuse by the older patient. Obviously, both of these can happen, but the immediate point is that there are older adults who doctor-shop and pharmacy-hop in order to get large amounts of psychoactive medications. As with all psychological disorders, substance abuse in later life can occur either because substance abusers get old or because some older adults develop substance abuse problems for the first time late in life.

There is also the case of unintentional misuse, when older clients misuse prescription medication through misunderstanding dosages and timings, inappropriately combining medications, or forgetting how much they have taken due to memory decline (Simoni-Wastila and Yang 2006). In these cases, there may be feelings of guilt on the part of the older person to realize that they themselves caused medication misuse. There is also the possibility that the older person is trying to maintain independence in the case of failing faculties, and has resisted assistance with medications because of a feeling (perhaps correct) that admitting difficulties in this realm might lead to institutionalization.

Substance abuse poses challenges for the clinician with respect to assessment, diagnosis, and treatment approaches. Factors associated with substance use and abuse vary widely with particular substances, but broadly speaking include male gender, social isolation, chronic physical illness and multiple comorbidities, a history of a psychiatric disorder or substance abuse, and medical exposure to prescription drugs with potential for abuse (Menninger 2002; Simoni-Wastila and Yang 2006). However, interestingly, although older men are more likely to drink to excess, older women are more likely than men to start drinking heavily in later life (Menninger 2002). In the case of social isolation as a potential risk factor worthy of investigation, it may be difficult for the clinician to obtain information if the patient is unable to give an accurate history. Life events such as retirement, major illness, and bereavement may trigger substance misuse. Chronic physical illness and multiple comorbidities often result in multiple medications, sometimes prescribed by different health care providers. Polypharmacy may lead to or exacerbate substance abuse issues, in part due to side effects of the medications. Older adults may also share medications among themselves, and may take OTC medications that their regular physicians know nothing about. All of these issues may lead to misuse and abuse of substances, as well as complicate treatment for these issues.

Generally speaking, substance abuse in later life is under-recognized, under-assessed, and under-treated (Barry and Blow 2010). Barriers to the recognition of substance abuse in later life include the low level of clinician alertness to this problem among older adults, with clinicians especially likely to overlook substance abuse in women, and in those with a higher level of education or income (Moore et al. 1989). Age-biases exist in the diagnostic criteria for substance dependence and abuse, as for many other disorders, and this can also be a barrier for correct diagnosis of older adults (Barry and Blow 2014). Some of the key diagnostic criteria, such as the development of tolerance for substances, getting in trouble with law enforcement, or problems relating to work or social interactions are less likely to be endorsed by older people (Blow and Barry 2012).

Up to this point in time, alcohol misuse and abuse have been relatively more common than abuse of other substances in later life (Blow and Barry 2012). As the Baby Boomer cohort ages, attitudes to substance use, as well as the types of substances used will change from earlier cohorts, and this presents an evolving landscape for the clinician, which may hinder recognition of substance abuse issues, especially if older adults are seen relatively rarely in the practice.

Increased alcohol intake has been linked to increased risk of dementia, depression, hypertension, and insomnia in older populations (Blow et al. 2000;

Chermack et al. 1996; Saunders et al. 1991). Often in older adults, it is difficult to ascertain whether depression is a cause or consequence of excessive drinking. Alcohol intake has been shown to negatively affect general health and physical functioning in older adults, as well as to increase risk of suicide (Blow et al. 2000; Blow et al. 2004). However, as the Baby Boomer generation ages, clinicians may see a wider spectrum of substances misused and abused among their older clients.

Prescription medication use is high among older adults, and one of the most common classes of medications prescribed in this population are sedative-hypnotics such as benzodiazepines (Llorente et al. 2000). These drugs are prescribed at a much higher rate in older adults than in younger adults (Colenda et al. 2002). In addition to the risk of falls and the adverse sequelae of falls (Neutel et al. 2002; Ray et al. 2000), benzodiazepines as prescribed for older adults are prone to misuse, particularly in individuals with insomnia and those in residential aged care. The use of sedative-hypnotics in residential aged care settings is high and often does not follow best practice guidelines with respect to contraindications and polypharmacy (Blogg, Suzuki, Roberts, and Clifford 2012). Benzodiazepines are often prescribed for continuous use when they may not be required, or when intermittent use might be more effective (Llorente et al. 2000).

Assessment in substance use cases

The initial clinical interview is of great importance in the assessment of substance use, as establishing rapport early on is critical to gaining insight about substance use; thus, gauging when and how to approach the topic should be done in a thoughtful manner. Asking about alcohol use in the context of general health behaviors (exercise, smoking) is one way to approach the issue (Blow and Barry 2012). If such an approach is used consistently as part of a general interview strategy, not only will the clinician not feel awkward, but all patients will be systematically screened for substance abuse, which is recommended for adults over age 60 (Center for Substance Abuse Treatment 1998).

It is important to note that many older adults may have difficulties related to substance dependence or abuse without meeting any formal diagnostic criteria. Thus, it is important to discuss patterns and levels of substance abuse in the interview, and attempt to gauge how these patterns fit into the current and historical contexts of use for that individual. How the older adult sees their use of substances is important, but gaining this perspective, again, depends on trust and rapport. The clinician should be alert to the fact that older adults with alcohol problems may initially present with relatively non-specific symptoms, such as falls, self-neglect, incontinence, and malnutrition (Black 1990). Clinicians who do not see older patients regularly may believe, incorrectly, that such symptoms are usual in later life and fail to explore them with the client.

There are several important behaviors to be explored in assessing substance use. These include excessive use of the substance beyond reasonable limits, experiencing periods of amnesia while drinking, and the inability of the older adult to curtail or stop using the substance. Physical cues to excess alcohol use may include anemia, abnormalities in liver chemistry laboratory results, and new seizure activity. Cognitive and behavioral cues include decreased cognitive functioning, and frequent falls or fractures (Menninger 2002).

When enquiring about alcohol consumption, the clinician may need to explain what a standard drink is, so that both parties are on the same page with respect to amounts and usage. It is worth noting that what a standard drink constitutes varies internationally, as does what is considered "normal" amounts to drink for individuals of specific genders and ages, what places and times of day are appropriate for alcohol consumption, and what the society as a whole views as appropriate use of alcohol. This is a particularly important consideration for individuals from different cultural and religious backgrounds who have immigrated into a society whose customs and expectations may be very different to their own.

In our experience, it is fairly common for clients to report drink quantities based on how much they pour into the glass, with "one drink" perhaps being the equivalent in ounces of three to five standard drinks. It is also important to note that the myth of persons with substance misuse or abuse being unable or unwilling to accurately report how much they are drinking is not supported by research (Barry 1997). The impact of the use of the substance on the person's physical, cognitive, emotional, and behavioral functioning, including risk-taking behavior, such as driving while intoxicated or mixing alcohol with prescription medications, are important to consider. The impact on nutrition (either in missed meals or lowered thiamine levels) should also be considered. Finally, the effect of use of the substance on interpersonal relationships, work or similar obligations, and finances, should be explored.

Barriers to assessment and screening include lack of information and pessimism on the part of health care providers about substance abuse treatment programs and the response of older adults to interventions (Menninger 2002). Both family and health professionals may prefer to explain away the behavior (e.g., "Mom is just drinking until she gets over Dad's death") or to assume it will resolve on its own. Finally, other aspects of the person's functioning, whether or not these may be related to the substance abuse in fact, may take precedence as a subject of intervention (e.g., instigation of memory testing, medical work-up for puzzling physical symptoms, restriction of activity levels in the face of frequent falls).

In older adults for whom substance abuse is an issue, getting a history of substance use and abuse over the lifespan is important background information for the therapy. This might also include a family history of substance use, if relevant. Table 7.1 offers the clinician a summary of relevant variables associated with early as opposed to late onset of problem drinking.

Table 7.1 Clinical characteristics of early and late onset problem drinkers.

Variable	Early Onset	Late Onset
Age at onset	Various, e.g., < 25, 40, 45	Various, e.g., > 55, 60, 65
Gender	Higher proportion of men than women	Higher proportion of women than men
Socioeconomic status	Tends to be lower	Tends to be higher
Drinking in response to stressors	Common	Common
Family history of alcoholism	More prevalent	Less prevalent
Extent and severity of alcohol problems	More psychosocial, legal problems, greater severity	Fewer psychosocial, legal problems, lesser severity
Alcohol-related chronic illness (e.g., cirrhosis, pancreatitis, cancers)	More common	Less common
Psychiatric comorbidities	Cognitive loss more severe, less reversible	Cognitive loss less severe, more reversible
Age-associated medical problems aggravated by alcohol (e.g., hypertension, diabetes mellitus, drug–alcohol interactions)	Common	Common
Treatment compliance and outcome	Possibly less compliant; Relapse rates do not vary by age of onset (Atkinson et al., 1990; Blow et al., 1997; Schonfeld and Dupree, 1991)	Possibly more compliant; Relapse rates do not vary by age of onset (Atkinson et al., 1990; Blow et al., 1997; Schonfeld and Dupree, 1991)

Reproduced from Center for Substance Abuse Treatment. Substance Abuse Among Older Adults. Treatment Improvement Protocol (TIP) Series, No. 26 (HHS Publication No. (SMA) 12-3918), p.21 © 1998, Substance Abuse and Mental Health Services Administration.

Comorbidities of note in the assessment of substance use disorders

Delirium is a reversible syndrome characterized by impaired mental status and caused by an underlying medical condition such as an infection, which can be reversed with medical treatment. It is important to note that any number of medical situations may cause delirium; infection is certainly one of the most common, but if an infection screen to detect the possible presence of a urinary tract infection comes up negative, for example, this is not in itself a reason to state that delirium is not present. If the symptoms of delirium are present, the potential probable causes in that individual (e.g., polypharmacy, metabolic disorder) should continue to be explored.

As mentioned, delirium has a range of causes, but benzodiazepine use prior to hospitalization has been shown to be a significant risk factor among hospitalized patients for the development of delirium. Given that benzodiazepine use is common in older adults (Blow and Barry 2012), noting the possibility of delirium in cases of use of this drug is important. With respect to assessment, the Confusion Assessment Method (CAM; Inouye et al. 1990) is a brief and reliable screening tool in such cases (see Chapter 5 for more information about the CAM and its use).

Depression and anxiety may act both as triggers for substance abuse, or be consequences of their use or cessation. Satre et al. (2011) noted that among older patients seeking treatment for depression, alcohol use in the prior month was reported by half the sample and cannabis use by 12% of the men. Misuse of sedatives in this study was reported by 12% of men and 9% of women. The assessment tools discussed in the relevant chapters in this text (e.g., the Geriatric Depression Scale, see Chapter 3), are therefore relevant for use with older adults in this context. Of particular note is the possibility of suicidal behavior with depression in those with comorbid past or current substance abuse. For example, risk of suicidal behaviors is elevated in older adults with alcohol use problems (Conwell 1991).

Clinical experience suggests that bipolar disorder and substance abuse are often comorbid, although it can also be unclear as to whether the apparent mood swings are primarily caused by the substance abuse. One older woman in her 70s, with a long history of bipolar disorder and possibly other serious mental illness, as well as a known early history of drug abuse, was discovered rather late in therapy (with BK) to be drinking quite heavily (see the Mildred case in Knight 1992, pp. 158). The assessment of substance use disorders is an important aspect of the overall assessment process. When mood swings not connected to stressors are common, substance abuse should be carefully considered (see also Chapter 9, "Bipolar Disorder and Psychosis").

Finally, pain and sleep disorders have been linked with alcohol and substance abuse in later life (Blow and Barry 2012; Barry and Blow 2014). Simoni-Wastila and Yang (2006) reported that 25% of older adults use prescription psychoactive medications that have the potential to be abused. Older adults often respond to disturbed sleep with an attempt to self-medicate, commonly with alcohol (Blow and Barry 2012). Medications for pain or sleep are one category of frequently misused medications and again are fairly commonly prescribed in later life. The long-term prescribing of these medications for chronic pain or insomnia may be the occasion for development of abuse or dependence. Physicians may also be unaware of changes in pharmacodynamics with age and may prescribe a higher than needed dose of sleeping medication, which can lead to dependence or addiction in an older adult.

Pain and insomnia symptoms can also be used (intentionally or otherwise) to obtain medications for over-use. Alcohol use contributes to insomnia and we know that addictive substances can reinforce pain behavior. Thus, the interrelationships are very complex and require careful exploration. On the plus side, interventions for psychological management of pain, including pain stemming from medical issues or chronic conditions, are effective with older adults (see Barlow et al. 2002; Keefe et al. 2005, for an overview).

Medications for pain and sleep may also be negatively affected by the consumption of alcohol. Use of self-reported pain or sleep screening instruments as appropriate may assist determining the impact of either or both on current substance use (please refer to Chapter 8 for more information on pain in the context of sleep disorders).

Clinical interview and screening

As mentioned at the beginning of "Assessment in substance use cases," the accuracy of data gathered with respect to substance abuse depends upon the relationship of the clinician to the patient. With increasing age, it may be that barriers are introduced that may hinder the clinical interview or weaken rapport. If the clinician is uncomfortable discussing substance abuse, feels that it is not a problem in older cohorts, or adopts a judgmental stance, the clinical interview is unlikely to proceed well. Similarly, if the older adult feels judged, misunderstands the nature and intent of questions, or believes that there may be adverse ramifications to answers about substance abuse (e.g., that they may be placed in a nursing home, or may have their ability to drive curtailed) then positive outcomes from the interview will be limited.

Diagnostic interview tools may be useful in ascertaining whether the criteria for substance dependence or abuse are met or not. The Structured Clinical Interview for DSM Disorders (First et al. 1996b) and the MINI (Lecrubier et al. 1997) may both be of use here, providing a more structured approach to a standard clinical interview. However, gathering pertinent background information in combination with a screening tool may be a better option for the clinician in practice. This is in part due to the often sensitive nature of enquiring about substance use, and potential misuse and abuse.

The Substance Abuse and Mental Health Services Administration (SAMHSA) publishes a Treatment Improvement Protocol (TIP) Series; one volume in the series deals with substance abuse among older adults (Blow 1998) and offers expert consensus guidelines on this topic. In this publication, the consensus is that every 60-year-old be screened for alcohol and prescription drug abuse as part of their regular visit to the family physician. This panel also recommends a line of questioning that is non-threatening and designed not to disrupt rapport. The advice provided to medical practitioners is to consider asking questions about whether medical conditions or medication side effects may be linked with substance abuse and also to avoid judgmental terms during the interview. Similarly, psychologists can link questions within their standard interview with use of substances, and be alert in the course of the interview for non-verbal cues from the patient signaling potential substance abuse (e.g., minimizing drinking behaviors, fidgeting at mention of substance use). When appropriate rapport has been established, it is useful to inquire about the size of drinks, as well as the number consumed. In several instances, we have found that "one or two drinks of an evening" refers to 8 oz glasses, not standard shots.

The TIP series on substance abuse from the Center for Substance Abuse Treatment (1998) suggests a number of useful approaches to screening for substance dependence and abuse in older adults. The guidelines emphasize that the clinician should not adopt a judgmental stance, and that questioning may be more or less direct, but should avoid the use of euphemisms, as these may simply serve to minimize the issues and may even encourage evasiveness on the part of the patient. The purpose of questions relating to substance use should be clearly related to the person's health or mental health concerns, as this serves as the context for the questions, rather than an abstract or potentially value-laden judgment on behaviors. Finally, both the interview questions, as well as any assessment tools, should be straightforward and easy to understand. In some cases (e.g., if the person is cognitively impaired and cannot self-report accurately) an informant may need to be sought. However, in using a family member or other informant, it is important to keep in mind that past substance abuse may have affected the relationship between the informant and the patient, such that the informant's report may be biased or describing past incidents.

Specific screening tools for use in older adults

There are several screening instruments that have been developed or adapted for use with older adults; alcohol screens will be discussed first. The CAGE questionnaire (Ewing 1984) is perhaps the best known of these. Very brief (four items), its simple yes–no self-report format and simply worded items make it appropriate even for those with relatively low literacy levels or mild cognitive impairment. A total score of 2 or more is considered clinically significant. However, it has been suggested that a single positively endorsed item may be enough to signal clinical significance in older adults (Conigliaro et al. 2000); subsequent research on use of the single item as a threshold found a sensitivity and specificity of 86% and 78%, respectively, in an outpatient medical setting (Buchsbaum et al. 1992). In a systematic review of the literature, Fiellin et al. (2000) found sensitivity for the CAGE questions ranging from 43% to 94% and specificity between 70% and 97% across studies and populations in a primary care setting. However, for the single study reviewed of those over age 60 in this setting, the figures reported were 14% sensitivity and 97% specificity. The CAGE then may not be the ideal screener, but is possibly better at confirming than identifying presence of alcohol abuse in older adults.

It is important to note that the CAGE measures lifetime drinking issues, rather than current concerns. In addition, and supportive of the sensitivity data presented above, there has been research suggesting that the CAGE is better suited to identifying more serious drinking problems, but somewhat less effective as a screen for women with drinking problems (Blow 1998).

The Michigan Alcoholism Screening Test—Geriatric Version (MAST-G; Blow et al. 1992) is a widely used alcohol screen with older cohorts. Considerably longer than the CAGE, the MAST-G has 24 items with a yes–no response format. The instrument has sound psychometric properties and like the CAGE has been translated into a number of languages. The MAST-G has been shown to be effective as a screen in both inpatient and outpatient contexts, including residential care facilities (Blow 1998); reported sensitivity and specificity for the MAST-G is 70% and 81%, respectively (Morton et al. 1996). A short version of the scale, the SMAST-G, has 10 items, and has been shown to have good sensitivity and specificity, and good acceptance by older populations (Blow et al. 1992).

A final alcohol screening tool in wide use is the Alcohol Use Disorders Identification Test (AUDIT; Babor et al. 2001. Developed by the WHO (manual available on the web at <http://whqlibdoc.who.int/hq/2001/who_msd_msb_01.6a.pdf>), the AUDIT is widely used in clinical research and is well-validated. It has particular psychometric strengths with culturally diverse groups (Frank et al. 2008) and is also brief (10 items), asking about drinking habits that are rated on a scale of frequency (e.g., how many times a week a person has needed a drink in the morning). However, data on its clinical use with older adult populations are lacking relative to the instruments discussed previously. In one study with a population older than 65 years, the AUDIT had a sensitivity of 33% and a specificity of 91% (Morton et al. 1996). It is also a more visually complex instrument, with a more complex response set, making it less well-suited to those with cognitive impairment. Of all the tools discussed, it looks the most like a detailed inventory of drinking habits, and may be more likely to provoke resistance or anxiety in clinical settings. A short version of the AUDIT (AUDIT-C) has been shown to have reasonable psychometric properties (Reinert and Allen 2002).

In general, there has been more research in older populations on the assessment and intervention of alcohol-related substance dependence and abuse than with other illicit substances or prescription medications. Drew et al. (2010) suggest a number of behaviors that may alert clinicians to potential substance misuse in their older clients, including:

- excessive worry about whether the medications are working;
- strong attachment to a particular psychoactive medication;
- resisting cessation or decreased doses of a prescribed psychoactive drug;
- excessive anxiety about the supply and timing of medications;
- decline in hygiene or grooming;
- sleeping during the daytime;
- medical symptoms, such as fatigue, weight loss, or insomnia;
- psychiatric symptoms, such as irritability, memory problems, or depression.

The last two items on the above list point out the differential diagnostic conundrums that may arise in the face of undetected substance misuse or abuse, particularly stemming from prescription or illicit substance use.

The US National Institute of Drug Abuse (NIDA) has developed a tool for measuring illicit drug abuse, known as ASSIST. It can be used to detect problems with alcohol, tobacco, prescription drug misuse, and use of illicit substances. The NIDA suite of substance use screeners includes a four-item quick screener, and then the longer ASSIST, which goes through lists of specific drugs in terms of frequency of use in the last 3 months as well as lifetime use. It gives a level of risk associated with substance use, and is relatively easy to score and interpret. ASSIST has been used with older adults with good results (Schonfeld et al. 2010).

Positive screening results should be followed-up with either a semi-structured or structured interview to confirm diagnosis, as well as discuss the implications of positive findings on the screening instruments. Again, sensitivity and an emphasis on the fact that substance use problems can respond well to treatment should be emphasized. Gauging willingness to address the problem is also important. Knowledge of community resources that can support and respond well to the needs of this cohort in managing substance abuse is important information to pass onto clients (see Case Example 7.1).

Case Example 7.1 Emily: assessment of substance abuse

Emily, age 77 years, was referred by her GP to a clinical psychologist for evaluation of potential dependence/abuse of alcohol. She had come to him for her annual check-up, but as her previous GP had retired, this patient was new to this physician. On this visit, a number of screening questions were administered as standard practice for new patients; one of these was a brief alcohol screen. The GP was struck by Emily's evasion and defensiveness around these questions. He noted that she had lost her husband a few years before and had refused pharmacological help, as well as counseling at that point, despite experiencing profound depression for over a year after his death. Her family had been concerned enough to contact the former GP (a friend of the family), but when pressed, Emily continued to deny any need for help, and eventually the problem appeared to pass. The physician spent a long time discussing Emily's health, impressing on her that he wanted to try to keep her active and healthy. He explained that he was worried about her being a candidate for developing congestive heart failure in the future, and was convinced that changes in certain lifestyle choices could keep her independent. As she treasured her independence, she reluctantly agreed to see the psychologist.

The therapist started the consultation by taking a detailed history and working hard to establish a rapport. Emily appeared to enjoy filling the psychologist in on her many ailments, major and minor, and her daily activities, which seemed to involve many mishaps and misadventures. However, Emily was often circuitous in her speech, and it seemed that these mishaps were more often the result of confusion or misunderstanding on her part. She became very tearful when talking about her husband who had passed away.

When asked about coping strategies she let down her guard and told of just sitting in her living room in the evening, with the TV on and a drink, until she fell asleep there, which appeared to be a daily habit. The therapist asked questions about her bad back with respect to this behavior, then moved the conversation carefully to the issue of the drinking at night. Emily stated she often had several drinks, but did not count them; "I just have a decanter in the refrigerator."

Given Emily's age and the fact that her GP had recently administered the CAGE test, which Emily refused to entirely complete, the psychologist administered the short version of MAST-G, SMAST-G. The psychologist was able to get Emily to complete this inventory, and also to agree to come back for a second session. SMAST-G was administered at the end of the interview. The only other measures completed were an MMSE and GDS (15-item version) completed together with the intake questionnaire at the very beginning of the session. Emily's MMSE was 27 out of 30; she missed the date, and two out of three of the recall questions. On the GDS she scored 8/15, and complained that many of the items were "just what you'd expect at my age." She did not endorse any items regarding suicide, and a few follow-up questions ascertained that this was not an area of current concern. Emily scored 4/10 on the SMAST-G, endorsing the items relating to skipping a meal after drinking, drinking to relax or calm her nerves, drinking when feeling lonely, and increased drinking after a loss.

This item, about increasing alcohol intake after a loss, was the item that caused her to become emotional. "I did start drinking more once Sam died—we always liked our parties and it has been such a struggle without him . . ." The therapist was able to frame the situation of increasing drinking after a loss as one that many people found themselves in, but that decreasing alcohol intake was also possible, with help. "I have tried to cut back but then I just feel so lonely in the evenings." Emily confined her drinking almost exclusively to her home, and drank primarily in the evenings, again a common pattern for older persons with alcohol abuse. Emily agreed to see the therapist over several sessions "for the sake of my health—Sam would not want to see me letting my health go downhill."

Psychotherapy with older adult substance abusers

Psychological treatments, in particular relatively brief targeted interventions, have been efficacious in addressing substance use issues in older populations (Whitlock et al. 2004). Group interventions for substance abuse in older adults have also been developed, many with good results (e.g., Center for Substance Abuse Treatment 2005). Involvement of partners, family, and caregivers, as appropriate, may assist with achieving good results with older alcohol and substance users (e.g., Simoni-Wastila and Yang 2006). Older adults have been found to do better in treatment than younger adults (Satre et al. 2012). Barriers to reaching a greater proportion of older adults with substance use issues include the stigma of seeking treatment for such disorders, a lack of mental health providers trained to deliver such interventions to older adults, and reimbursement issues (Blow and Barry 2012).

The treatment of the medical side of substance abuse disorders requires age-appropriate interventions as well, just as the psychological side of treatment. For example, benzodiazepine withdrawal symptoms differ between younger and older adults (Curran et al. 2003). Generally, benzodiazepine withdrawal is seen as more problematic in older patients (Holden et al. 1994); yet the potential for significant cognitive and functional improvement after withdrawal makes this avenue worth pursuing if possible (Curran et al. 2003). However, especially with frailer older persons, detox interventions may not be straightforward. For example, medical comorbidities or other physiological considerations make opioid detoxification generally a matter of an inpatient stay for older patients (Menninger 2002).

As mentioned in the "Clinical Interview and Screening" section, a useful resource for approaching interventions for older adult substance misuse and abuse is the SAMSHA Treatment Improvement Protocol (TIP) series on *Substance Use Among Older Adults* (Center for Substance Abuse Treatment 1998). Among the suggestions offered in this resource (pp. xxi) is a general list of suggestions for consideration when embarking on interventions for substance use with older clients:

- age-specific group treatment that is supportive and non-confrontational, and aims to build or rebuild the patient's self-esteem;
- a focus on coping with depression, loneliness, and loss (e.g., death of a spouse, retirement);
- a focus on rebuilding the client's social support network;
- a pace and content of treatment appropriate for the older person;
- staff members who are interested and experienced in working with older adults;
- linkages with medical services, services for the aging, and institutional settings for referral into and out of treatment, as well as case management.

Developmental influences on substance abuse

A typical developmental pattern with substance abuse is a beginning in adolescence or young adulthood with experimentation with different substances. Longitudinal studies suggest lessened drinking and a greater percentage of abstinence as people age (Satre 2013). Patterns of heavy drinking seem to change over this phase of development, with young drinkers tending toward binge drinking, and middle-aged and older drinkers having settled into a pattern of more frequent, but less heavy drinking. It often takes until middle adulthood for problems to be recognized. It appears to take a number of substance-related problems or crises for abusers to recognize the problem. It is also common to need more than one treatment attempt to be successful at stopping or controlling the abuse. These repetitions take time and mean that many of those who are successful in achieving sobriety or control will be in middle to older age at that point.

These changes in use are probably due in part to developmental aging. With biological aging, the body's uptake, and metabolism of alcohol and other drugs changes—less is needed to produce the same effects. Those individuals who monitor their reactions to alcohol may well reduce their intake to maintain the same level of intoxication. Those who do not self-monitor may slip into problem drinking while maintaining their typical levels of drinking. It can take longer to eliminate the substances from the body; idiosyncratic reactions become more common, as do side effects and interactions with other medications.

These physical changes with age can mean that amounts of alcohol and other drugs that used to be tolerated well can lead to problems for the first time in later life, even without changes in the older adult's consumption patterns. (See Case

Example 7.2) However, the great majority (two-thirds or more) of older adults with alcohol use disorders are early onset users, and so are individuals who have not learned from the changes in their bodies; nor have they developed more effective coping skills in response to experiences within their life. With biological aging also leading to increased prevalence of chronic physical conditions in later life, the older adult is also more likely to be more sensitive to the effects of alcohol due to increased physical frailty and to be taking other prescription medications that can interact with alcohol and recreational drugs. Older adults who are health conscious are likely to reduce or cease alcohol use for these reasons. The desire to do so is a common reason for older clients to seek psychological help to control alcohol use. Health problems and falls are common reasons for referrals from physicians or family for the older substance abuser.

> **Case Example 7.2 Identifying substance abuse issues in therapy for depression**
>
> One woman in her 80s had been referred for help with a long-term recurrent depression, which she related to chronic loneliness. The loneliness and depression had been much worse in the decade since her husband had died. Most of their social contacts had been through his initiative; she saw herself as a lifelong loner. During a third visit time was spent exploring how she spent her day. She described the two rather strong cocktails she had each evening, and said that she looked forward to these drinks all day long. We discussed the likelihood that age and illness had changed the likely impact of this decades-long drinking pattern. Her physician, contacted with her permission, was unaware of this pattern. She did, however, immediately see the importance for the patient's antidepressants.

On the other hand, as noted in Chapter 1, coping skills tend to improve with developmental aging, and so middle-aged and older adults are more likely to have improved coping abilities with less reliance on avoidant coping strategies such as getting intoxicated as a way of responding to life's stresses. This improvement in coping skills may be one of the reasons that substance abuse is lower in later life. The reduced reliance on avoidant coping, which is generally ineffective, and greater use of active coping and acceptance coping styles (or positive emotion regulation), are also assets for those in treatment for substance abuse.

Social context and later life substance abuse

In earlier phases of life, substance abuse problems are often brought to the attention of the abuser by other people, including their spouse, other family members, employers, and sometimes the police. Older adults with substance abuse problems, however, are often retired and may have more limited contact with family relative to their child raising days. Older adults also seem less likely to engage in behavior while intoxicated that attracts the attention of the police. Thus, some of the external sources for recognizing substance abuse are not present in later life. In the same way, this reduction in number of contacts can mean less feedback to the older person about a developing substance abuse problem. The exception to this may be substance abuse in nursing home settings, as discussed later in "Working with alcohol and substance use in the nursing home", where multiple actors are involved in supplying, detecting, preventing, and advising on alcohol and alcohol-related matters with respect to the patient. Here, as in other nursing home issues, ensuring that the clinician understands the wishes, needs, and context of the older adult is key to finding a workable way forward.

Older adults are likely to have more contact with health care providers, and those who decide to stop their drinking or drug use often cite health reasons for doing so. The likelihood of physicians recognizing and confronting older adults about substance abuse appears to be uneven, although the newer standards encouraging assessment of drinking behavior may change this in the future.

The lack of time structure in the post-retirement lifestyle can also lead to increased drinking for some older adults. Simply put, if one never drank until after work during working life, then after retirement drinking can start earlier and earlier in the day. The increased contact with physicians and pharmacies may increase the opportunity and appeal of abuse of prescription medications. Self-medicating or the use of prescription medications for pain related to illnesses of later life may lead to addiction as well.

Working with alcohol and substance use in the nursing home

Residents of nursing facilities have been noted to have relatively high rates of alcohol dependency and abuse (Joseph et al. 1995). Oslin et al. (1997) found 29% of residents of nursing homes have a lifetime diagnosis of alcohol abuse. A recent survey found relatively declining rates of alcohol use and increasing rates of drug use disorder in younger nursing home residents (Lemke and Shaefer 2010). It should be noted, however, that screening and diagnosis of substance dependency and misuse in residential care facilities can be uneven at best. Institutions may vary widely in their policies and practices with regard to alcohol consumption on site. Some facilities may offer wine with meals or even have a bar area where alcohol is served in a social setting, with the idea of increasing casual socializing, as well as offering a less institutional setting for residents to socialize with friends and family. Some institutions may limit alcohol consumption on medical grounds; some may require residents to have a physician's permission to consume alcohol. Family can themselves contribute to both confusion and abuse by covertly providing alcohol to residents, which may also have adverse effects on medications and side effects that can be serious if the situation goes unchecked.

Attitudes of staff may play a role in the nursing home as well, with respect to use of alcohol and other substances. As alluded to earlier, some might feel that alcohol consumption in later life, including within the institutional context, is a "last pleasure" that should be encouraged. Others may view drinking in later life, particularly within the long-term care medical setting, with suspicion and with the view that it may exacerbate existing substance abuse issues (Klein and Jess 2002). Staff holding opposing viewpoints and then acting on these is not only confusing for patients and their families, but may result in unintended negative side effects and interactions with medication regimes.

In the experience of NP, substance use in general and addictive behavior in particular can elicit extreme reactions in nursing care staff, and even opposing reactions among staff at the same facility toward the same patients. Several of her consult liaison team's consultations to nursing care facilities were triggered by exacerbations of behaviors of concern among persons with dementia that stemmed directly from substance use. One common scenario is when a resident with a chronic alcohol problem is given no alcohol on site, but is taken out for lunch on a regular basis by their spouse and given excessive amounts of alcohol. This causes a rift between family members and the care staff, and has implications for risk management. It is also incredibly confusing for the patient. Family meetings, in some cases, have worked to set ground rules.

Similar scenarios have emerged with smoking, with staff either facilitating or inhibiting smoking on site, and anger and aggressive behaviors resulting when access to cigarettes is withdrawn. Here, NP's team often finds staff split on how to handle the smoker, again with some facilitating and some denying access to cigarettes (although in one such facility, staff were allowed to smoke in the supposedly non-smoking nursing home). It is striking in both cases:

- how the rights of the person with dementia to pursue the behavior or the medical implications of pursuing the behavior take a back seat to battles over which party gets to control the behavior;
- how difficult it is to assess what is really happening, especially in a consult-liaison framework.

NP's team has found that talking to the maximum number of persons involved in the case is vital to understanding what is really happening in situ. Then, with respect to our observations, assessments, and recommendations, findings are sent to all parties concerned, including primary care physicians and family members. This serves two purposes. First, all parties will be on the same page with respect to the findings and recommendations. Secondly, because it is up to the staff at the facility to implement the recommendations, there is very little our team can do to make change happen, but if all parties are aware of the recommendations as well as lack of progress on follow-up consultation, then others (e.g., GP, family) can lobby for action to be taken (see Case Example 7.3).

> ### Case Example 7.3 Handling substance abuse in nursing home setting
>
> An interesting case arose during one such assessment of an individual with bipolar disorder and a long-standing substance abuse disorder. The patient was quite insistent on alcohol with meals, but her behavior deteriorated when she was given alcohol, since she would not be able to stop at one or even three glasses of wine. Staff were split over what should be done; some wanted no alcohol, others preferred that she drink rather than become aggressive toward other residents and destructive of property (a wine bottle had been thrown on one occasion). The current situation consisted of inconsistent provision of alcohol, and much ill-feeling between staff and the resident and also among staff, and fractious mealtimes for the other residents.
>
> The occupational therapist on our team suggested a novel intervention—a careful history had revealed a fondness for a particular type of wine that came in a distinctive bottle. A mock alcoholic beverage was decanted into the bottle and the bottle presented to the patient; she consumed the non-alcoholic beverage with gusto, and upon finishing the bottle was content to be led to her room for an afternoon nap. This ruse was embraced by the staff and was put into practice with the blessing as well as the financial assistance of the resident's family. Although the patient's husband insisted on buying her "the real deal" on their weekend Sunday lunch outside the facility, staff were not overly concerned by this since the patient's behavior was greatly improved within the facility. This case underscores the value of careful history-taking, a creative approach to care management, and getting all parties on side with the intervention.

Cohort and cultural effects on substance abuse

The largest cohort effect of which we are aware is the greater prevalence of alcohol use disorders in Baby Boomers compared with earlier born cohorts. Baby Boomers also have a larger prevalence of illicit drugs use in their earlier years, and a higher prevalence of cannabis use in middle age and the young-old years (Satre 2013; Wu and Blazer 2011).

The preference for particular types of alcohol (e.g., beer, wine, cocktails) tends to change somewhat from cohort to cohort. Cohorts also vary in the overall acceptability of drinking by women. Members of some earlier born cohorts consider only "hard liquor" to be problematic, with wine and beer not seen as serious drinking, even in large quantities. The same is true with the acceptability of different types of recreational drugs and types of prescription drugs to abuse. Women in some earlier born cohorts have been taking very strong tranquilizers or barbiturates for decades without perceiving their use as a problem.

A cohort difference frequently cited by current cohorts of older adults with some exposure to treatment programs is that earlier born cohorts more typically have abused alcohol only, whereas Baby Boomer and later cohorts have tended to be multiple substance abusers. To the extent that the earlier cohorts see alcohol abuse as distinct and, for their cohort, more socially acceptable, they may find mixing with younger drug users uncomfortable to unacceptable. However, as with all complaints about treatment, this can be a sincere reaction and/or a rationale for discontinuing therapy.

Cultural groups also show some variation in types of alcohol preferred and types of drugs to abuse. Risk varies by ethnicity with Whites, Latinos, and Native Americans showing higher rates than Black and Asian Americans (Satre 2013). The role of alcohol across cultures can be varied in terms of how common it is at family mealtimes, the extent to which moderate consumption is modeled for children within families, and the extent to which obvious drunkenness is tolerated. In working with clients with substance abuse issues, getting the client's perception of how their cohort and cultural background affects the meaning of the drug of choice in their lives is useful background information for the therapy. This is considered especially relevant with regard to any perceptions of differences in attitude with members of later born cohorts in their families, and with health care providers of differing cohort and cultural backgrounds. Cultural attitudes toward aging and drinking may also prevent identification of alcohol abuse, with several cultural groups being inclined to defend the attitude that drinking in old age is natural and that there are few other enjoyments in later life.

Issues in substance abuse treatment with older adults

A key difference in work with people with substance abuse issues is that they are more likely to be minimizing their problems than are clients with depression and anxiety. The therapist needs an attitude of compassionate skepticism to work effectively with substance abuse clients. That is, neither believing everything the client says nor getting angry about being misled, is helpful when working with substance abusers.

The positive attitudes toward older adults held by most therapists seeking to work with them can interfere with recognizing the substance abuse itself and with recognizing that the older client is lying. This basic difference in evaluating what clients are saying may be one reason why substance abuse intervention is often a separate specialty. In fact, there is some basis for seeing the typical supportive interaction style that is quite effective in working with depression and anxiety as being counterproductive in working with substance abuse treatment.

Ideally, therapists working with older adults who need substance abuse treatment will have competence in both treatment of addictions and in geropsychology. When that combination is not available, choices need to be made about which competency is more critical at a particular point. One older client in his 70s described using AA for his drinking problem and psychotherapy for his thinking problem. That is, for this man, sobriety solved many of his difficulties in life, but he still had automatic negative thoughts and self-schema that led to a chronic depressed mood even when sober.

The older adult with a substance abuse problem is likely to have a long history with the drug of choice, whether the history of abuse per se is long or more recently developed. Getting a sense of the history of use, and especially of prior attempts to control use or to stop is an important first step. The prior record of success and failure can give the therapist and the client a good sense of what strategies are most likely to work, and which are not worth trying. It is important in evaluating that history to keep in mind and to point out to the client that overcoming abuse often has to involve multiple attempts, and so simple lack of success on a prior try is not in itself reason not to try again. That is, the choice is likely to be the best among a set of previously failed options, rather than being able to pick an ideal, successful alternative.

Twelve-step programs are a common alternative in most communities. It is helpful for the therapist to have enough understanding of Twelve-step programs to be able to make an intelligent guess as to when a client is reporting accurately on problems in local meetings, and when the reasons given for not going are spurious. In general, there are usually enough meetings around and enough variety in them that clients can be advised to try several before reaching a conclusion. In our experience, clients often bring up the religious or "focus on a higher power" aspect of Twelve-step programs as a reason why they do not fit in. It is helpful to know that, in general, groups are very flexible about how the higher power is defined; being traditionally religious is not a requirement. However, there are some meetings where a majority of attendees are very religious, and tend to push their own approach to religion and spirituality.

Similarly, concerns about finding an age-appropriate meeting are often resistance, rather than reality. Discussing what in particular the client finds off-putting about the age mix can be helpful. Expecting an older adult to attend and gain benefit from a group comprised mainly of teens is pointless, but the older adult expectation of finding a group comprised only of age peers with very similar life concerns is likely to be resistance on the client's part. This may be followed-up by suggesting that different groups be tried or by exploring with the client the other contexts in their life in which age-integrated interactions occur and are helpful. It may also require some discussion of what to focus on in the groups and what to ignore.

Detoxification, when needed, will need medical supervision, probably undertaken in an inpatient setting. If the older adult is physically healthy otherwise, this may be fairly easy to arrange. When the older adult is physically or cognitively frail, or has multiple medical comorbidities, finding a setting that can handle both the detox and the medical/nursing care needed may be impossible in many localities. An increased chance of delirium in older adults undergoing detoxification has been noted (Kraemer et al. 1997).

Outpatient therapy can also be an important part of the treatment process and is likely to be different depending on where the client is in the sequence of controlling the addiction. Motivational interviewing is a recommended strategy for those uncertain about starting therapy for addiction and for enhancing commitment to the process of change throughout therapy. Evaluations have shown motivational interviewing to be effective with older adults (Satre 2013). Cognitive behavioral strategies aimed at behavior change have also been successful in therapy for substance abuse with older adults (Satre 2013; Cummings et al. 2008), and have been adapted to relapse prevention, a key issue in treatment of addictions (Dupree et al. 2008). As noted earlier in this chapter, therapists should consider their level of competency when working with clients with addictions, and not simply assume that success with therapy for emotional disorders will translate into success with addictions.

Summary

Therapy, and particularly assessment, with older adults around issues of substance abuse is often overlooked in clinical practice, particularly by practitioners with less experience with older persons. Questions around substance use must be broached in a forthright yet sensitive manner; tying the clinical interview questions to concerns about health and functioning is useful. Therapy approaches can be relatively brief and targeted. In the future, there may be an increasing role for psychologists to conduct such interventions from a primary care base.

In the next chapter, we explore working with sleep disorders. Complaints about sleep are very common in older adults. They frequently co-occur with many of the psychological disorders discussed in this book, but are perhaps most often associated with depression and anxiety disorders. Some familiarity with sleep disorders and basic approaches to working with common sleep complaints is essential to skillful work with older adult clients.

Chapter 8

Sleep disorders and complaints in later life

Introduction to sleep disorders and complaints in later life

Complaints about quality and quantity of sleep are very common in later life. Prevalence estimates for insomnia in later life are above 30% for older adults, compared with about 5% for those under 30 (Morgan 2000). Sleeping medications are used by many in this group—10-20% of community-dwelling older adults and up to 40% of those in institutions report their use (Buysse and Reynolds 2000). Typically, the use of such medications is long term, even though the research base is largely comprised of studies of short-term use, and many sleeping medications actually interfere with sleep when used for longer periods of time. Such perpetual, unreviewed pharmacological interventions unfortunately appear typical in older adults—witness unreviewed neuroleptic and sedative–hypnotic medication use in older adults, particularly those dwelling in nursing homes.

Problems with sleep had been seen as symptoms of other primary mental health disorders, including depression and anxiety, but more recently, sleep disorders were viewed as a primary disorder and a possible causal precursor of disorders such as depression and anxiety (Smith 2010). Primary sleep disorders in older adults included obstructive sleep apnea, periodic limb movements during sleep, and restless legs syndrome; common secondary causes of sleep disturbance in this age group include medical illnesses (e.g., renal disease, gastrointestinal disease, respiratory disorders, cardiovascular disease, and chronic arthritis), or pharmacological interactions or side effects (Crowley 2011). While this distinction between primary and secondary sleep disorders had been used in recent research, in the DSM-5, sleep disorders are now called sleep–wake disorders, and the distinction between primary and secondary sleep disorders has been eliminated (American Psychiatric Association 2013).

Chronic sleep disturbance can significantly contribute to excessive daytime sleepiness, which may result in attentional and general cognitive declines, which can then affect activities of daily living such as driving. Difficulties with sleep may also foreshadow more general declines in overall physical health (Driscoll et al. 2008), and as such should be investigated and treated if at all possible.

Although research appears to support the idea that healthy older adults, despite having somewhat lighter, more easily disturbed sleep, appear to fall back asleep as quickly as younger adults (Klerman et al. 2004), ill-health (including mental health concerns) and environmental conditions, can conspire to interfere with sleep in older adults. Significantly fragmented sleep in older adults over age 75 has been linked to increased risk of medical illness and depression (Dew et al. 1994). Older adults with sleep difficulties report high incidences of problems with balance, ambulation, and visual difficulties, even after adjustment for medication use (Brassington et al. 2000). Achieving quality sleep in light of such concerns is therefore a primary focus of sleep interventions.

Insomnia in older people is associated with reduced quality of life (Zammit et al. 1999) and increased health service utilization (Novak et al. 2004). Insomnia is often comorbid with medical conditions such as arthritis, malignancies, neurological disorders (including Parkinson's disease, stroke, and dementia), and chronic conditions such as pulmonary disease and congestive heart failure (Ancoli-Israel 2000). A bi-directional association exists between insomnia and depression, with depression increasing the risk of insomnia and vice versa in older adults (Buysse 2004). Insomnia has also been linked with both depression and anxiety in older adults (Barbar et al. 2000; Riedel et al. 2001).

Sleep disturbance is present in many forms of dementia. It can cause significant caregiver burden, and is often cited as a contributing factor for nursing home admission for the person with dementia (Crowley 2011). Patients with Alzheimer's disease (McCurry et al. 2000), Parkinson's disease (Zoccolella et al. 2010), and stroke (Johnson and Johnson 2010) may all experience disturbed sleep via primary (e.g., sleep apnea or neurobiological mechanisms such as disruption of circadian rhythms) or secondary (e.g., polypharmacy, pain) mechanisms. In Alzheimer's disease and Parkinson's disease, sleep disturbance tends to worsen as the disease progresses; in the former, it is also associated with night-time wandering (Crowley 2011). Treatment of disturbed breathing affecting sleep in persons with stroke has been shown to result in positive outcomes with respect to subjective well-being and mood (Johansson et al. 2009).

A range of social and behavioral factors may increase the risk of insomnia in later life. These include bereavement, retirement, decreased physical activity, low social support, and unrealistic beliefs about sleep and sleep habits (Morin and Espie 2003; Wolkove et al. 2007). There is some evidence that having good perceived social support is linked to better sleep in older persons, both with and without insomnia (Troxel et al. 2010). While there are many possible explanations for this, the authors speculate that better sleep leads to better functionality, including better social functioning, rather than social support being an active protective factor for good sleep in later life. Pain, particularly poorly controlled chronic pain, and sleep disturbance are also related, and there is some evidence that the relationship between chronic pain and insomnia is bi-directional (Smith and Haythornthwaite 2004). Many medications frequently used by older adults can also increase the risk of insomnia, including antidepressants, opiates, antihistamines, non-steroidal anti-inflammatories, and corticosteroids (Bliwise 1993). The number of medications used by an older individual correlates with sleep disturbance, with increasing numbers of medications associated with increasing likelihood of insomnia (Crowley 2011). Use of nicotine, caffeine, and alcohol may also have a negative impact on sleep in later life, as older adults are more susceptible to the stimulant effects of such substances than younger adults. However, in older adults, medical conditions remain the strongest predictors of the incidence and persistence of insomnia (Gureje et al. 2011).

In particular in later life, older adults report sleep-maintenance insomnia (an inability to maintain sleep throughout the night) and early-morning insomnia (waking early in the morning with an inability to return to sleep; Ancoli-Israel 2000). In order to effectively treat older adults with complaints about poor sleep, an understanding of typical changes to the quality and patterns of sleep with advancing age is essential. The criteria of ≥31 minutes of sleep onset latency (SOL) or wake time after sleep onset (WASO), and experiencing these symptoms three nights a week, for 6 months or longer, appears to best separate older adults with insomnia from normal sleepers (Lichstein et al. 2003). Insomnia is more prevalent in women than men, but for both genders, age remains the greatest risk factor for the development of insomnia (Foley et al. 2004). Difficulties sleeping may well be multifactorial in older adults, and so careful assessment is required of the circumstances, natural history, and context of sleep patterns themselves, as well as potential contributors to poor sleep, such as medical and psychiatric conditions, medications, substance use and use of stimulants, and their interactions.

Research suggests that only a small fraction of persons with chronic insomnia receive treatment (Morin and Espie 2003). Untreated chronic insomnia has been reported to increase the risk of nursing home placement in those with co-morbid cognitive impairment (Pollak et al. 1990), and is associated with increased morbidity and mortality in older adults (Crowley 2011; Dew et al. 2003).

Assessing sleep and related symptoms of insomnia

As mentioned in "Introduction to sleep disorders and complaints in later life", insomnia in older adults is probably associated with factors conspiring to increase the *risk* of sleep disorders brought about by age-associated changes and circumstances regarding sleep, into an actual sleep disorder requiring treatment. Poor health, polypharmacy, mental health, and social and environmental disturbances, all may contribute to the development of insomnia in later life (Monk et al. 2006; Ohayon 2004; Ohayon et al. 2001), as mentioned previously. Capturing these factors, as well as any prior treatments for sleep disturbance, is essential in the interview. In order to assess, diagnose, and chart out a potential treatment plan for older clients, a detailed clinical interview as well as collateral information about sleep patterns is important.

Undiagnosed sleep apnea may be as high as 29% in older adults with sleep complaints, and will probably require medical or sleep specialist interventions. A key assessment question with regard to sleep disorders is being able to recognize when the sleep disorder goes beyond complaints and simple insomnia, to more complex sleep disorders that require sleep laboratory assessment and are likely to require more sophisticated interventions.

Clinical interview

An interview is important for correct diagnosis of sleep disorders. As part of the interview, it is important to accurately capture the history of current physical and psychiatric disorders, and any attendant medications taken, both prescribed and over-the-counter medications. It is also important to review the client's everyday activities and habits that might inadvertently interfere with what is generally regarded as good *sleep hygiene* practices. For example, many older adults take a glass of wine or other alcoholic beverage in the evening, either out of habit or believing that this will help them get to sleep. In fact, drinking an alcoholic beverage before bed has mixed effects. According to a meta-analysis (Ebrahim et al. 2013), alcohol taken before sleep has the effect of decreasing sleep latency in the first half of sleep, irrespective of dose. However, the second half of sleep is often experienced as more disrupted. Similarly, ingesting coffee or other caffeinated beverages before bedtime can interfere with sleep, and there is evidence that sensitivity to caffeine increases with age.

There are a variety of structured and semi-structured diagnostic interview tools appropriate to use with older adults that may be useful in arriving at a diagnosis of insomnia. These include the Structured Clinical Interview for DSM Disorders (SCID) (First et al. 1996b) and the MINI (Lecrubier et al. 1997). The latter is compatible with both DSM-IV and ICD-10 diagnostic systems, neither of which have had much detail about age-related changes to sleep in relation to diagnosis, although this has been suggested by the sleep research community for the latest iterations of each (Reynolds and Redline 2010). The MINI is considerably shorter (15–20 minutes to administer) than the much longer SCID, with a simpler response format, which is useful if cognitive impairment is an issue in older clients. For older adults, the MINI would be the instrument of choice for a structured interview for use in clinical practice.

Across these various diagnostic systems, the main components essential to an insomnia diagnosis include a subjective complaint of difficulty sleeping, which occurs despite adequate opportunity to sleep, resulting in impairment in functioning during waking hours. The duration and quality of sleep is a difficult aspect of everyday functioning to report on. Often clients will claim to go for long periods of time with no sleep at all, although the sleep literature suggests that such long periods without sleep are associated with severely impaired functioning (Morin and Espie 2003). Both older and younger adults may find it hard to estimate actual time asleep, especially in the face of chronic sleep difficulties, which impact negatively on cognition and probably also impact negatively on the ability to self-report on sleep accurately. In fact, excessive thinking about sleep (or lack thereof) has been identified as a key target in intervention strategies for sleep difficulties. In other words, obsessive reflection on sleep and sleep duration is bad for inducing sleep. If the sleep problems are comorbid with dementia, self-reporting will be difficult and probably inaccurate. Getting an informant (hopefully one acquainted with the patient's long-standing sleep cycles, such as a spouse or partner) can provide crucial data to assist with charting how sleep is being affected, and how this differs from earlier sleep patterns.

It is important in the interview to establish what sleep patterns were like earlier in life, and note any changes in diet, environment, life circumstances, illness, or medications that might be linked to a negative change in sleep pattern for the individual (see Case Example 8.1A). Life events or other interpersonal issues may also play a role, and may or may not always be appreciated as potentially linked to lack of sleep. Furthermore, if the individual experiences no internal or external event to interfere with sleep, but simply actively resists the normal biologically driven changes in the sleep–wake cycle, disrupted sleep may occur. Along with gathering evidence about an individual's perceived sleep cycle, and their own feelings and thoughts about this, some psychoeducation about normal sleep changes with age may be warranted. There are many myths about sleep and how much is "best" or "required," and this early conversation can be very illuminating.

Case Example 8.1A Nora: assessment of sleeping difficulties

Nora was referred by her GP to a clinical psychologist for sleep difficulties. Nora and her husband Tom, both aged 70, appeared at the psychologists office 30 minutes before the appointment, with both looking quite tired and anxious. It was quickly apparent they felt that neither had had a good night's sleep in quite some time. Tom had a diagnosis of sleep apnea, but before receiving this diagnosis he disclosed that his fragmented sleep and sudden breathless awakenings had quite disturbed Nora's sleep. With the use of a CPAP

> machine, his sleep had improved, while Nora's had become even more fragmented and unsatisfactory. Other than Tom's sleep apnea and Nora's rheumatoid arthritis, both were in generally good health.
>
> Nora relayed how very anxious she had been about Tom's frequent night-time awakenings. "I really thought many times he was going to just die!" Nora described herself as "never a great sleeper—always up early..."
>
> Tom and Nora had run a local nursery together for many years; they had planned on continuing to run it part-time into their retirement, but a severe thunderstorm had resulted in a flood, which had inundated their property and at that stage they decided to sell their property, rather than rebuild. They had moved about 5 years ago from a small home at the back of a large property where they had had their nursery, into the city, where they could be closer to their daughter and grandchildren.
>
> Tom's sleep apnea had been diagnosed just after their move into the city and his sleep had continued to improve over the intervening years. Nora's sleep had been disturbed while they had lived in their home in the country, but despite the improvements in Tom's sleep, her own sleep had seemed to deteriorate since they moved into the city.
>
> "I find it hard to get to sleep with the noises of cars and buses late at night" she reported. Tom and Nora had wanted to rely more on public transportation since they moved to the city, and so had chosen an apartment in a central part of town next to amenities and public transportation.
>
> "We thought now we could stay out late and sleep late—that is always how I viewed my retirement" said Tom. Tom had grown up on a large farm in another state, and had helped his parents around the farm from an early age. "Cows do not wait to be milked!" joked Tom. He reported always waking early, and this pattern had continued while he and Nora had tended their nursery. In the evenings they had read and tended to their two children, who were born relatively late in life. Both of their children had married and moved to the city in their late 20's to pursue their professional careers. They each had two children on whom Tom and Nora doted.
>
> "We were really keen to help our kids out when we moved to the city to be closer to them. We could babysit and let them enjoy more time with their friends." Unfortunately, this had entailed many late nights, due to a desire to take public transportation, rather than driving across town. "I can't sleep at night and then I'm sleepy all day—I'm forgetting things and have had to give up my book club, which I really enjoyed. I can't even read in bed at night anymore, I'm so distracted..."

Interestingly, research suggests that despite poor sleep and insomnia being reported as an extremely common symptom in large surveys of older adults (e.g., Morin and Espie 2003), many older adults are not distressed about their sleep, despite not experiencing good quality sleep (McCrae et al. 2005). In those that report distress, however, excessive sleepiness during the day and worries about their sleep are common complaints (Riedel and Lichstein 2000). Studies about the beliefs and attitudes about sleep of older adults with and without insomnia have revealed interesting findings. Morin et al. (1993) found that older adults with insomnia held more dysfunctional beliefs generally about the consequences of lack of sleep than did self-identified good sleepers. Moreover, these beliefs played an important role in maintaining and reinforcing poor sleep.

Assessment instruments targeting sleep

Although not often incorporated among formal sleep measures, some exploration of beliefs and attitudes about sleep may be pertinent both in assessing and treating insomnia in older adults. The Dysfunctional Beliefs and Attitudes about Sleep (DBAS) Scale (Morin 1993) may be of use to clinicians interested in exploring attitudes about sleep in their clients. This scale has 30 items rated on 100-mm visual analog scales. A briefer 16-item version with a simpler 0–10 Likert scale response format and good psychometric properties may be more amenable for use in regular clinical practice (Morin et al. 2007). Morin and colleagues have demonstrated improved attitudes toward sleep in patients with insomnia treated with both cognitive behavioral therapy (CBT), and combined CBT and pharmacotherapy approaches compared with pharmacotherapy alone or placebo (Morin et al. 2002). The scale can thus serve to point out beliefs and attitudes that could be addressed during treatment, and also document improvements and changes in attitudes toward sleep pre- and post-treatment.

There are several self-report measures of sleep and sleep-related issues that have been used with older populations; a few have been developed specifically for older adult populations. These include measures of sleep dysfunction, daytime sleepiness, and measures of related sleep issues such as sleep apnea.

The Epworth Sleepiness Scale (ESS; Johns 1991) measures daytime sleepiness by asking for ratings of the probability of falling asleep in eight common relatively quiet situations; the scale ranges from 0 (would never doze) to 3 (high chance of dozing). Everyday situations surveyed include sitting and reading, and watching television. This scale has been used with older populations (e.g., Lichstein et al. 1999). Ratings on this scale can be used to help gauge level of dysfunction during the day due to sleepiness. Daytime sleepiness also carries a risk of potential harm via accidents, particularly motor vehicle crashes (Smith et al. 2009).

The Pittsburgh Sleep Quality Index (PSQI; Buysse et al. 1989) is a brief subjective measure of sleep quality in older adults. Its nine items ask about sleep patterns (e.g., "When do you usually go to bed?") and ask for ratings of frequency of sleep issues (e.g., "Cannot get to sleep within 30 minutes"). It also asks for an overall self-rating of sleep quality. This instrument has been used in a variety of studies internationally (translated into 56 languages) and has very good psychometric properties. It is easy to administer and score in both clinical and research situations.

The Stanford Sleep Questionnaire and Assessment of Wakefulness (SQAW; Miles 1982) includes items on sleep habits, sleep problems, and daytime alertness, as well as items canvassing mood, memory, and sexual behavior. The scale also examines four specific sleep complaints:

- difficulty falling asleep;
- frequent nocturnal awakenings;
- early awakenings;
- non-restorative sleep.

The Stanford scale is comprehensive and easy to use. It has been used in intervention and survey studies, and has been translated into several languages. The Sleep Disorders Questionnaire (SDQ; Douglass et al. 1994) is a brief screening questionnaire, derived from the SQAW, to identify patients with high-risk sleep disorders. The SDQ contains four diagnostic scales, for sleep apnea, narcolepsy, psychiatric sleep disorders, and periodic limb movement disorder. Undiagnosed sleep apnea may be as high as 29% in older adults with sleep complaints (Gooneratne et al. 2006), so use of such a screening tool may serve as an important detection function in clinical settings. The SDQ is designed for use by a range of health professionals and is written in simple language (eighth grade reading level). Stanford University's Center for Sleep Sciences and Medicine has links to much useful research and clinical information about sleep disorders (< http://sleep.stanford.edu/>).

Aside from formal scales, use of sleep diaries may assist both the assessment process as well as evaluating the effectiveness of interventions. Typical sleep diaries include the recording of time of going to bed, time of rising from bed, total time in bed (both awake and asleep, which can be used as a measure of sleep efficiency), estimated sleep-onset latency, time(s) awake after sleep onset, medication intake, and so forth. Sleep diaries are frequently used in intervention research as a means of prospectively monitoring sleep in the client's home environment. Over time, sleep diary data reflects an important dimension of chronic insomnia, namely the patient's subjective perception of their own sleep, and how it is changing (or failing to change), and is an important tool to consider using in clinical practice.

Sleep diaries may be quite useful in helping the older adult gather information for the clinician. An example of a sleep diary (from Carney et al. 2012) is given in Table 8.1, but the clinician can tailor the format to best suit their clients.

Table 8.1 Consensus sleep diary. This tool is distributed under the terms of an Attribution Non-Commercial license (<http://creativecommons.org/licenses/by-nc-nd/3.0/legalcode>). Unrestricted use is granted to individual practicing clinicians. Industry, organizations, or researchers wishing to use this questionnaire should contact Dr Colleen Carney (ccarney@psych.ryerson.ca).

Consensus Sleep Diary-Core ID/Name: _____

	Sample							
Today's date	4/5/11							
1. What time did you get into bed?	10:15 p.m.							
2. What time did you try to go to sleep?	11:30 p.m.							
3. How long did it take you to fall asleep?	55 min.							
4. How many times did you wake up, not counting your final awakening?	3 times							
5. In total, how long did these awakenings last?	1 hour 10 min.							
6. What time was your final awakening?	6:35 a.m.							
7. What time did you get out of bed for the day?	7:20 a.m.							
8. How would you rate the quality of your sleep?	☐ Very poor ☑ Poor ☐ Fair ☐ Good ☐ Very good	☐ Very poor ☐ Poor ☐ Fair ☐ Good ☐ Very good	☐ Very poor ☐ Poor ☐ Fair ☐ Good ☐ Very good	☐ Very poor ☐ Poor ☐ Fair ☐ Good ☐ Very good	☐ Very poor ☐ Poor ☐ Fair ☐ Good ☐ Very good	☐ Very poor ☐ Poor ☐ Fair ☐ Good ☐ Very good	☐ Very poor ☐ Poor ☐ Fair ☐ Good ☐ Very good	☐ Very poor ☐ Poor ☐ Fair ☐ Good ☐ Very good
9. Comments (if applicable)	I have a cold							

Given that common daytime functioning impairments reported as a consequence of poor sleep include fatigue, poor concentration and reaction time, depressed mood, and impaired cognitive functioning (Riedel and Lichstein 2000), it is very important to assess depressive symptoms in the course of assessing sleep complaints. There is some indication of comorbidity among both younger (Buysse et al. 2008) as well as older (Buysse 2004) patients with respect to insomnia and depression. More specific studies detailing relationships between insomnia and lifetime versus late-onset depression have yet to be undertaken. Measures used to screen and assess suspected depression are detailed in Chapter 3. Decisions on which depression screen to use probably are best dictated by the client's issues and concerns, but in general the Geriatric Depression Scale (GDS; Yesavage et al. 1982) would be appropriate.

Similarly, screening for anxiety is useful in assessing insomnia, especially given the strong probability of worry about sleep, and possibly more generalized worry and anxiety presenting as well. Again, measures used to screen and assess suspected anxiety are detailed in Chapter 4, and instrument use is best guided by client concerns. However, either the full 20-item Geriatric Anxiety Inventory (GAI; Pachana et al. 2007) or the briefer 5 item version (Byrne and Pachana 2011) would be appropriate. Similar to late-onset depression, there has not been extensive research on sleep and anxiety disorders in later life. However, some links between anxiety state and insomnia in older adults have been established (Riedel et al. 2001). Certainly, since anxiety is relatively common in later life, and can contribute directly *to* sleep difficulties as well as result *from* sleep problems, a screen for potentially undetected clinically significant anxiety in the face of a presentation of insomnia in an older adult is warranted (see Case Example 8.1B).

Case Example 8.1B Nora: assessment of sleeping difficulty

Given this couple's level of distress about their sleep, the therapist saw Tom and Nora together to try to piece together aspects of both of their sleep patterns, as well as potential issues and circumstances that might be combining to interfere with sleep. A thorough medical and psychological and family history, including personal and family history of sleep disturbance, was obtained for both. A detailed description of Nora's primary sleep complaint was obtained, both in the interview as well as via the ESS and SQAW. These revealed difficulty initiating and maintaining sleep, together with the feeling of non-productive (non-restorative) sleep and greatly increased daytime sleepiness. Indeed, she felt so sleepy at times that she was beginning to restrict her activities outside the home. Upon close examination of the timeline of sleep changes, it appeared that prior to Tom's diagnosis and treatment for sleep apnea, worries about Tom's health had become an increasing preoccupation before going to sleep. This had resulted in increasing difficulty for Nora in falling asleep, but on nights where Tom's sudden awakening had not roused her, Nora reported (and Tom confirmed) that Nora had for most nights been able to sleep through the night, with minimal impact on wakefulness the following day.

However, since moving to the city, even though Tom's sleep was relatively undisturbed, it appeared that Nora's sleep had become worse. She cited the noise of traffic, ambient light from streetlights, and noise from neighbors as contributing to a negative stream of thinking when lying in bed preparing for sleep. "Why do the upstairs people have to stomp about? I'll never get used to this traffic. I am sure that I will never be able to fall asleep. Tomorrow will be another day wasted if I can't get a good night's sleep tonight." Also, since moving to the city and joining a book club, Nora felt pressure to keep up with the reading in order to be able to participate at the club's meetings. However, her inattention during the day often meant she put off reading until evening. Then being behind in her reading (which she often did in bed) became another source of stress and concern.

On a subsequent visit Nora returned with completed sleep diaries, which pointed to an average of 45–90 minutes in bed before sleep virtually every night, and waking up for 30–45 minutes several times a night on three nights in the previous week. Her score on the Geriatric Depression Scale (15-item version) was 4, and her score on the Geriatric Anxiety Inventory was 7, suggesting that at this time depression and anxiety were mild.

Her score on the Dysfunctional Beliefs and Attitudes about Sleep Scale, however, revealed the extent of her dysfunctional beliefs surrounding her sleep, including an extremely rigid set of beliefs about what constituted "normal" sleep and what one should do to obtain better sleep. Her beliefs were what had prevented her GP from prescribing sleeping medications. These same beliefs had seen her resist "giving in" to the slowly increasing sleepiness earlier in the evening, which had begun while they were still living in the country. She felt that now that she was retired and could order her own schedule, that sleep was something that should "just happen when I want it. If I want to sleep late, I should just be able to sleep in—I deserve it after so many days of waking up early to tend our plants in the nursery!" Nora had fallen into a pattern of obsessing about the consequences of a poor night's sleep, and despite Tom's urging, felt a short nap during the day was "unnatural" and was also linked in her mind to scenes of her aunt, whom she had visited in a nursing facility for many years, who "was always sleeping in the afternoon—I am still too young to do that."

Nora was not taking any medication other than a non-steroidal anti-inflammatory drug for her arthritis. Her family, personal medical, and psychiatric history was unremarkable, and she reported no family history of insomnia or other sleep disorders, such as sleep apnea or narcolepsy. On the MMSE she scored 28/30, although on selected subtests of the Wechsler Memory Scale, her performance in the low average range reflected her own complaints of poor memory over the past few years. Psychoeducational materials given to the couple in the first session had been eagerly digested, and the couple had purchased a "white noise" machine, which Nora reported as "soothing." Nora was very eager to explore a non-pharmacologic approach to her sleep difficulties.

The therapist reflected back to the couple that their story was not an uncommon one for older persons, where a series of events (changes in residence, onset of sleep apnea) may lead to dramatic changes in sleep efficacy.

It is possible to combine various forms of self-reported sleep issues and diary-keeping with actigraphy to obtain data about actual sleep patterns in patients. Actigraphy is a method of inferring wakefulness and sleep from the presence or absence of limb movement (most often the wrist) (Lichstein et al. 2006). Data derived from an actigraph are more sensitive than sleep diaries for documenting sleep fragmentation, and are non-invasive, less expensive, and more conducive to repeated measures than polysomnography (PSG; Kushida et al. 2001). Actigraphy could be useful in documenting sleep in persons with mild cognitive impairment, as well as persons in long-term care settings, but more clinical research addressing these populations is required. The actigraph can also be used with people who cannot fill out sleep logs, such as infants and adults who cannot read or write.

Increasingly, actigraphy is within the reach of the average person, courtesy of a variety of off-the-shelf health monitoring devices, including pedometers and even applications available for use on smart phones. Such devices can provide objective data on sleep cycles and also, as a benefit, give the clinician and patient a way to actually chart positive changes in sleep due to treatment. It is probable that such devices will be increasingly incorporated into the assessment and treatment of insomnia in older adults.

Medication use and insomnia in older adults

The use of prescription medications for insomnia in older adults is widespread. In recent surveys between 5% and 33% of older adults in North America and the United Kingdom were prescribed a benzodiazepine or a benzodiazepine receptor agonist for sleep difficulties (Aparasu et al. 2003; Craig et al. 2003), with differences in rates dependent on location (Europe versus the USA) and setting (community vs residential aged care). The use of benzodiazepines is particularly associated with risk of falls in older adults (Neutel et al. 2002; Ray et al. 2000). A recent review of the risks and benefits of benzodiazepine use in older adults for sleep complaints concluded that while improvements in sleep were statistically significant across a range of studies, the magnitude of effect sizes was small, with a significant risk of adverse events, including falls, in people over the age of 60 (Glass et al. 2005).

There are a range of medications commonly used in older adults that have a side effect profile that includes insomnia. These include corticosteroids, and various cardiac and allergy medications. For a review of common medications related to insomnia, please see Roux and Kryger (2010).

Psychotherapy for insomnia

There are several established psychological interventions for late-life insomnia. The evidence base is strongest for sleep restriction/sleep compression therapy and for multi-component cognitive behavioral therapy for sleep disorders (Dillon et al. 2012). Other psychological interventions have promise, but do not have the number of systematic studies needed to be defined as evidence-based, in some instances because they are often included as part of multi-component interventions. These include stimulus control, sleep hygiene, and relaxation training (Dillon et al. 2012).

When older clients complain about sleep-related problems, it is always useful to start by exploring what the typical sleeping pattern is like. For reasons described in the first part of this chapter, it is common for older adults to expect, or at least to wish, to sleep more hours than adults need to sleep. A fairly common, minimal intervention is discovering that the client is getting 6–7 hours sleep per night, just as they did earlier in life and then educating the client that this is as much as they can expect.

Sleep hygiene also includes discussion of the effects of caffeine consumption, smoking, and alcohol on sleep. The discussion of these factors will often need to involve the reminder that the body handles these substances differently as we age. Therefore, long-established patterns of drinking coffee, alcohol, or smoking, that did not appear to cause problems in the past, may disrupt sleep in later life due to physical changes in response to these substances, or in the speed with which they are metabolized. The effects of alcohol on sleep disruption can be deceptive, since it often improves the ability to fall asleep, but then makes early waking more likely by interfering with the second half of the sleep cycle. Exploring how much liquid of any kind is drunk after late afternoon can be a helpful part of increasing restful sleep time. Waking in order to go to the bathroom is a common event in later life and decreasing the number of awakenings is also useful as part of sleep hygiene. For a good general review of sleep hygiene in the treatment of insomnia, see Stepanski and Wyatt (2003).

Wakefulness often has a cognitive component with the client becoming caught up in repetitive worrying, which then keeps them awake. Finding ways to break this habitual pattern can be an important element in helping the client sleep. In general, it involves finding substitute thoughts to replace the worries (Morin et al. 2000). Planning other activities that are mentally engaging and that distract from worry until sleep comes is one useful strategy, and can involve reading, watching TV, listening to the radio, etc. In selecting the activity, it must be engaging enough to distract from worry, but not so intriguing as to keep the client awake. Thus, clients may be encouraged to deliberately select bland to boring television programs, or reading that is somewhat difficult and unexciting.

Doing work or other tasks while lying in bed may interfere with sleep; the general thinking here is that the association between bed and sleep is weakened with these multiple uses for this space. Stimulus control approaches are helpful for promoting sleep (Bootzin and Epstein 2000). Encourage clients to get out of bed when it becomes obvious that sleep will not return soon and wait somewhere else in the home for sleepiness to return. The waiting period should not involve activity that will tend to keep the client awake, but may need to involve some distraction from worry if that is part of the picture. Helping clients problem solve about other aspects of their lives that may influence sleep can also be useful.

More complex sleep interventions, such as systematic approaches to sleep restriction/sleep compression therapy and multi-component CBT for insomnia are best undertaken by people with specific training in these approaches. Ideally, they should be done in conjunction with sleep laboratory assessment. Of course, these resources are not available everywhere.

Developmental effects on sleep

As described in a review by Morgan (2000), there are a number of changes in sleep with aging. The high prevalence rate of insomnia among older adults appears to be due to an accumulation of this often chronic disorder over the adult lifespan, rather than a sharp increase in later life, given that incidence rates appear not to increase much from early adulthood to old age. This is in contrast with the typical belief that sleep changes more abruptly in later life, which may discourage both patients and health care professionals from pursuing potential causes and interventions for insomnia later in life.

Generally, sleep patterns change in predictable ways with age. Neurobiological changes in the hypothalamus result in a shift in the sleep–wake cycle such that with age, the onset of sleepiness occurs earlier, with a concomitant shift to an earlier waking time (Monk 2005). Total sleep time (e.g., total time spent asleep) decreases with age (Ohayon et al. 2004). Although generally the amount of sleep is still roughly comparable with that in younger adults (Foley et al. 2004), on average it drops from about 7 hours in middle age to slightly less than 6 hours in later life. The structure of sleep often changes with more frequent arousals and shifts from one stage of sleep to another with aging. The percentage of time spent in deep (delta wave) sleep, the most restful part of the sleep cycle, appears to decrease on average. Circadian rhythms shift, with older adults tending to shift both sleep onset and waking times earlier in the day, in contrast to the shift in the opposite direction seen in adolescence (Lichstein 2014).

Older adults generally experience their sleep as more easily disrupted compared with when they were younger. A large meta-analysis of sleep patterns in healthy community-dwelling older persons revealed that most age-related changes in sleep occur by the age of 60, after which (in this healthy population) only minimal changes occurred (Ohayon et al. 2004). In this same study, changes in sleep patterns, including lighter sleep experienced with age, were more pronounced in women than in men. A meta-analysis by Zhang and Wing

(2006) of gender differences in insomnia found women at an overall greater risk of developing insomnia, which was exacerbated with increasing age.

To date, it is unclear how much of the changes in sleep related to age are primary developmental changes in sleep processes per se and how much may be due to the effects of changes in health that are associated with age. Increased pain can obviously interfere with sleep. Many chronic physical conditions of later life can also interfere with sleep, especially restless leg syndrome, apnea, and other sleep-related respiratory disorders. Medications taken for the treatment of common medical problems in later life can interfere with sleep. Dementia also increases these changes in sleep structure and can lead to disruption of sleep.

An important component of understanding changes in sleep and helping clients deal with problems related to sleep is educating the client about normal changes in sleep. In some instances, older adult clients have unrealistic expectations that sleep should remain the same as it was in younger years. If these expectations become sources of worry, the ruminative worry and related anxiety can exacerbate the sleep problems.

A key issue in working with older adults with sleep disorders or with sleep-related complaints is helping them understand what is known from their health care providers about the causes of their sleep-related problems. In turn, they may not realize how aspects of their illness or the illness of the person they are caring for (e.g., motor changes related to Parkinson's disease) may be interfering with their sleep. Again, education about these issues, together with liaising with the patient's health care specialists, may assist in formulating a sensible treatment plan going forward.

Social context effects on sleep

The most dramatic effects of social context on sleep arise in group care of the elderly, when the care facility wants to have the older residents asleep for 10–12 hours per day for the convenience of staff. The same situation can occur in family care of older adults when the caregiver wants the frail older adult to sleep for longer periods of time than would be normal for their age. In both institutional and home care situations, caregivers often tolerate or even encourage daytime napping, which then makes nighttime sleep less likely.

Institutional environments also tend to be noisier and more brightly lit than residences are at nighttime. This higher level of stimulation is, of course, likely to interfere with sleep. Disruptive events during the night can be moderately common in nursing homes and other residential facilities for older adults, as residents can have health crises that require nighttime assistance by staff, or that require attendance by an ambulance and hospitalization. Nighttime wandering by residents also requires staff intervention. While all of these situations require activity on behalf of the affected person, they also disrupt the sleep of the other residents. Basically, if the residents are sharing rooms, then the other person's habits or conditions (e.g., snoring) may also disrupt sleep.

Another common context effect creating sleep complaints is when older adults find their social environment unchallenging and boring, and attempt to turn to sleeping long hours as a way to pass the time. As with externally imposed demands for long hours of sleep, these expectations to pass the time by sleeping 10 or more hours per day are unlikely to work, and often result in being awake during even less intrinsically interesting parts of the day.

Finally, a lack of physical exercise or exposure to daylight (with its regulating effects on circadian rhythms) may also serve to interfere with good sleep in nursing home residents. In general, older adults whose days are spent in low energy expenditure ways, even when remaining awake throughout the day, are likely to experience difficulties staying asleep at night. Simply put, if one rests throughout the day, getting restful sleep at night is unlikely.

Cohort and cultural effects on sleep

To our knowledge, there is little consideration of potential cohort and cultural differences with regard to sleep disorders and aging. Worthman (2011) brings an ecobiocultural perspective to the study of potential cultural influences on sleep, but limits the discussion to minor children and their parents. In general, she finds that many non-Western cultures have very different patterns for sleep, including commonly sleeping with others, no expectation of quietness, flexibility in timing of sleep, and a combination of nighttime sleep and daytime napping. Jean-Louis et al. (2007) summarize comparisons of African Americans and Whites with regard to sleep, using some data based on older adult samples by noting that African Americans complain less about sleep problems, although objective evidence suggests that Whites get more sleep. It seems plausible that different generational cohort groups and different cultures will have distinctive ideas about the role of sleep in life and particularly in the lives of older adults. Jean-Louis et al. (2007) further noted that sleep time per night appeared to have decreased over time over the preceding 40 years, a finding that could certainly contribute to age-cohort differences in expectancies about sleep. Attitudes toward exercise, activity, and daytime napping are likely to differ across cohorts and cultural groups. Aerobic exercise, for example, has proven effective in improving self-reported sleep and quality of life in older adults (Reid et al. 2010). The clinician suggesting exercise as a part of an intervention for sleep problems may wish to consider how appealing or relevant this suggestion will seem to different cohorts or cultural groups. Not enough research on sleep disorders has included cultural or cohort distinctions, and so at present the nature of those cohort differences is largely unknown.

Issues in working on sleep disorders with older clients

Sleep hygiene education is a straightforward, but important part of sleep interventions (Riedel 2000). Discussing napping and exercise as components of the client's daily schedule is one aspect of sleep hygiene that can arise more often in later life because post-retirement life has few schedule constraints and napping regularly is an easy habit to acquire. It is fairly frequently the case that daytime napping has become a common part of the daily routine, and that the total amount of daytime napping and nighttime sleep is in the same range as during middle age. A common reframing of the sleep complaint is urging the view that 7 hours per 24-hour period (or whatever amount was common in mid-life) is what can be expected, and what the client can control is which hours they will spend asleep. More physical activity during the day, and decreasing or eliminating napping are key behavioral changes than can improve nighttime sleep quality.

Schedule readjustment can also be more of an issue in later life, without time constraints imposed by work and family obligation. The change strategy may be mainly cognitive, such as challenging the thought "I go to bed at 8 p.m. because there's nothing interesting on TV," by pointing out that TV viewing options are even worse at 3 a.m. when they wake up again. If the sleep schedule is in part maintained by sleeping late or by daytime sleeping, setting an alarm, or using exercise and other methods to avoid daytime napping will be part of the behavior change intervention (see Case Example 8.2). Obviously, a theme winding through

---

Case Example 8.2 Working on readjusting the sleep schedule

One client in her 70s had sleeping problems as one of her principal complaints. She was unsure how long she slept each night, but reported feeling fatigued every day, and often sleeping an hour or more in the afternoons. After keeping track of her sleep pattern for a week, it was clear when we reviewed the notes in therapy that she got about 7 hours per day total, and typically slept from about 8:30 or 9 p.m. to around 3 a.m.. She was then unable to go back to sleep until the afternoon nap. She found evenings alone boring and somewhat depressing, and so went to bed early. She acknowledged finding the wakeful early morning hours even more boring and often spent the time thinking about what had gone wrong in her life.

With frequent reminders from the therapist that the goal was hers and the object was to avoid the early morning wakeful times, she found ways to avoid daytime napping, including taking short walks in the neighborhood in the afternoon. With the therapist, she identified some activities that would keep her awake without making her so agitated that she would not be able to fall asleep—generally a couple of hours of reading or sewing, followed by listening to music. She shifted her sleeping time to 11 p.m. until 6 or 6:30 a.m.. The tendency toward negatively toned life review vanished with the changed sleep schedule, and she spontaneously added increased daytime activity and social contact as she felt more energetic with better sleep.

all of this is how the client spends their time, and finding ways acceptable to the client to make waking hours more interesting and more physically active.

When the sleep issues focus on problems falling asleep or going back to sleep after waking, some form of relaxation therapy is often helpful. This can take the form of progressive relaxation, breathing exercises, or other passive relaxation approaches familiar to the client. Occasionally, clients report not being able to complete the relaxation because they fall asleep. It can be useful to point out in advance that this is a success in reaching the goal, rather than a failure to complete the exercise.

While sleep change recommendations are generally straightforward and fairly simple to explain to clients, actually achieving the change can be more complex, largely due to client's resistance to changing the behavior patterns that result in poor sleep (see Case Example 8.3).

Case Example 8.3 Negotiating sleep change with the client

One client in her 90s brought up as a major concern that she woke up so late in the day and then took so much time getting ready to go out due to various physical frailties, that in winter it was dark by the time she was ready to leave home. She also reported falling asleep while doing things in the late evening at home, which frustrated her because she did not complete the activity and because she often woke in discomfort. She often sent e-mails and wrote on her blog in the late evening, and would fall asleep over the keyboard, for example. She was highly resistant to changing her sleep schedule because she had always been "a night owl" and also saw it as part of her artistic, somewhat bohemian lifestyle. Some progress was made by the therapist being clear that unlike her physician and her friends, the therapist was suggesting that she try to go to sleep about 2 a.m. and wake up by 10 a.m., rather than adopting a more normal sleeping pattern. The therapist also kept bringing the client back to what her own goals were in changing her sleep pattern and so side-stepped the resistance to taking advice from others that characterized a lot of the client's life. The therapist also worked on helping the client recognize signs of sleepiness and take that as a cue to go to bed, rather than pushing herself to keep working on e-mail and her blog.

Summary

Sleep disorders are relatively common later in life, and may result from a combination of biological, psychosocial, and environmental factors. Often education about how sleep changes with normal aging is an important step toward resolving sleep issues. Careful assessment, particularly keeping a sleep diary, can be useful in informing intervention strategies. Cultural and cohort effects influencing both the incidence of sleep disorders and the efficacy of treatment approaches are areas requiring further research.

Up to this point in the book, we have focused on disorders that tend to be relatively short term and whose onset can occur at any point in adult life. Chapters 9 and 10 focus on two disorders that tend to last for decades, rather than months and years: psychoses and personality disorders. As with the other diagnoses considered in this book, these can present somewhat differently and pose different challenges in later life, even though the onset is usually in early adulthood for these disorders, and so the client has an adult lifelong history with the disorder and often with its treatment.

Chapter 9

Psychosis and bipolar disorder

Introduction to psychosis and bipolar disorder

People with schizophrenia, paranoid psychoses, bipolar disorder, and other psychoses grow old as do the rest of us. Psychotic disorders in later life have been less well-recognized than manifestations of the disorders at younger ages, and consequently older adults with such presentations did not (and to a certain extent still may not) receive the support they need to maintain functionality and quality of life, either in the community or in institutional settings (Bartels 2002). Both current and past diagnostic criteria also remain problematic for these groups (Jeste et al. 2007).

With respect to treatment, both the quality of mental health services and adequate numbers of geriatric-trained mental health professionals within such services for older adults lag behind those services catering for mostly younger and middle-aged patients (Bartels 2003). Schizophrenia and psychotic and bipolar disorders in later life are grouped together in this chapter, due to similarities in functionality and sequelae of the disorders in late-life and later-onset groups.

Schizophrenia and psychosis in later life

The great majority of older adults with a psychotic disorder will have long histories of the illness, with early adulthood onset and usually a long history of treatment for the illness (Whitbourne and Meeks 2011). Older adults with schizophrenia represent a large proportion of those with serious mental illness later in life of an origin not related to dementia (Cohen et al. 2000). With respect to schizophrenia, 75% of older patients with schizophrenia will have experienced the onset of the disorder in early and mid-life, and 25% in later life (Jeste et al. 1999). In British psychiatry, this late-life onset profile has been recognized for several decades and often called paraphrenia (Clare and Giblin 2008). The two groups tend to differ in symptom profiles, with early-onset older schizophrenics having mostly negative symptoms in later life, whereas the late-onset schizophrenics are more likely to have hallucinations and delusions, with delusions of the paranoid type being most common (Clare and Giblin 2008).

For those in treatment, over the course of several decades treatment is likely to lead to better, although not necessarily normal, functioning. People with psychoses also learn from their experiences about how to manage the illness and avoid distressing relapses. Coping strategies appear in some studies to evolve and improve with age (e.g., Cohen 1993). Shepherd et al. (2012) reported on a qualitative study of interviews with older schizophrenics who recalled the early history of their disease as a time of confusion and distress, but saw themselves as having achieved greater understanding of the disorder and mastery of symptoms over time. There were differences among them in their distress over the contrast between what their life with psychosis had been versus their aspirations when younger, with some having achieved some acceptance and others still in despair.

Thus, most older adults with psychosis are likely to have reached a chronic, residual level of illness largely without obvious positive symptoms of mental illness. Yet their illness may have left them vulnerable to further disability in their later years. For example, late-onset schizophrenia has been identified as a potential risk factor for dementia (Brodaty et al. 2003). In our experience, irrespective of whether their psychotic disorder is comorbid with some form of dementia, such older individuals are sometimes perceived in long-term care settings and community-based aging services settings as eccentric or depressed, rather than as having a serious mental illness. Therefore, they may not receive appropriate care; at times they are perceived as simply manifesting behavioral and psychological symptoms of dementia, and again may not be adequately treated.

That said, even older adults with histories of psychosis and with years of functioning at a chronic, residual level, without obvious signs of illness, can decompensate dramatically under stress and have full-fledged psychotic breaks. These episodes are likely to be quite startling to the aging services system professionals or long-term care settings where the older adult resides. The episodes are likely to require crisis intervention and psychiatric hospitalization in a center that has competence in working with older adults with mental illness. If gradually escalating symptoms are recognized quickly enough, they can be handled on an outpatient basis and in situ, but our experience is that the symptoms are seldom recognized and responded to quickly enough in aging services and long-term care settings. Age-appropriate outpatient or residential treatment programs for older chronic psychiatric patients remain relatively rare (Cohen et al. 2000).

The dangers of increased morbidity and mortality from over-medication or inappropriate use of antipsychotics are very real for older adults (Karim and Byrne 2005). Older women are particularly vulnerable to extrapyramidal side effects from antipsychotic medications (Kane et al. 1992). Older adults in general are also at increased risk of falls when on antipsychotic medications (Lindsey 2009). Antipsychotic drugs are associated with both somatic and neurological side effects, in addition to increased all-cause mortality and sudden cardiac death in older populations (Leon et al. 2010). Tardive dyskinesia is not only more likely (up to 5–6 times more likely) in older adults taking such medications, but is less likely to remit; in this respect, new atypical antipsychotics have a better side effect profile (Jeste et al. 2008). The current need for more health care professionals with geriatric skill and experience (Jeste et al. 1999), particularly in emergency rooms and in consultation and liaison psychiatric teams that often encounter older individuals with psychotic symptom profiles, is underscored by the confusion and the often inadequate treatment occasioned by the presentation of an older adult with psychosis. This inadequate treatment may include missing signs and symptoms of health-related conditions, which is not helped by the fact that neuroleptic medications may reduce pain sensitivities, and cognitive impairments may reduce both reporting and insight into medical complaints in later life (Cohen et al. 2000).

While the majority of older adults with a history of serious psychotic and related disorders will also have had experience with treatment, there are some who have managed to avoid treatment by only discussing their hallucinations and delusions with sympathetic family and friends. They found ways to support themselves that were not stressful and where contact with others is limited such that their symptoms did not lead to problems at work. Untreated psychotic and related disorders for those older adults with more serious manifestations of these disorders may result in impaired community functioning, cognitive impairment, poorer quality of life, heightened caregiver distress, and increased morbidity and mortality (US Department of Health and Human Services 1999). Lack of treatment in later life also increases the risk of nursing home placement in this group (Bartels et al. 1997).

Bipolar disorders in later life

According to the Epidemiological Catchment Data Survey (Weissman et al. 1988), bipolar disorder occurs at a 1-year prevalence rate of 0.1% in adults aged 65 and over, relatively low compared with rates in the same data set for schizophrenia and depression in this age group (roughly three and 14 times that of bipolar disorder, respectively). Subsequent studies have found similarly low rates for bipolar disorder in those over 65 in outpatient samples (e.g., Hirschfield et al. 2003a, with their finding of 0.05%). In samples from inpatients, the rates were considerably higher, ranging from 4.7% (Yassa et al. 1988) to 18.5% (Moak 1990), with a mean prevalence in a large critical review of 61 studies of 8.7% in inpatient psychiatry settings and 6.1% in outpatient psychiatry settings

(Depp and Jeste 2004). The gender ratio for bipolar and schizophrenia in older adults is roughly two to three females per male (Depp and Jeste 2004; Keith et al. 1991).

In terms of age of onset of disease, the proportion of late-onset bipolar disorder among older individuals who have had the disorder for some time ranges from 6.1% to 11% (Almeida and Fenner 2002; Cassidy and Carroll 2002; Clayton 1983; Goodwin and Jamison 1990; Sajatovic et al. 2005a), among older individuals aged 60 and over. Depp and Jeste (2004) report in their large review that the majority of studies found gender ratios to be equivalent between early- and late-onset groups, and greater risk of comorbid neurological illness and less risk of comorbid substance abuse in late onset as opposed to early-onset mania and bipolar disorders. Bipolar patients have increased neuropsychological deficits compared with non-psychiatric populations, particularly in information processing speed and executive functioning (Gildengers et al. 2012). Bipolar patients also have an increased risk of developing dementia later in life (Kessing and Anderson 2004). In Depp and Jeste's (2004) study, prior family history of psychiatric disturbance, lack of social supports, and the presence or absence of psychotic features were inconsistently linked with either early- or late-onset bipolar disorders across studies. Moreover, they also found that the definition of early and late onset varied considerably between studies. In subsequent research (e.g., Chu et al. 2010), examination of differences between early- and late-onset bipolar disorder, in terms of such variables as psychiatric comorbidity and medical burden, showed few clinically useful differences between these groups.

With respect to recovery from later onset bipolar disorders, while the long-term outcome of early-onset bipolar disorder showed that the majority have recurring or residual symptoms, far fewer patients with later onset bipolar disorder show full functional recovery from their illness (Depp and Jeste 2004). Older bipolar patients appear similar to older patients with schizophrenia in terms of disability and functional status (Depp et al. 2006). For example, older adults with mania have greater psychosocial deficits and poorer outcomes than similarly aged depressed and control groups (Berrios and Bakshi 1991). However, persons experiencing a later onset of bipolar disorder may experience fewer health issues in later life; Schurhoff et al. (2000) reported that individuals diagnosed with bipolar disorder after age 40 experienced less severe forms of the illness, with fewer psychotic features and decreased comorbidities.

Older patients with bipolar disorder are high consumers of health and mental health services. Older bipolar patients use almost four times the total mental health services and are four times more likely to be hospitalized compared with similar aged patients with unipolar depression (Bartels et al. 2000). Older bipolar patients tend to have longer hospital stays and increased use of outpatient services (Sajatovic et al. 2004). Again, age of onset plays a role in health service use. Individuals with late-onset bipolar disorder tend to have less mental and medical services outpatient visits than earlier onset groups (Meeks 1999; Sajatovic et al. 2005b).

Increased morbidity and mortality in older bipolar patients from both physical illnesses, such as circulatory disorders, as well as suicide, remains a concern (Angst et al. 2002). Tsai et al. (2002), in a study of suicide in bipolar disorder across the lifespan, found that the highest risk for completed suicide was between 7 and 12 years post-onset in those under age 35, roughly similar to the relationship between age and suicide in those with schizophrenia (Pinkahana et al. 2003). Older early-onset bipolar patients may thus belong to what could be termed a "survivor cohort" (Depp and Jeste 2004, p. 360).

Assessment of schizophrenia and bipolar disorder

Assessment of older adults with schizophrenia, other forms of psychosis, mania, and bipolar disorders is aimed at ascertaining the nature and extent of symptomatology, as well as arriving at a differential diagnosis. Common differential diagnoses of psychosis in older populations (adapted from Targum 2001) are given in Box 9.1.

Box 9.1 Common differential diagnoses for psychosis in later life

- Delirium.
- Dementia.
- Major depression.
- Mania.
- Substance-induced psychosis.
- Delusional disorder.
- Schizophrenia.

Obtaining collateral information as part of the assessment can be extremely useful, but may also be less likely if family members are estranged as a result of ruptured interpersonal relations due to the mental illness. A medical history, including medication history, with information on what medications have been used in the past and which have or have not been effective, is important information to obtain, and will facilitate liaising with other health care professionals and planning intervention strategies.

Clinical interview and differential diagnoses

In light of the possibility of delirium, depression, or dementia underlying a psychosis-like or manic presentation, it is important to be mindful of this when conducting the clinical interview and selecting an assessment strategy. Here, past personal history of depression or a family history of either depression or dementia would be important to ascertain. Obvious medical causes for delirium and a waxing and waning presentation of symptoms would suggest that the possibility of a delirium at least be considered. Delusions in older adults with depression are usually mood-congruent and contain common themes of guilt, persecution, and nihilism (Webster and Grossberg 1998). Suicide attempts are more common in older depressed individuals who experience delusions (Lacro and Jeste 1997), hence a careful risk assessment is warranted.

Risk factors for psychosis in later life (adapted from Targum 2001; Targum and Abbott 1999), arguably one of the more vexing differential diagnostic challenges among older adults, are given in Box 9.2.

Box 9.2 Risk factors for psychosis in later life

- Female gender.
- Cognitive impairment.
- Co-morbid medical conditions.
- Medications (particularly those with dopaminergic or anticholinergic properties).
- Substance abuse.
- Sensory deficits.
- Social isolation.
- Pre-morbid personality traits (particularly paranoia).
- Family history of psychosis.

In light of these risk factors, careful inquiry into current and past substance abuse is prudent (refer to Chapter 7 in this text for relevant substance abuse assessment strategies). Social isolation may be missed by the interviewer with less experience of older adults, who may be more inclined to view increasing social isolation as "normal" in later life. This is an erroneous assumption. Premorbid expressions of paranoia as a personality trait may be difficult to ascertain if informants are either not familiar with the patient, or if informants are family members who have conflicting views of the client or views colored by interpersonal conflict.

Structured or semi-structured interviews such as the MINI (Lecrubier et al. 1997) may be productively used in clinical interviews with older adults with suspected psychosis or bipolar disorder. Combining such a structured interview with a thorough history-taking may help, particularly as ascertaining which disorder may be manifesting often can be quite obscure. Here, gathering evidence from multiple sources is key. An inexperienced or time-pressed clinician may be tempted to rely on only one informant's view of the symptoms of purported psychosis or bipolar presentation; this may distort the picture of the patient's behavior. For example, in the nursing home the patient may be described as having a delusion that their belongings are being stolen. However, given both the tendency for objects to go missing in nursing home settings and the very real probability that other residents may indeed be taking objects from the patient's room, getting a clear picture of the behaviors is essential. Especially in residential aged care settings, multiple informants should be interviewed.

An important differential diagnosis with respect to psychosis is delirium. The prevalence of delirium in older hospital patients has been reported as ranging from 11% to 24%, with higher rates found in post-surgical patients (Fann 2000). As noted in Chapter 5, the Confusional Assessment Method (CAM; Inouye 2003) is the preferred tool for ascertaining presence of delirium. The CAM can be administered in about 5 minutes and has good sensitivity and specificity (94–100% and 90–95%, respectively; Inouye 2003). The CAM has two parts: part I is an assessment screen for overall cognitive impairment, while part II includes only those four items found to have the greatest ability to distinguish delirium from other disorders. Unfortunately, in clinical practice delirium often goes undetected. A wrong diagnosis of a psychotic disorder when delirium is present may:

- exacerbate the delirium;
- result in inappropriate medication and perhaps restraint;
- result in increased risk of self-harm due to the confusional state of delirium;

In sum, untreated delirium carries significant risk of negative outcomes for patients, including older adults.

Assessing symptoms of psychosis and bipolar disorder

Despite the increased amount of research on psychosis in later life, instruments specifically developed for older populations are still lacking. The Brief Psychiatric Rating Scale (BPRS; Overall and Gorham 1962), although not developed specifically for use in older adults, nevertheless has been widely used in this population. The BPRS is the classic example of a test designed at a time when clinical rating scales and screens were scarce; it was an attempt to facilitate systematic collection of psychiatric data on psychiatric inpatients. Since its introduction, the items themselves as well as the response scale have undergone numerous revisions and elaborations. Several versions of the scale exist; for example, one 24-item version rates 24 symptoms (e.g., bizarre behavior, blunted affect) using a Likert scale with simple anchor points ranging from "not present" through to "very severe." Other versions of the scale include more detailed descriptors of the symptoms themselves; for example, "blunted affect" is described as "reduced emotional tone; apparent lack of normal feeling or involvement." The so-called Hillside Hospital anchors for the scale attempt greater clarity with respect to the severity ratings, again offering brief elaborations on the anchor items; modest improvements in reliability are reported in these versions (Woerner et al. 1988). Nevertheless, research has reported an alarmingly low inter-rater reliability for raters without training or retraining on this measure (Bark et al. 2011).

Brief screens such as the MMSE and BPRS, in versions with more detailed instructions, tend to produce more reliable results, if the assessor is trained on the "standardized" version. Given the balance of evidence to date, the 24-item BPRS with better described anchors than the "Hillside Hospital" version is thus recommended both for improved psychometric characteristics, but also its potential to curtail "drift" and poor inter-rater reliability (Ventura et al. 1993).

The MMPI 2 is a general measure of psychopathology in adults that has very good reliability and validity. The normative sample includes adults up to age 85, and it is considered to be valid with older adults (Graham 2006; Segal et al. 2006). However, it is often discounted for use with older adults based on its length. BK has used it selectively with older adults and has not found the length to be a problem, nor does the test typically take longer with older adults. This experience is based on selected clients who were not cognitively impaired and for whom diagnosis was unclear, when based on history and shorter screening tools. The MMPI 2 was given after the client had been seen at least a few times and a rapport had been established. The MMPI 2-RF was based on the same normative sample and in principle should also be useful with older adults (Ben-Porath 2012), but we have no direct experience with its use.

There are a few rating scales explicitly designed for patients with mania that have been used in studies with older individuals. The Modified Manic State Scale (MMSS; Blackburn et al. 1977) was used with older adults in a study by Broadhead and Jacoby 1990). The Bech-Rafaelson Mania Scale (BRMS; Bech et al. 1978) was used by Tariot et al. (2001) with older persons. The Neuropsychiatric Inventory (NPI; Cummings et al. 1994) would be of use with patients with dementia displaying either psychotic or bipolar symptoms.

Finally, the Mood Disorder Questionnaire (MDQ; Phelps and Ghaemi 2006; Twiss et al. 2008) is a self-report screening tool for older patients with suspected bipolar disorder (see Case Example 9.1). The MDQ has a simple yes–no response

> **Case Example 9.1 Phillip: assessment of bipolar disorder**
>
> Phillip was a 68-year-old man who looked much older than his stated age, seen by the consult-liaison psychiatry team at a local nursing home in an outlying suburban setting of a large city. Phillip was very loud and restless, constantly "pestering" the other patients and staff, as described by the nursing home manager. Phillip had only moved into the facility just over a month ago; he had already alienated several staff and residents refused to eat with him at mealtimes. Phillip had moved into the facility after a long inpatient stay for recurrent diverticulitis. During this time he had undergone surgery on his bowel, contracted a severe infection, and had needed to be weaned off all medications.
>
> Staff suspected that he had chronic mental illness, but Phillip was a very poor historian and had no family, being divorced for over 20 years and without children. The team psychologist administered the Mood Disorders Questionnaire (MDQ) after taking time to build a rapport with Phillip; the psychologist also chose to interview Phillip just after the mid-afternoon snack, as staff reported that this was when he was calmest. Phillip was surprisingly open and articulate, outlining a long history of inpatient stays due to "my ideas not being fashionable, I guess." On the MDQ Phillip endorsed 10 of the 13 symptoms on item 1 of the inventory, and confirmed in item 2 that he had often experienced multiple symptoms at the same time. He rated the symptoms as causing him moderate problems, but clarified that this was mostly due to the reactions of other people.
>
> The combination of seven or more symptoms being endorsed, coupled with positive answers on items 2 and 3, indicated possible bipolar disorder. This was confirmed through the history and from the medical records eventually forwarded by Phillip's psychiatrist. Phillip often went off his medications for short stretches of time and one of these had coincided with his admission to the hospital for diverticulitis. When he was unexpectedly discharged to a nursing home, his medications did not include the drug lithium, which had been best able to control his symptoms.
>
> The team used the MDQ data not only to diagnose Phillip, but also to give the nursing home a baseline of behaviors to monitor, to ascertain whether the addition of lithium helped with symptom management, and whether Phillip's behavior would improve further through targeted behavioral and psychosocial interventions.

format when asking about the presence or absence of 13 specific symptoms (such as feeling irritable, being easily distracted, and being more interested in sex than usual) It also has a 4-point Likert scale for indicating the amount of distress the symptoms cause. Sensitivity and specificity of this instrument vary considerably with population type. For example, the sensitivity and specificity of the MDQ in the general population is 28% and 97%, respectively (Hirschfield 2002), whereas in an outpatient clinic serving primarily a mood disorder population, the sensitivity and specificity were 73% and 90%, respectively (Hirschfield et al. 2000). With low to moderate sensitivity and relatively high specificity, the MDQ is better at confirming bipolar disorder than detecting it (Hirschfield et al. 2003b; Phelps and Ghaemi 2006).

Therapy with persons with schizophrenia and bipolar disorder

Given the fact that older persons with chronic mental illness may have made gains in adaptations to life with their illness as they have become older, group approaches with such patients may be particularly efficacious. For example, a behavioral group intervention called Functional Adaptations and Skills Training (FAST) was the subject of a randomized trial (Patterson et al. 2006) in middle-aged and older adults (mean age 50 and 51 years, in the control and intervention groups, respectively) with schizophrenia. The FAST program is described by the authors of the trial as a 'manualized behavioral intervention' based upon Social Cognitive Theory (Bandura 1989) and Liberman's Social and Independent Living Skills Program (Psychiatric Rehabilitation Consultants 1991). The FAST program targets six areas of everyday functioning—medication management, social skills, communication, organization and planning, transportation, and financial management. The intervention groups met once a week for 24 weeks for 2 hours in a group format (see Patterson et al. 2003, for a full description of FAST). Compared with an attentional control condition, the FAST participants who attended at least 25% of the sessions demonstrated significant improvement in everyday living (organization, planning, transport, and finances), communication, and social skills, but not medication management skills.

Similarly, McQuaid and colleagues (2000) developed and trialed an integrated cognitive behavioral and social skills training intervention for older patients with schizophrenia. Although only a modest pilot ($n = 10$; mean age = 62.6), the intervention was well-tolerated by the patients, who met as a group for 1-hour sessions over 12 sessions. This manualized approach included sessions on basic thought-challenging skills, symptom self-management, and communication skills. The group format of the intervention was noted as a particular strength by the participants. An increased research focus on such group interventions for late-life schizophrenia should be ongoing.

Finally, Bauer and McBride (2003) have developed and published a structured, manual-based group intervention for older adults with bipolar disorder. They incorporate a psychoeducational, problem-solving approach with the aim of improving illness-management skills. Their Life Goals Program incorporates elements of CBT as well as motivational interviewing techniques (Miller and Rollnick 2002). Encouraging active self-management in a supportive group environment can offer individuals the chance to better manage both the psychiatric and medical components of their illness.

Developmental influences

The developmental trajectories of people with schizophrenia appear to be varied across domains of functioning. Jeste et al. (2011) reported that biological aging seems to proceed faster among schizophrenics, with disease and frailty setting in earlier in life. Casey et al. (2011) noted that older schizophrenics have higher rates of diabetes and cardiovascular disease, are more likely to be obese, and to smoke or have long histories of smoking. Health-related quality of life appears to be lower in older bipolar patients (Leon et al. 2010). The quality of medical care received in all of these patient groups appears to be lower than for patients of similar age without chronic mental illness. However, an interesting finding is that older persons are more likely than younger persons to adhere to a regime of mood-stabilizing medications (Berk et al. 2004), and this may be reinforced to the patient's advantage by the therapist who is cognizant of such age-related influences and behaviors.

The normal developmental trend in schizophrenics aging with the disease is the reduction of positive symptoms in later life (Angst 1988; McGlashan 1988). The increase in prominence of negative symptoms of chronic schizophrenia in later life remains a subject of debate in the literature (e.g., McGlashan and Fenton 1992). Part of the difficulty in studying negative symptoms in later life is uncertainty of the degree to which such symptoms represent the disease process, long-term medication side effects, negative sequelae of institutionalization, or poorer socioeconomic levels and outlooks (Davidson et al. 1995). In addition, up to two-thirds of older adults with chronic schizophrenia also manifest comorbid depressive symptoms or diagnoses, and this comorbidity is linked to poorer physical health and reduced social networks (Cohen et al. 1996). Reduced social networks are related to increased loneliness and decreased quality of life in older persons with schizophrenia (Cohen et al. 1997).

In general, symptoms of schizophrenia and psychoses are less severe in later life. Changes in the brain with aging may ameliorate symptoms. For example, decreases in dopamine with aging can reduce positive symptoms related to excessive dopamine in the brain (e.g., Finch and Morgan, 1987). To the extent that aging brings lower arousal levels and increasing physical frailty, older adults with psychosis are generally less threatening to others than when they were younger.

However, the exception here is cognitive decline, which may be amplified in older adults with schizophrenia. Many aspects of the disease combine to bring about this situation, including cognitive sequelae of the disorder, medication side effects, institutionalization, lower educational and employment opportunities, and the aging process itself (Cohen et al. 2000). These cognitive changes may also negatively impact on social relationships and functioning (Harvey et al. 1998). This is unfortunate, since social support is highly predictive of positive adaptations to the illness in later life (Meeks et al. 1990).

Cognitive aging seems to proceed at a similar rate of decline among schizophrenics as in normal aging. However, early onset schizophrenics show cognitive deficits from around the beginning of the illness (Jeste et al. 2011). Throughout life, people with schizophrenia show some deficits in cognitive functioning, especially in attention and other executive functioning. Long-term treatment can also leave clients with side effects from the medication that can have an impact on appearance and functioning (e.g., tardive dyskinesia), and sometimes on cognitive functioning. Although the side effects of medications such as lithium are not as severe for patients with bipolar disorders, cognitive declines are apparent in patients with late-onset bipolar disorder above and beyond what would be expected with normal aging (Depp and Jeste 2004).

In contrast, emotional and social functioning tend to improve over time in schizophrenia and bipolar disorder, although are likely to remain at a lower level than for those aging without psychosis. Greater social supports may have many benefits for the older individual, as well as assist with the therapy process, but one stumbling block, particularly for older individuals who have coped with chronic mental illness for most of their life, is that their social networks, even family ties, may be frayed. Assisting with social ties may form one goal of the therapy.

As noted in the introductory comments, like the rest of us, older people with psychoses accumulate experience and learn from their experiences. In general, they tend to mature in their coping styles, experience some reduction in negative emotionality, and some reduction in general arousal levels (Jeste et al. 2011). Cohen et al. (2011) found a similar structure of coping styles among older schizophrenics as in community elderly of similar age, with the use of active cognitive coping styles, rather than the avoidance predominant among older adults with schizophrenia (Case Example 9.2). All such adaptation and slow accumulation of coping strategies occurs within the context of their illness, and its particular influence on their lives, and in the context of contacts with the mental health system and attempts to treat their illness. The availability or lack of social support networks may also influence coping, for better or worse. Thus, their overall level of functioning is generally lower than that of people without psychosis, and their lives have been more chaotic with the interruptions of psychotic episodes and treatment for them.

Case Example 9.2 Sophia: therapy with person with paranoid schizophrenia

Sophia was over 70 and a cultured, well-groomed Polish-American woman. She moved and spoke with great dignity. She was well-educated for her cohort with some post-secondary education. She had been married to a professional man and her son was an engineer who was doing well. Her husband had died more than 10 years earlier, and she described a normal if difficult grieving process. She had moved to Chicago and lived in the Polish community there for several years, returning to California about 3 years prior to our first contact. She had not done well since her return. In the previous year, she had been kicked out of three residential care facilities for hostility or bizarre behavior, and had been admitted to the county inpatient psychiatric unit each time and to the state hospital twice. It was felt that she had finally been stabilized on antipsychotic medication during this last admission.

There were disputes with landlords and neighbors, then she moved into residential care, and experienced a number of arguments and fights there. Most of these disputes involved her confronting people whom she knew were conspiring to kill her, kidnap her, or who were poisoning her food. She was anti-Semitic and still quite fearful of Nazis. Her delusions centered on plots by Jews, the FBI, and the Gestapo.

Since she had been primed by her counselor at the hospital for our relationship, she virtually instantly formed a strong attachment for BK. She was impressed by my specializing in working with older people and by my educational background. She had also decided, after the multiple hospitalizations, that she needed to take her "nerve medication."

Her conversations were often quite normal and free from distortion. We discussed her problems in adjusting to the residential care home in which she lived. She had some normal disagreements and conflicts with other residents. She felt a sense of loss over her declining social status. We discussed in some detail her past in Poland and in southern California while her husband still lived. She was surprised, hurt, and saddened to find herself a psychiatric patient living in residential care homes.

With her permission, I accompanied her into the psychiatrist's office, and described her increasing nervousness as she got into conflicts with residents or the owners. She was always more candid about her delusions with me than with the psychiatrist. She frequently began to wonder if the owners had connections to the Gestapo. At one point she became convinced that they were operating a house of prostitution with the other female residents (all over 75, and either demented or chronically mentally ill) as the "girls." Changes in medication generally reduced these concerns within the week. Our visits continued on a once or twice per month basis.

She drew a great sense of security from our visits and from our relationship. She tended to view me as a powerful and protective person. Gradually, she came to accept my advice about the reality of some of her fears or at least the likelihood that she was in immediate danger. When she was becoming more delusional, her comfort was often simply in the equally delusional conviction that I was a powerful and protective authority who could hold the FBI at bay.

In working with older adults with chronic mental illness, drawing on this past experience of how they have come to understand their illness and what they have learned from past treatment efforts, both positive and negative, is a rich resource for intervention. Stresses and novel social situations in later life may require new problem solving as well, but drawing on past experience can guide the solution and provide the client with confidence in their ability to cope with the new problems.

Social contexts

For older adults with psychosis, if the physical changes or social circumstances of later life necessitate a move into a senior housing environment, the increased contact with others can be a stress that can upset even a decades-long adjustment. Many older adults whose psychosis is under a fair degree of control manage moderately well with minimal social contact, or with contact with people who are well known to them and who understand their illness. Living in congregate housing environments of any type, from independent living to skilled nursing care, puts the older person with psychosis into increased contact with others, which can be stressful in itself. The other older adults in the senior housing environment may not be tolerant of the eccentricities of a person with chronic residual psychosis, and are certainly likely to react poorly to positive symptoms of psychosis.

The lack of understanding of serious mental illness on the part of many staff members working in senior housing environments often leads to evolving problems being ignored until a crisis point is reached. Once the crisis is reached, the desire is often to have the older person with psychosis removed from the setting. It can take several repeated examples of this pattern for a mental health consultant to educate staff that problems can often be ameliorated with much less stress for all concerned if the request for mental health consultation comes early in the process. Staff in senior settings are likely to need education in recognizing early warning signs of escalating psychosis, and education and reassurance about their ability to cope with such presentations when they arise.

Cohort issues

Cohort issues specific to older adults often arise from their experiences of mental health treatment in earlier decades (see Case Example 9.3). Mental health policy and treatment changes over time. Within the memory of older mental health clients, the United States has moved from state psychiatric hospital care with long stays, to community-based care and short inpatient admissions, to massive cutbacks in the mental health system. In other countries, health care systems reorganized in part as a reaction to the 2008 global financial crisis. In addition,

Case Example 9.3 Mildred: cohort issues in working with long-term seriously mentally ill person

BK first met Mildred while running a satellite outreach office in a Housing Authority apartment building on the lower income side of town. She came to see me in some distress, and very concerned that she would be labeled as "crazy" and put away. Her concern was somewhat vague in focus, but she felt that one of her current caseworkers for an aging support services program did not like her very much and might try to have her institutionalized because of her mental health treatment background.

In fact, Mildred had spent a number of years of her life in mental health treatment. She had been in and out of state psychiatric hospitals throughout her adult life. The episodes of treatment had lasted from weeks to years. Her recollection was that she had usually been diagnosed as suffering from depression, but had also been labeled as having schizophrenia several times and once as being retarded.

At the time that BK first met her, she had not been in the state facility in more than 10 years and had been hospitalized once or twice during that time for a few days each time in the county psychiatric ward. She had lived in various board and care homes, and had follow-up psychiatric care for medication, as well as follow-up casework through a special program for persons released from psychiatric inpatient hospitals. At this time, she was not on medication, and was living in a subsidized apartment with in-home supportive services and had caseworkers in both of those programs.

One of her concerns was over the likelihood of being readmitted to the state hospital. I reassured her that this was considerably more difficult at the present than it had been at the time of her last admission. I further explained how such decisions were made and that, unless the circumstances were extreme, as her therapist I would effectively have veto power over an attempt to admit her. This information was highly reassuring for her.

In this context, we discussed her prior admissions to state hospitals. She had been admitted once by her father when she was a young woman. She professed to have no idea why this admission had taken place. One of her husbands (she had been married and divorced four times) had dropped her off at the hospital as they were breaking up after a stormy relationship. She had been admitted once after an overdose. Her more recent admissions for short stays had generally involved arguments with people where she was staying. Although always charming with me, she clearly had a tendency to get into disagreements with other people that accelerated rapidly into agitated confrontations. She had, however, never hit anyone nor been hit during one of these arguments.

With the immediate crisis resolved, Mildred then became quite depressed. She was acutely aware of being labeled as a mental patient. I was surprised by the latter because unlike some other older people with long histories of psychiatric treatment, there was nothing in her appearance or mannerisms to suggest long-term mental illness. She revealed to me that she often volunteered the information to people as she got to know them, sometimes in initial conversations. She would then be insulted or hurt by the remarks people made or by their withdrawal.

I suggested that there was really no point in bringing up her history. After discussing the injustice and the inaccuracy of the stigma at some length, she acknowledged that it was unlikely that she would change anyone's mind, and that her goal should be improved contact with people. She reduced the frequency of her self-disclosure, and her daily interactions with people improved rather dramatically over the next several months.

> With the concern about the labeling and stereotyping by others out of the way, her own negative self-evaluation came to the foreground. Mildred was seriously distressed by her chaotic and unsuccessful life. She had been quite bright and attractive as a young woman. She had worked in the civil service at one time and had wanted to complete college. Instead, she had four ex-husbands and, she revealed at this point, a daughter in a neighboring state from whom she was estranged for reasons she either did not know or did not want to discuss.
>
> She had multiple psychiatric hospital admissions and had lived on disability due to psychiatric problems most of her life. She had felt most productive and most "at home" during one admission lasting several years when she had a responsible job in the state hospital laundry and a good relationship with one of the psychiatrists. Out of the hospital, her life had been spent in marginal jobs (she bragged of having once been a "taxi dancer"), residential care homes, or single room occupancy hotels, and sometimes lying about suicidal impulses or hearing voices to get back in the hospital.

new medications are discovered and come into use, the side effects of old ones become obvious with widespread use over time, and some fall out of favor. The use of electric shock therapy was common with diagnoses of psychosis in the middle of the twentieth century, fell out of favor almost entirely, and then returned with different procedures and a more narrowly defined scope of use (usually restricted to depression now). Psychosurgery was used more in the mid-twentieth century than in the early twenty-first century. Older clients will remember this history, many will have experienced it, and may have lasting effects from it, good or bad. It may be important to acknowledge these problematic contacts with the mental health system in the patient's past.

Clients can also gain confidence and increased understanding from life review that includes their experience with their illness and its treatment. Mental health treatments have changed over the decades, and so these life histories often include important past experiences with treatments no longer considered effective or appropriate. This can include medications that were eventually found to have severe side effects and are no longer used, the closing of some psychiatric hospitals, and in some cases use of electroshock or insulin shock treatments. Some of these treatments and the patient's reactions to them may have generalized to mental health practitioners in general – an idea that the psychologist should be cognizant of. Helping clients put their own experience with these discontinued treatments into historical perspective can be useful to them.

Cultural issues

While professionals certainly need to aware of the cultural context of clients and be alert to any tendency to interpret cultural differences as due to mental disorders (e.g., a certain degree of suspiciousness in social situations and in dealing with authorities for many disadvantaged cultural minorities is probably realism, rather than paranoia), the opposite tendency is also a problem in accurate diagnosis (see Case Example 9.4). Symptoms of mental disorder may be incorrectly attributed to cultural differences. In our experience, the combination of age and cultural differences may make this particularly likely.

> **Case Example 9.4 Sam: recognizing paranoid disorder in near homeless African-American client**
>
> Sam was a 71-year-old African American who lived in a single room occupancy hotel near Skid Row in Los Angeles. He had been referred for depression by his caseworker in a social services program for older adults. His trainee therapist had seen him for several months, developed a good relationship, and was using CBT methods to work on improving his mood. The goals involved both increasing pleasant activities and working on his thoughts about interpersonal interactions, which were often negative. In fact, as time went on, a recurrent theme in his interactions with others was suspicion that they were going to steal from him or that they were thinking negative or hostile thoughts about him. After an argument with a bus driver apparently got very heated and resulted in Sam being put off the bus, we began to re-evaluate his diagnosis and consider the likelihood that he had a long-term psychosis with paranoid symptoms. His history of mental health diagnoses or treatment was unknown to us, although Sam readily admitted having had several therapists and having been in therapy much of his adult life. He had never married and had seldom held a job. He had lived on a disability pension prior to changing over to an age-based pension. He was evasive about the nature of the disability. In Sam's case, his African-American background and his immersion in a subculture of poverty in the Skid Row area seemed to disguise his mental disorder for caseworkers and others in his environment.

In countries with large immigrant populations, issues of acculturation and varying degrees of acculturation between family members may also be an issue. In working with families of persons with bipolar disorder or psychosis, for whom acculturation may be an issue, sensitivities to mental illness as a stigma may vary among family members, as may an individual's embrace of Western treatment approaches.

Issues in therapy with older adults with bipolar disorder and psychoses

Psychotropic medications will, of course, be a major element of the treatment of psychosis in older adults. The medications can also become a focus of the client's thinking about what is wrong with their lives. In a pattern also often seen in people with chronic physical illness, the client may blame the medication for making them ill or the medications may become part of the delusional system. Once a rapport is established, the psychotherapist can play a role in helping clients to think more realistically about the medication. As in the example of Sophia, the therapist may play a role in conveying symptom changes to the prescribing psychiatrist and also in helping the client to see a role for the medication in her treatment.

Psychological interventions with older adults with serious mental illness can take the form of organized psychosocial programs, with a focus on psychoeducation about the disorder and on building social skills (McCarthy et al. 2008). These approaches are common with younger adults with serious mental illness, but some adaptations with older persons can be useful. As noted by McCarthy et al. (2008), these adaptations can include changes in scheduling to accommodate older adults' more limited mobility and difficulties using public transportation, changes to adjust to older adults' sensory changes, and a greater focus on dealing with the health care system and health care professionals as part of the social skills training classes. Given the physical medical problems experienced by older schizophrenics, a greater focus on physical medical assessment and management of physical illnesses is also an important age adjustment.

On an individual therapy basis, there is evidence for the effectiveness of cognitive therapy for older people with psychosis (Kingdon et al. 2008). The work requires starting with the client's understanding of their problems and symptoms, and then working with them to learn the antecedents, beliefs, and consequences that seem to be associated with the hallucinations or delusions. The work requires flexibility on the therapist's part in responding to changes in topic due to the client's shifting attentional focus or to manage the client's level of distress when discussing difficult topics (Kingdon et al. 2008). As with the psychosocial programs, some focus on helping the client understand the condition and its role in their lives, in terms that the individual client can understand and find acceptable, is important.

A key difference in working with people with psychosis is that the nature of the therapeutic relationship can be quite distinct. The warmth and empathic understanding that is a common part of therapy with clients who have depression or anxiety can be anxiety-arousing for people with psychosis. The therapist is kind, but needs to read the client's non-verbal cues carefully and may need to be more reserved than with other types of clients. Staying calm, and projecting confidence and strength, no matter how bizarre the client's thinking or behavior, can be more important than warmth.

In general, it is important not to lie to clients, especially those with paranoid ideation. Learning to avoid arguing about delusions and hallucinations, while also not appearing to endorse their reality is an important skill in working with psychosis. In most instances, the scattered thinking of loose associations and the bizarre thinking of delusions and hallucinations are best handled by remaining quiet but attentive and by responding verbally to the more reality oriented and understandable elements of the client's conversation.

Psychological intervention often involves a combination of stress management training and problem solving in order to help clients avoid levels of stress that set up acute episodes, and to handle the vicissitudes of life with a chronic psychosis. The triggers for stress are likely to be much less intense than for other clients and may be based in unrealistic perceptions of the world. For Sophia, her stress over feeling that she was living in a house of prostitution was alleviated by focusing on the fact that she was not being asked to sell herself personally. Given the overall lower level of functioning, the problem solving is likely to be about more basic issues of life than is often true with older clients without psychosis. For Sam, the problem solving focused on what he could do to be able to continue to take the bus and how he could react differently when he felt a bus driver might have a bad opinion of him.

Summary

Advances in the assessment and treatment of older persons with psychotic disorders and bipolar disorders have lagged behind advances in assessment and intervention with other disorders, such as anxiety and depression. Often health care professionals are poorly informed about the presentations of psychotic disorders and bipolar disorders in later life. Social support networks for these individuals are often poor and present a challenge for the therapist. More research on such disorders, as well as longitudinal studies examining trajectories and impacts on health and well-being over the lifespan, is needed in this area.

In the next chapter, we move on to the discussion of personality disorders. Long-standing personality issues are often the reason that therapy for depression, anxiety, and other disorders may become more difficult and take longer.

Chapter 10

Personality disorders in older adults

Introduction to personality disorders in older adults

Personality disorders were first located on a separate axis for diagnostic purposes in the third edition of the American Psychiatric Association's Diagnostic and Statistical Manual of Mental Disorders (DSM-III; American Psychiatric Association 1980), although the first appearance of personality disorders was in 1952, in the first edition of the DSM. The original rationale for this placement on a separate axis was to encourage clinicians to consider the possibility of the influence of a personality disorder on the psychiatric symptoms of all of their patients presenting for interview, and was congruent with an idea current at the time that such personality disorders were more common than suspected and that disturbances in personality significantly influenced presentations of other Axis I disorders (Frances 1980). The separate axis for personality disorders was retained in iterations of DSM-IV, but was abandoned in DSM-5 (American Psychological Association 2013). One problem that remains in the DSM-5 is the considerable overlap in the criterion for the various personality disorders discussed in the literature (e.g., Farmer 2000).

In early work on personality disorders in later life, Abrams and Horowitz (1999) reported the overall prevalence of personality disorders at approximately 10% in persons over the age of 50. Schuster et al. (2013) used data from the National Epidemiological Survey on Alcohol and Related Conditions to examine the prevalence and medical and psychosocial correlates of personality disorders on older Americans aged over 65 years. They found that just over 8% of their sample of 8205 adults presented with at least one personality disorder, with obsessive-compulsive personality disorder being the most prevalent (5.25%); see Table 10.1 for the prevalence of all personality disorders in the survey. Men were significantly more likely than women to have antisocial or schizoid personality disorders. Marriage or cohabitation appeared to lower risk of personality disorders in later life, with never-married persons more at risk for avoidant or schizoid personality disorders, divorced persons more at risk for paranoid or histrionic personality disorders, and widowed

Table 10.1 Prevalence of lifetime DSM-IV personality disorders in individuals aged 65 years and older in the National Epidemiological Survey on alcohol and related conditions.

Personality Disorders	N	Percent	SE
Avoidant	68	0.81	0.11
Dependent	23	0.29	0.07
Obsessive—compulsive	392	5.25	0.30
Paranoid	166	1.75	0.17
Schizoid	149	1.70	0.17
Histrionic	51	0.58	0.09
Antisocial	41	0.60	0.12

Note: Percentages are weighted values.

Reprinted from American Journal of Geriatric Psychiatry, 21, Schuster, J.-P., Hoertel, N., Le Strat, Y., Manetti, A., & Limosin, F., Personality disorders in older adults: Findings from the national epidemiological survey on alcohol and related conditions, 757-768, Copyright (2013), with permission from Elsevier.

persons more at risk for obsessive compulsive or paranoid personality disorders. A variety of cardiac and gastrointestinal disorders were associated with specific personality disorders, and overall older persons with personality disorders (except for those with histrionic and antisocial personality disorders), were more likely than those without a personality disorder to report higher scores on a mental disability scale (the Short-Form 12 Health Survey, version 2; Ware et al. 2002).

Van Alphen et al. (2006a) reported that the prevalence of personality disorders in later life ranged from 2.8% to 13% in community settings, from 5% to 33% among outpatients, and from 7% to 61.5% among inpatients. This latter data on older persons in inpatient and outpatient settings echoes the Schuster et al. (2013) finding of poorer mental and physical health associated with the presence of a personality disorder diagnosis later in life.

Personality disorders in later life have begun to attract more significant research efforts. More work in this area is badly needed, particularly with respect to refinements in diagnostic criteria and assessment measures that may be applied to older adults (Oltmanns and Balsis 2011). Yet despite this increase in scrutiny, many clinically relevant aspects of personality disorders have not received the attention they should. For example, the cross-cultural validity of the criteria for personality disorders as well as the instruments that purport to measure them is relatively inadequate (Okazaki et al. 2002). Existing cross-cultural studies are mainly confined to documenting differences in presentations rather than the mechanisms underlying variations in the presentations of personality disorders (Okazaki et al. 2002; Widiger and Samuel 2005). Age-biases within diagnostic criteria for personality disorders have not received as much attention as is warranted; for example, the dependency exhibited in older adults with chronic illness might be inappropriately labeled as reflecting a dependent personality disorder, whereas many of the more extreme behaviors evident in younger persons with a personality disorder may be muted in older persons due to lower energy levels, physical frailty, etc. (Abrams 1991).

Age of onset of personality disorders is in late adolescence and early adulthood (American Psychological Association 2013). At the time of diagnosis, irrespective of age, the clinician should be mindful that the symptoms of another psychiatric condition (e.g., mood or substance abuse disorder) may be confounded with symptoms of a personality disorder, that personality disorders may be comorbid with a range of psychiatric conditions, and that in turn the presence of a personality disorder can make it much more difficult to accurately diagnose a psychiatric condition such as a mood or substance abuse disorder (Dolan-Sewell et al. 2001; Farmer 2000; Widiger and Coker 2002). If a patient presents with a high degree of distress, it may be difficult to ascertain the characteristic modes of approaching others and that could signal the presence of a personality disorder.

Personality disorders, because of their persistence and their disruptive influence on interpersonal, occupational, and functional capacity, can have profound effects on health and well-being (Agronin and Maletta 2000). Personality disorders in older adults result in increased use of health and mental health systems (Rosowsky and Gurian 1992). Adjusting and adapting to the sequelae of aging may also be hampered by the presence of a personality disorder (Agronin and Maletta 2000). Longitudinal research suggests a reduction in prevalence of personality disorders in later life, possibly due in part to a maturing, softening stance with respect to interactions with the environment (Kenan et al. 2000; Paris 2003). However, as with other disorders such as depression, it may be that the expression of symptoms of personality disorders varies across the lifespan, and that diagnostic criteria and assessment tools to date remain only modestly capable of capturing this diversity.

The assessment of personality disorders in older adults has received specific attention relatively recently, although assessment tools in particular lag behind geriatric assessment tools for other psychiatric disorders (Agronin and Maletta 2000). Accurate detection of personality disorders in later life has not been helped by age-biases in diagnostic criteria, as well as the lack of instruments to accurately assess personality disorders in this cohort (Oltmanns and Balsis 2011). An additional concern when testing older cohorts has been the length of self-report instruments, and the time-consuming and user-unfriendly nature (e.g., modern or abstract language) of the structured and semi-structured instruments, which were largely designed to detect disordered personality in younger populations (van Alphen et al. 2006b).

Balsis et al. (2007) conducted a large, cross-sectional study in the general population (age range 18–98 years) using item-response theory; their analyses demonstrated that 29% of the DSM-IV-TR criteria for personality disorders lead to measurement errors when applied to older people. Such data is discouraging, to say the least. Yet accurate assessment of personality disorders is vital if effective treatments for patients, as well as accurate advice for referring health care professionals, are to be provided. Clearly, more research on assessment of personality disorders in geriatric populations is required.

In outpatient practice, the presence of a personality disorder may be recognized in early sessions of therapy when the client's history is characterized by decades-long problems in interpersonal functioning. More frequently in our experience, the personality disorder becomes apparent after working with a client on depression or anxiety for several weeks, and noting that little progress is being made and the therapeutic relationship with the client is more complex or demanding than usual.

In some settings there may be a reluctance to diagnose personality disorders in older adults. The combination of the perceived intractability of personality disorders combined with a person of advanced age, leading to assumptions about the limited nature and efficacy of treatment options, has been suggested to lead to such a diagnostic bias (e.g., Rose et al. 1993). In older adults with multiple comorbidities of physical, neurological, and psychiatric disorders, the signs of a personality disorder may become lost against this background noise. In addition, some of the hallmarks of personality disorders, such as eccentric behaviors or social withdrawal, may be mistaken by professional staff, as well as patients and their families, as being more easily ascribed to growing older, rather than to psychiatric disturbance (Segal and Coolidge 2001).

Personality disorders can also be encountered in consultations regarding difficult patients of physicians or difficult residents in 24-hour care settings or group residences of any kind for older adults. However, clinicians should be alert to the possibility of both failing to detect a pre-existing personality disorder, as well as potentially mislabeling aberrant behavior as a personality disorder. A difficult patient's behavior (e.g., dependency, aggressiveness) may be labeled by the staff as stemming from a personality disorder, in the absence of corroborating symptoms, but particularly the lack of any indication of an onset of the personality disorder in late adolescence or early adulthood. Labeling a patient as "narcissistic," "dependent," or "borderline" may serve as an effective rationale for staff in residential care settings to not look for environmental triggers and instead essentially blame the person with dementia for behaviors. This is not to say that patients with a pre-existing personality disorder are somehow absent in long-term care settings.

While certainly not the only cause underlying behaviors of concern, personality disorders may contribute to why the patient or resident is being perceived as difficult in ways that the referring person has difficulty articulating. In all cases, but particularly in 24-hour care settings, insisting upon some evidence of the presence of disturbed personality functioning in late adolescence or young adulthood is one means of ensuring the accuracy of such a diagnosis, or clarifying that it may be another psychiatric disorder mimicking a personality disorder (Triebwasser and Shea 1996). While issues such as disentangling potential comorbid psychiatric disorders and personality disturbance may be an issue at any age, in older adults with additional comorbid medical illnesses and potentially poorly documented early history, this task is more complicated still.

Assessment of personality disorders in late life

Assessment of older adults with personality disorder should, in principle, follow what is both a general assessment strategy for detecting psychopathology, but also one endorsed by those writing about personality disorder assessment more particularly: namely, it is sensible to first screen for presence of signs of the disorder, then assess more specifically with specialized instruments. This view has been articulated in several chapters in this book. That is, when evaluating depression, a screening instrument such as the Geriatric Depression Scale (GDS: Yesavage et al. 1982) might be followed, for example, by a lengthier, structured clinical interview, if warranted by the screening results, so as to ascertain a diagnosis. Self-report screens and such brief symptom-based measures are useful for detection, as well as documenting changes to symptom levels over time and certainly over the course of treatment. With regard to personality disorders in later life, this approach is hampered by the lack of adequate screening tools for this population.

In the case of personality disorders, ideally, a brief self-report inventory designed to gauge disturbance of personality functioning should be followed, if needed, by a semi-structured or structured interview to confirm the diagnosis of a particular personality disorder (Widiger 2002). The use of semi-structured and structured interviews greatly increases the reliability of the diagnosis of personality disorders (Segal and Coolidge 2003; Wood et al. 2002). Examples of well-validated, longer, structured clinical interviews include the Structured Clinical Interview for DSM-IV Personality Disorders (SCID-II; First et al. 1997) and the Structured Interview for DSM-IV Personality (SIDP-IV; Pfohl et al. 1997). Such structured interviews are lengthy (typically 50–90 minutes), hence the attraction of a briefer screening tool, particularly in a busy clinical practice environment.

However, to date a reliable screening tool, particularly for use with older adults with a suspected personality disorder, has yet to emerge. Furthermore, although it might seem that reliance on a screen initially may result in missed diagnoses of a personality disorder, on the whole, such screens have been shown to result in more false-positives (Widiger and Coker 2002). Finally, given that most persons with a personality disorder may lack insight into the nature of their disorder and consequences of their behaviors, measures that are heavily reliant on self-report may be suspect in such circumstances (Segal and Coolidge 2001).

For a full discussion of the relative merits and short-comings of structured, semi-structured, and self-report measures, the interested reader is referred to Widiger and Samuels (2005). In essence, Widiger and Samuels consider the indices of reliability and validity of general measures of personality disorders for all age groups, in light of the high level of overlap in the criteria for specific personality disorders, as well as the presence in studies to date of participants with multiple comorbid personality disorders. A conclusion reached by these and other authors is that the high level of overlap in symptomatology presents significant challenges to the clinician wishing to accurately assess for the presence of a personality disorder (see Case Example 10.1A).

Case Example 10.1A Ms. H: assessment of personality disorder

Ms. H was in her 60s and had been laid off from her work 15 years before being seen in therapy. She also had multiple physical problems and was severely depressed. While some of the physical problems were diagnosed and being treated by physicians, she was generally dissatisfied with treatment and tended to have severe side effects with most treatment regimens. In addition to these problems, she frequently had additional symptoms for which she sought diagnoses and treatments, many of which led to stressful diagnostic procedures and null results. Others would lead to a period of active treatment that made her feel even worse due to her reactions to the medications. Her history of medical illness with unsatisfactory resolution was now complicated by disorders associated with later life such as arthritis, which were causing decreasing quality of life.

Ms. H had never been married and had a limited history of relationships of any kind. She reported being raised by parents who were emotionally cold and hypercritical. Earlier in life, she had maintained only superficial relationships with other people, and had changed jobs and cities on a fairly regular basis. Currently, she reported being almost completely socially isolated with little contact with people other than her physicians. Her expectations of care and caring from the physicians were unrealistically high, and led to constant disappointment and feelings of being rejected by them when diagnosis or treatment did not go well. She acknowledged that part of her expectations stemmed from an idea that "I'm too old to put up with this pain anymore—I need results from these people, not excuses." It appeared that her pain levels were increasing, and her family physician speculated that this might be driving her increasing medical visits.

The referral for Ms. H. had mentioned only depression, but in the initial interview the psychologist felt that Ms. H's answers to questions about her social and occupational history suggested the possibility of an underlying personality disorder. For example, Ms. H described herself as never "taking" to people, to having few acquaintances and no close friends, and to working largely in jobs where contact with others was minimized. She viewed herself as socially inept and actively avoided activities where she felt she could be embarrassed in front of others. The psychologist felt that the reported levels of social isolation and generally a low level of functionality most probably reflected an avoidant personality disorder. The psychologist felt a need to explore the potential issue of a personality disorder in the initial assessment, especially given the lack of progress with treatment for depression in a recent inpatient stay. However, because of Ms. H's multiple medical problems, which included severe fatigue as well as pain, he felt she would not tolerate a longer personality interview.

With respect to structured clinical interviews, the SCID–II has a solid empirical base with respect to reliability and validity (First et al. 1997). The SCID–II also requires that each diagnostic criterion be evident over a 5-year period, which goes some way toward establishing the presence of the personality disorder prior to the current episode of distress. Since it includes screening questions that allow interviewers to focus only on those personality disorders that seem indicated, the SCID-II could be used effectively in clinical practice provided the clinician takes the time to avail themselves of the available training materials.

The SIDP-IV takes 60–90 minutes to administer, compared with an average of 50 minutes for the SCID-II. The items are generally open-ended and are scored on a four-point Likert scale. The SIDP-IV also includes a 20-minute informant interview. The literature suggests that agreement between patient- and informant-descriptions of symptoms of personality disorders is largely only poor to adequate, with levels of agreement varying considerably between specific personality disorders (Klonsky et al. 2002). However, Klonsky and colleagues also point out that despite levels of disagreement, the patient and a reliable informant may both contribute unique and valuable information to an assessment of personality disorder. Such information from an informant may assist in overcoming both constraints on the ability to self-reflect, as well as the tendency to give socially acceptable responses on assessment (Kane 2000). While information from collateral sources can help resolve issues of past behavior and can assist in differential diagnoses (Segal and Coolidge 2001), this again lengthens the interview process. The SIDP-IV requires that a personality trait be prominent for most of the preceding 5 years to be considered part of the individual's personality functioning style. Like the SCID-II, the SIDP-IV has solid psychometric properties (Pfohl et al. 1997). However, all of these clinical interviews require significant investment of time, as well as significant clinical experience and judgment to achieve high diagnostic fidelity (Segal and Coolidge 2001).

Yet it must be said that shorter instruments may be particularly problematic with regard to diagnosing personality disorders accurately. As one research team suggests of screening instruments versus longer assessment tools to measure personality disorders, "those that are reliable are not quick and those that are quick are not reliable . . ." (Van Horn et al. 2000, p. 29).

Given the desire in many settings for a briefer initial screening of personality disorders, use of such tools naturally appeals to the geropsychologist. However, there are few screening tools for personality disorders that have been developed and validated for use in older persons. For example, the Gerontological Personality Disorders Scale (GPS) was developed specifically to screen for personality disorders in older adults (van Alphen et al. 2006a,b). The instrument consists of two parts, one self-report and the other completed by an informant—the response format is simply yes or no. In the original sample, the items were administered to patients in their Dutch care settings via questions written on cards (see Box 10.1 for sample items from the scale). The instrument shows some promise, but psychometric issues including low sensitivity (45%) could be further examined and possibly improved. An additional limitation is that specific personality disorders cannot be assessed with this instrument.

Box 10.1 Sample of items from the Gerontological Personality Disorders Scale

- I don't like growing older because I become less attractive.
- I'm often afraid of losing those who care for me, such as members of the family or my partner.
- At important times in my life I've had a lot of trouble with nerves, stress, or moodiness.
- At the most I've only had one acquaintance or friend in my life.

An alternate choice of a relatively brief means of evaluating the presence of personality disorders in older adults is the use of a shortened structured clinical interview, which although potentially more time-consuming than a very brief screener, still requires less administration time than longer instruments such as the SCID-II discussed above. Examples of such interviews include the short version of the SCID-II (10 SCID-II; Germans et al. 2010); the Standardized

Assessment of Personality—Abbreviated Scale (SAPAS; Moran et al. 2003); and the Iowa Personality Disorder Screen (IPDS; Langbehn et al. 1999). However, to date to our knowledge there have been no studies on the reliability and validity of these shorter inventories on older adult populations specifically.

Given the dearth of instruments, clinicians are faced with several choices. Although not yet validated with older adults, the IPDS has the advantage of structured interview questions that take approximately 5 minutes to administer (Langbehn et al. 1999). Sensitivity and specificity of the IPDS are reported by Langbehn and colleagues in the original development study as 92% and 79%, respectively. The SAPAS has not been validated with older populations specifically, but is in increasingly wide use, with robust psychometric properties (94% sensitivity and 85% specificity) and good mapping onto personality clusters (Hesse and Moran 2010). The eight items on this measure are taken from the Standardized Assessment of Personality scale (SAP; Mann et al. 1981) and have a simple yes–no response set. A score of 3 or above was reported by Moran et al. (2003) to correctly identify the presence of a personality disorder in 90% of their clinical sample. Germans et al. (2010) report quite good sensitivity and specificity (78% each) for the shortened SCID-II screener in a direct comparison with the full SCID-II as the gold standard, using a cut-off score of 4; using this cut-off correctly classified 78% of the patients. The authors concluded that this brief screening test had good utility in outpatient psychiatric samples, and given the very good psychometric properties of the SCID-II, which has been used successfully with older populations (e.g., Devanand et al. 2000), this brief test could reasonably be applied to older patients (see Case Example 10.1B). It should be stated that the three brief screens described here are designed to be used to detect the presence of *any* personality disorder, rather than to diagnose either a specific personality disorder or personality disorder not otherwise specified (NOS).

> **Case Example 10.1B Ms. H: assessment of personality disorder (continued)**
>
> The psychologist administered the short version of the SCID-II personality disorders screen as he was conscious of Ms. H's medical conditions and tendency to fatigue easily. The screen suggested the presence of a personality disorder. Because of her lack of social supports due to a lifelong truncated social network, and her recent gravitation to a range of health practitioners due to her concerns about her various medical conditions, Ms. H. was not in a position to most effectively navigate her health care needs. Her medical carers felt put upon and unable to satisfy her demands, which in part stemmed from her maladaptive coping strategies. The psychologist, with permission, was able to contact Ms. H's key providers, inform them about her personality disorder, and also give them helpful strategies for managing her many requests. In therapy, Ms. H. worked on maintaining realistic expectations about what her medical providers could and could not assist with.

Part of her therapy aimed at improving her depression was to increase pleasant events, which included increasing her activities both on her own and with other people. Ms. H. had earlier in life been an active walker and she began to take up modest walking again. She also began volunteering 2 days a month in her local library branch, where she had gone for years as a patron. Finally, she negotiated with the therapist putting into practice more realistic expectations of the kinds of support she could and could not expect from her health care specialists. Although still generally avoidant in her dealings with persons other than her medical specialists, her care providers reported a decrease in her demands, as well as her overall number of contacts with their services. In addition, her depressive symptoms decreased over a period of several months.

The Millon Clinical Multiaxial Inventory–III (MCMI–III; Millon et al. 1997) is a general, broad-based measure of personality disorders that appears to be little affected by age and to have good clinical utility (Edelstein and Segal 2011). The Narcissistic, Histrionic, and Compulsive scales show a slight increase in scores with age, and all other scales show a small decrease (Edelstein and Segal 2011). It should be kept in mind, however, that it was designed for use in mental health settings and may yield a more pathological picture than is accurate when used in non-mental health settings, such as medical clinics and long-term care for the elderly. BK has used the scale with older adults in outpatient mental health settings to clarify suspected personality disorders. The test has often been useful in guiding approaches to difficult clients and in reframing perceived personality styles. In general, the results have tended to point to personality disorders or traits that were different from those suspected based on therapy sessions (e.g., diagnosis of dependent and avoidant traits in a difficult client who had been seen as possibly having borderline personality disorder).

There are no assessment tools to ascertain diagnosis of a personality disorder that have been developed and normed specifically for an older population. Age biases in diagnostic criteria, which appear to be largely unchanged in the DSM-5 (American Psychological Association 2013), coupled with the lack of even brief screening tools, hamper efforts on the diagnostic front. Nevertheless, if a clinician wishes to use tools designed for younger populations, they would be wise to keep in mind that these tools have not been validated on an older population, and hence their use and the conclusions drawn from them must be approached with caution.

What are some of the pitfalls of not having a geriatric-specific personality disorder screen or assessment inventory? For one thing, personality assessment tools that have been developed for younger adults, operating within a younger adult context, may not be appropriate for older adults operating within different contexts. On this point, Oltmanns and Balsis (2011) state that context (i.e., rarely leaving the home, no longer engaged in full time employment) will result in different answers to questions relevant to personality disorders, such as discomfort in being around others or whether behaviors interfere with occupational functioning. Current personality instruments lack face validity for older adults, which in turn affects how they respond to questions, thereby influencing reliability, validity, and utility more broadly (Balsis et al. 2009).

Therapy with older adults with a personality disorder

Developmental influences on personality disorders

Prevalence studies have generally led to the conclusion that personality disorders are less common in later life (e.g., Segal et al. 2006; Schuster et al. 2013; Zweig and Hillman 1999). Several researchers have observed that certain personality disorders associated with increased impulsiveness, such as antisocial personality disorder or borderline personality disorder, decrease in severity with increasing age (Arens et al. 2013; Paris and Zweig-Frank 2001, Stevenson et al. 2003). There have also been suggestions that some of the personality disorders characterized by high levels of risk taking (antisocial, borderline) make it less likely that those persons will live into old age. In any case, there is a fairly widespread clinical consensus that the personality disorders that manifest as behavior problems (e.g., borderline, narcissistic, antisocial) tend to lessen somewhat in severity with age.

In general, consistent with the positivity effect and generally better proactive emotion regulation with aging, the arousal dimension of emotions tends to decrease with aging, which could well tend to "dampen down" the intensity of the sadness or anger that drives these behavior problems (Charles 2011). However, it is also true that once in high arousal situations, older adults have more trouble down-regulating the arousal. There is also considerable evidence that most people develop improved coping skills with aging, in large part by giving up on ineffective coping strategies (e.g., Aldwin et al. 2007). Since personality disorders tend to be characterized in part by very poor outcomes in interpersonal relationships, decades of life experience can result in somewhat improved functioning (see Case Example 10.2). That is, while it is a characteristic of many personality disorders that the affected person does not readily learn from experience, they are often merely slow learners, rather than unable to learn at all. These observations are not meant to imply that the personality disorder is entirely resolved by life experience, but that the problem behaviors can be less extreme in later life than in younger adulthood. Thus, developmental considerations per se would seem to suggest that personality disorders would not worsen over time, and would likely show some improvement.

> **Case Example 10.2 Mrs. Q: improvement in personality disorder over adult lifespan**
>
> Mrs. Q, for example, was over 80 years old and was still working part time as a teacher. When she started therapy, she was involved in complex legal actions to try and keep her job. In her own descriptions of the work situation in therapy sessions, she was simultaneously angry about administrators' reluctance to assign classes to her and highly anxious about returning to teaching. At the same time, she had marital difficulties and at times considered herself separated while sharing living space with her husband, and considered eating out with him as one of the high points of her social life. Her history was characterized by multiple types of work over the decades, and an overall career that she saw as artistic and often rebellious with regard to employers and society more broadly. Her relationship history was also tumultuous, and her current marriage had been difficult from about 6 months after the marriage began. Although she was still having significant problems with relationships and a chaotic emotional life, her history suggested that she was doing better than she had as a younger woman.

On the other hand, the disorders that lead to withdrawal and passivity (e.g., avoidant, dependent) or to minimal interactions with others (schizoid, paranoid), may by their nature evade the kind of experiential learning that would help ameliorate the problems over time. Some older clients who are referred for depression are revealed over time to have these kinds of long-standing personality disorders. Many of the health care and aging services professionals who work with older adults overlook these kinds of problems, assuming that the social isolation of older clients is due to having outlived friends and family. While certainly possible, externally caused isolation in older adults is overestimated, and many older adults who are alone are those who have alienated or worn out friends and family with extreme dependency demands or passive self-defeating behavior.

To the extent that developmental aging is associated with higher risk for physical health declines and associated disability, with a resulting need to depend more on others, this increased dependency can exacerbate personality disorders of all kinds. The impact of late-life dependency on each personality disorder is a recurring theme in Segal et al.'s (2006) *Personality Disorders and Older Adults: Diagnosis, assessment and treatment*. As noted by Charles (2011), the vulnerabilities of chronic illness and disability tend to overwhelm the typical strengths of enhanced emotion regulation, even in healthy older adults.

Social context influences

One of the most dramatic social context changes for some older adults is the move into a group-living situation with other older adults. These can range from independent living, to assisted living, to skilled nursing care. The levels of care are distinct and, in general, as the level of care increases, so does the degree to which the older resident is interacting with staff for care needs, and is subject to more structure in the daily schedule, including more rules about behavior.

This move into group-living situations is a major transition for most people who enter a senior residence of some kind, especially those who have lived in their own single-unit housing for several decades. The increased social contact with other older adults and with staff can be especially difficult for older adults with personality disorders, who may well have reached a balance in their independent lives that involved limiting contact with others to those who were relatively accepting of their needs and behaviors. They may in fact have reached a successful balance that actually depended on a fairly high level of social isolation. Since the move into senior residential living is often related to the need for assistance and care, this higher level of dependence on others will be in direct conflict with the previous, and possibly successful, strategy of selective contact with others.

Requests for psychological consultations from staff are fairly often prompted by older adults with more manipulative styles of personality disorders or by those with dependent personality disorder (see Case Example 10.3). The former often cause problems by starting interpersonal conflicts (i.e., playing "Let's you and her fight.") and pitting residents and/or staff one against another, or family

> **Case Example 10.3 Mrs. M: personality disorder and life-long depression**
>
> Mrs. M was in her 80s and was being seen for depression. She had an adult life-long history of episodic depressions, including some brief hospitalizations. She was generally motivated and cooperative with outpatient therapy. Her life history was presented as one of life-long emotionally abusive relationships, first with an angry and critical mother, then with a husband (deceased several years at the time of the therapy) who was alcoholic, angry, and verbally abusive. She was passive and dependent, and devoutly religious. She lived in an independent living unit in a multi-level care residence for older adults, and took meals in the dining hall. Periodically, she had incidents in which she exploded in anger at another resident when she was frustrated by them. She found these incidents surprising and difficult to explain. In general, they seemed to be precipitated by criticism from other residents or by competition from other residents (e.g., for a specific seat in the dining hall). Her past history of being a victim, and her passivity and dependence on others led to her being very nice and helpful to others until she reached her limit, which she herself was largely unaware of. Her daughter would call the therapist to report the explosive incidents, together with the concern that her mother might be asked to leave the residence. Mrs. M's relationship with her daughter was complicated by a tendency to interpret criticism from the daughter as being like her late husband's anger at her.

members against staff. Those with dependent personality disorders are often initially liked, and find staff or residents who wish to help them out. Problems ensue when the need for help goes on and on, and overwhelms the helpers. Typically, staff are more emotional than usual about the consultation referral and either angry with, or overwhelmed and confused by, the resident being referred.

Cohort and cultural influences

Given the very limited research on personality disorders in general and the absence of longitudinal research, it is not surprising that there has been no attention to cohort differences, which require the more complex research designs of lifespan developmental psychology. Given the presumed connections between the Big Five personality factors and personality disorders (McCrae 2009; Widiger 1998), the existing evidence that there are cohort differences in levels of Big Five factors (e.g., Mroczek et al. 2006) suggests that cohort differences in personality disorders are likely. Following the same line of reasoning, the consistency of the Big Five factors across cultures (McCrae 2009) suggests that cultural differences in personality disorders may be relatively small. However, both of these potential influences need much more attention both in research studies and in careful clinical consideration that goes beyond the very common assertion that culture should be taken into account with respect to personality disorders.

Issues in working with older adults with personality disorders

A fairly common reaction to the idea of working with older adults with personality disorders is that the work will be very difficult if not impossible because of the length of time that the client has had the problem. On the other hand, the challenges of later life (illness, disability, caregiving, grief) and the different social environment of the post-retirement life style bring a lot of changes both within and outside of the person that can serve to motivate self-transformation in therapy. Also, as noted earlier, lowered emotional arousal levels and the accumulation of decades of life experience with the personality disorder can lead the older adult to both a desire and the ability to make changes. The awareness of death being near can also motivate the client to take steps to take care of unfinished business and to mend important relationships. That said, it is characteristic of personality disorders that they complicate therapy for depression and anxiety, and that they are slower to respond to intervention than depression and anxiety without comorbid personality disorder (Gradman et al. 1999).

Working with personality disorder often puts even more demand on the therapist to guide the therapeutic conversation, and to give the client negative feedback about aspects of their behavior, the way they relate to others, and so forth. Therapists in general, and younger therapists in particular, are often more reluctant to provide confrontive interpretations with older clients. In part, this is motivated by the training we get as children to be respectful and polite with our elders. It may also be rooted in a fear of hurting frail older adults. For some, it may grow out of a general therapeutic nihilism where older people are concerned, a feeling that they are unable or unwilling to change. On the whole, older adults are somewhat more responsive to such input than younger people with personality disorders. Of course, as with any client, a strong therapeutic relationship and good timing of the interpretations are key to the success of this strategy.

In general, working with personality disorders with older adults will change the focus of therapy to working on self-schema, rather than day-to-day thoughts and behaviors. With the much longer life history of the older client, there are a lot of examples to work with, and this can make it easier for both client and therapist to perceive patterns across relationships and problem situations that have arisen multiple times across the decades. On the other hand, the wealth of life history material provides the resistant client with the option of providing a lot of information, while omitting key aspects of life that may be very important to therapeutic progress. As with clients of any age, paying attention to shifts in topic or responses that seem somewhat tangential to the questions asked can be helpful. With older clients, it is also useful to keep track of which decades of life the client has talked about in depth, and which ones have been omitted or glossed over. It can also be useful to think about which thematic areas of life have been covered and which have not (e.g., work history, the history of family of origin and of adult life families, love and sex, religious or spiritual life, friendships, etc.).

Cheavens and Lynch (2008) note that in adapting dialectical behavior therapy to the treatment of older adults with depression and personality disorder, they found that older clients reported an over-reliance on past problem-solving strategies and information, and so they added a module on "Radical Openness." This involved a focus on the present, new information, and a "fresh, fixed, and fluid mind." They also added a focus on reducing bitterness through forgiving oneself and others.

As noted by James (2008), challenges of working at the schema level with personality disorder include the likelihood that the client has not had experience of life without the schema being active and so there are no counter-examples from the past to use in challenging schema. Mrs. M (described in "Social context influences" section) had a life-long conviction that no one had loved her and there must be something terribly wrong with her. She was unable to think of any counter-examples, and the therapist had only the daughter as a potential counter-example. Mrs. M was more focused on needing the love of a parent or a spouse. She also questioned the daughter's love due to the daughter's impatience with her, when in fact the daughter was overly stressed by work and caring for her mother.

There is also no prior experience with what the end goal of therapy would be like. It is likely that the client has relied on strategies such as maintenance (e.g., selecting relationships with people who do not elicit the schema), avoidance (e.g., not getting into situations that activate the schema), and compensation (e.g., acting inconsistently with the schema, but in ways that avoid activating it). In working with a man in his late 60s with long-standing depression and a combination of schizoid and avoidant personality disorders, we found that when the depression lifted, he did not recognize what being free of depression was like. It took additional work to get him to the point of being able to give up the self-schema of being a depressed person, and accepting his new life and image. The reluctance was motivated in part by a schema level belief that feeling happy would lead to negative consequences and so being depressed was self-protective.

Summary

Working with persons with personality disorders is challenging at any age. There may actually be some advantages in working with such patients later in the life course, as their emotional reactivity may be lessened while a willingness to tackle the personality disorder may be strong. Assessment with older adults with a suspected personality disorder is an area that greatly deserves more research, but progress is also predicated on better descriptions of the progression and presentations of personality disorders in later life.

Once one has experience and expertise in working with older adults, the training of the next generations of clinical geropsychologists becomes an important focus. Also, colleagues with more limited experience with older adult clients will ask for advice and assistance. Chapter 11 deals with supervision and consultation issues in the practice of geropsychology.

Chapter 11

Supervision and consultation in clinical geropsychology

Introduction to supervision and consultation in clinical geropsychology

Supervision in clinical psychology is an integral part of all aspects of a professional career, irrespective of what settings the psychologist practices in. From early steps in learning how to administer a Wechsler intelligence test, to later stages in a career where supervision of psychologists in training and consulting with new and established colleagues is common, supervision and consultation are important for all parties involved. The general goal in supervision is to insure ethical and competent treatment of the client, and to promote skills and professional development in the person being supervised (Reese et al. 2009). Supervision in clinical geropsychology may be more complex. As Qualls et al. (1995) noted, "The scope of supervision may be broader in geropsychology than in other specializations within psychology because the clients are so diverse, the supervisees often come from several disciplines with several levels of competence and expertise, and the settings are diverse" (p. 124).

In the general competencies model that describes competencies as involving attitudes, knowledge, and skills (e.g., Rodolfa et al. 2005), clinical supervision is critically involved in the development of attitudes and skills. While knowledge acquisition may also be a part of supervision, knowledge can also be acquired in classes, continuing education programs, and other didactic settings. Importantly, supervised clinical experience is the training method that assures that the knowledge base is applied in the clinical setting. Duffy and Morales (1997) noted: "Although important knowledge about aging processes may be efficiently provided in academic courses, effective learning is often limited by lack of clinical experience" (p. 373). They further note that "... there is a vast difference between supervised experience and experience alone" (p. 374).

With respect to geropsychology, we believe that supervision is critical for professional development. Often, first exposure to the field comes via supervision; this was the case for NP, who had not considered working with older adults until a geropsychology rotation in her internship year. In that year, working with an experienced geropsychology supervisor and an interdisciplinary geriatric team led to immersion in the field, and subsequent postdoctoral geropsychology experiences. For BK, while the initial interest in clinical geropsychology started in graduate school and focused first on didactics and knowledge acquisition, clinical supervision during internship and postdoctoral training was key to developing skills and attitudes in clinical geropsychology. The specific clinical skills for geropsychology practice, the introduction to the multiple settings of geropsychology practice, the skills for interprofessional teamwork essential to geropsychology practice, and the monitoring of the development of those skills and of the attitude competencies critical to effective practice with a wide range of older adults are all learned in supervision.

Consultation can cover a variety of activities in clinical geropsychology as in professional psychology more generally. In this chapter, we are using the term to refer to case consultation with colleagues about geropsychology issues. That process involves many of the same skills and activities as supervision, but without the professional oversight implied in supervision, since it occurs in a peer to peer context. We discuss case consultation specifically at the end of this chapter, but would note here that much of what we say about supervision throughout the chapter will also apply to peer consultation.

Competency in professional geropsychology training and practice

In a bid to more clearly articulate the competencies required both in training and practice in geropsychology, a set of competencies for professional geropsychology practice were developed during the National Conference on Training in Professional Geropsychology in 2006. This conference of expert clinicians and researchers in the geropsychology field, held in Colorado Springs, USA, produced the Pikes Peak Model for Geropsychology Training (Knight et al. 2009). Taken together, the competencies are aspirational in nature, rather than being required of any particular psychologist in order to practice with older adults. The Pikes Peak conference also led to the creation of the Council of Professional Geropsychology Training Programs (CoPGTP), based in the USA, but also comprised of foreign affiliate training programs. CoPGTP developed a competency evaluation tool for educators, supervisors, and practitioners to have a measure by which to gauge competence in serving older adults (Karel et al. 2010a).

The 50-item Pikes Peak Geropsychology Competency Assessment Tool is available in paper format and online (<http://www.gerocentral.org/copgtp/ppcat.php>) as a self-assessment for psychologists and trainees to evaluate their perceived competence in clinical practice with older adults. Each Pikes Peak geropsychology knowledge and skill competency is specified by behaviorally descriptive items, and can be rated along a continuum ranging from novice to expert. Areas of competency covered range across several domains, and include foundations of adult development and aging, geropsychology professional practice, assessment, intervention, and consultation. The tool is designed to evaluate the learner's knowledge base and skill set separately for the same domains, as the awareness of information, and the ability or experience to applying it in clinical contexts may differ. A preliminary validation of the Pikes Peak tool found that total scores differentiated well between professional geropsychologists and psychology graduate students (Karel et al. 2012). In a cross-national study of clinical psychology students' perceived competencies using the Pikes Peak tool, students enrolled in training programs with specialty geropsychology tracks, generally perceived themselves as being in the intermediate to advanced range of competence. Ratings from students not enrolled in training programs with such specialty tracks were significantly lower and were generally in the novice to intermediate range (Woodhead et al. 2013).

Attitude competencies in geropsychology training

The Pikes Peak model, like most discussions of competency-based training, divides competencies into attitude, knowledge, and skills competencies. Attitudes toward aging are an essential underlying element of competency to work with older adults. In general, people electing to focus on specialty training in geropsychology tend to have positive attitudes toward older adults. There are exceptions, however, and some combination of screening out those with inappropriate negative attitudes, and providing corrective teaching and experiences in supervision, are key elements of good training. In BK's experience, negative attitudes toward older adults most commonly arise in trainees who believe that an interest in geropsychology may improve their image given an otherwise lackluster preparation for graduate training in professional psychology. People who are drafted into working with older adults, or compelled by professional and economic circumstances to start working with older clients, can also have particularly negative attitudes.

Negative attitudes toward aging are widespread, however, and even among those choosing geropsychology, it is not uncommon to hear trainees (and colleagues for that matter) express commonly held negative attitudes toward the aging process. BK fairly frequently comments on trainees expressing a negative attitude toward growing older themselves with the reminder that geropsychologists should be looking forward to growing older, often with some reference to advantages of aging into the post-retirement lifestyle or the acquiring of more mature coping styles and emotion regulation abilities. NP has often been amazed at the tolerance of clinical colleagues for ageist comments by trainees, where such tolerance would not be in evidence in the face of racist or sexist remarks.

The positive attitudes held by the great majority of our trainees can pose their own issues for correction in supervision. Positive stereotyping, after all, still fails to attend to the specific individuality of the older adult. Common issues related to positive attitudes can include (but are not limited to) a reluctance to perceive and diagnose dementia, substance abuse, and personality disorders. Positive attitudes toward aging can also lead to a reluctance to interrupt older clients, keep them focused on important therapy themes, follow-up effectively on missed therapy homework, and confront older clients on sensitive issues in therapy. These are common elements of supervision with trainees in geropsychology, and should come with explanations of why it is important to recognize and actively treat problems of aging, rather than to simply radiate positive feelings toward older clients.

Older adults are defined, as are we all, in multiple ways and not solely by age. An important part of supervising trainees for work with older clients is to insure that they have experience with, and guidance in thinking about, the array of individual diversity in later life. In the nature of work with older adults, this will include understanding ways in which age- and birth-cohort membership affects the experience of other sources of diversity. Different cohorts of women have distinct experiences of what it has meant to grow up female and different experiences of the changes in gender roles over the twentieth century. Working with women who had virtually no control over deciding to have children and limited to no choices in work can be challenging for trainees who have known a much different sociopolitical environment for women.

Different cohorts of ethnic minority groups have distinct experiences of what it means to grow up as a minority person in the USA. Even trainees with a decent intellectual understanding of US history, for example, can be surprised to find themselves working with an older African-American client who grew up in the segregated South. Trainees may be even more surprised to discover that some White older adults grew up with minority status and social discrimination (e.g., Italian Americans, Polish Australians, and so forth). The religious experience and training of earlier born clients can also be quite different from those of later born trainees.

The experience of being gay or lesbian is quite different for clients who came of age well before there was a gay rights movement of any substance. This difference can include meeting gay older men who were married to a woman for much of their lives, for example. These differences are often surprising to trainee therapists and certainly there is a distinction between knowing about such potential differences and experiencing them with clients in the close relationship of psychotherapy. Arranging those experiences and helping the trainee examine them and integrate them into their understanding of aging is a key part of supervising new geropsychologists.

We would note that attention to attitudinal competencies requires some direct observation of the trainee's work. In 35 years of experience supervising clinical work with older adults, BK has never had a trainee or a colleague seeking assistance verbally report having said something ageist in a supervision session. Most ageism is unintentional, and grows out of common social beliefs and feelings about older adults that are thought of by the trainee as simply true. As with racism and sexism, many professionals believe that if they do not actively dislike the group in question they are free from bias. This belief fails to recognize the negative impact of incorrect beliefs about, and of common behaviors toward, older adults.

Addressing attitude competencies in supervision requires both the opportunity and ability to recognize problematic attitudes toward older clients and the supervisor's readiness to address them. Attitude competencies are a key component of the ability to build therapeutic relationships with clients, to accurately assess their psychological issues, and to help them overcome psychological disorders.

This aspect of supervision may be more challenging for the supervisor than imparting knowledge, or teaching and modeling clinical skills. The conversation about attitude competencies touches on more personal aspects of the trainee, and requires diplomacy, tact, a supervisory relationship that is safe for the trainee and encourages openness about such issues, and probably self-disclosure on the supervisor's part.

In the course of supervising a therapy case, BK was struck by how often the client seemed to make extremely poor decisions and also by the client's concern that others would think that she was stupid. When BK suggested to the trainee that the client might well be below normal in IQ, the trainee was distressed because she liked the client, felt that seeing an older adult as possibly developmentally disabled was insulting to the client, and was also concerned about potential racial implications, since the client was African-American. In addition to laying out the reasons why he suspected low IQ, BK made it clear that he did not see this as detracting from the client's value as a human being, discussed some positive experiences with developmentally disabled people, and then encouraged the trainee to discuss her own feelings about intelligence. Some of her feelings came from being highly intelligent and knowing it was impolite to call attention to it when one is smarter than others. She also was not explicitly thinking through how the intervention would need to be explained differently to someone less intelligent than she, in this case substantially so.

We then discussed ways to shape the therapy using this knowledge without confronting the client with it. This feedback and the focus on the attitudes involved led to a clearer understanding of the client and her concerns, and eventually toward progress on key issues around her decision making. In essence, approaches based on assuming normal to higher intelligence had not been working and adopting strategies that assumed a lower level of comprehension of problem situations and the ability to see alternatives was more successful.

NP has also found it useful to discuss potential ageist attitudes in the supervision both of the case formulations as well as the research projects of clinical trainees, where often hypotheses may be at least partly informed by the student's own biases, and stereotypical ways of viewing older adults and the aging process. For example, assumptions about how often older persons will show cognitive deterioration, psychiatric symptoms, deficits in coping or interpersonal relationships often get factored into both clinical case management as well as research designs—the vigilant supervisor will encourage students to check their assumptions against the literature first.

Having the opportunity to interact with a socially diverse group of older adults (including socioeconomic background, race/ethnicity, gender, sexual orientation) may be useful in extending knowledge as well as improving attitudes toward older adults (Hinrichsen et al. 2010). NP often exhorts her clinical students to spend time with older adults in non-clinical settings, to gain familiarity with interacting with older persons in non-clinical settings, as well as to gain insight into the settings and contexts in which older people live their lives.

Knowledge competencies in geropsychology

Providing a thorough grounding in the knowledge base of professional geropsychology is likely to be a particular strength of doctoral program training. Understanding what changes are and are not attributable to normal aging facilitates accurate assessment of older clients and provides a solid background for helping older clients comprehend their own aging experience. Such knowledge also helps to distinguish between individual changes that are attributable to aging, and those that are due to physical disease and/or psychological disorders. When these knowledge competencies are not acquired in a doctoral program, for example, it is important that clinical supervisors find ways to insure that trainees can acquire the knowledge base through readings, in-service training courses, didactic continuing education programs, and so forth.

An understanding of lifespan developmental psychology methodology and the ways in which aging effects, cohort effects, and time of measurement effects are disentangled can also be used to help older clients understand when they are incorrectly attributing differences between themselves and younger persons in their lives to aging, rather than to cohort differences. A few years ago BK provided clinical supervision to a student in our program who was not pursuing a focus in clinical geropsychology, but was seeing older clients as part of her therapy training. At one point, I heard the trainee agreeing with the client when the client expressed the view that growing older meant becoming progressively more frail and old-fashioned compared with the young people around her. An appropriate depth of knowledge competence in psychology and aging would have led her to explore both of these assumptions in more detail and to challenge their accuracy. The client was healthy, free of any progressive chronic diseases, and the differences with younger people around her were common ones that could have been seen as reflecting strengths of the earlier born cohort.

Building a rapport and accurately understanding older adult clients can depend on one's ability to get outside of one's own cohort perspective, and to understand the point of view of people born and raised in another time and place. This requires some sense of historical changes over time, but more particularly it requires the ability to learn the client's perspective on what it has been like to be a member of that cohort. Transcending the values and perspectives of one's own cohort can be as difficult as becoming aware of cultural biases and unquestioned assumptions. Earlier born cohorts can have very different typical life histories. In order to understand how a client's life has been normative or differs from the usual experience of that cohort, one must have some knowledge base regarding the sociohistorical framework within which the client grew up and became an adult.

A thorough grounding in mental health and aging knowledge is essential to understanding what is and is not different about psychological assessment and treatment of older clients. Familiarity with the current knowledge base about psychopathology of late life, the principles and instruments for assessment of older adults, and the knowledge base for psychological intervention with older adults is, of course, indispensable for work in professional geropsychology.

In BK's view, much of what goes wrong in work with older adults by psychologists without geropsychology competencies results from the lack of these knowledge competencies and the resultant reliance on conventional wisdom about aging, and one's own personal and familial experience of aging. Without appropriate depth of knowledge in mental health and aging, clinicians tend to be overly certain of assessment judgments based on initial screenings with simple instruments, and make treatment decisions based on personal beliefs, rather than evidence.

This can be as basic as having a good knowledge base concerning dementia in later life. BK was once startled (and appalled) when during a question and answer period following a continuing education event, one person identified himself as having worked in long-term care for about 6 years, and asked if we were saying that there were people with dementia in long-term care and if there were screening instruments to help identify them. The lack of knowledge competency can also lead to interpreting mental status screening tools too literally: "a score of X or less means dementia, a score greater than X means normal." More commonly at this point in time, it can lead to only thinking of older adult psychological disorders as dementia and depression, and not considering the other possible diagnoses (or even the possibility of no diagnosis). It can also lead to limited and stereotypical treatment goals for older clients, rather than truly individualized treatment planning.

Skills competencies in professional geropsychology

In general, supervision is most likely to involve observation of whole sessions (either directly or through recordings) and a higher ratio of supervision time to client contact time in the early phases of training such as doctoral program clinics and externships. The use of extensive direct observation and the ratio of supervision time to client contact time tends to decrease over the course of training in psychology. This is in part a recognition of the trainee's increasing competence, and partly a reflection of the resources and goals of the training environments. What exactly can be done will depend on the resources of the program and of the community in which it exists. Important goals include exposure to a range of problems in older clients so that the trainee can begin to accumulate experience and skills in distinguishing between the dementias, emotional disorders, substance abuse, and psychological consequences of medical problems and their treatments. Similarly, some range of experience in psychological intervention with a range of client problems is very useful.

Knight (2010) provided discussion of common issues that arise in supervision that involve specific geropsychology skills that trainees need to acquire. For assessment, these include a nuanced view of diagnosis that goes beyond the not uncommon practice in aging and mental health of relying on short screening questionnaires and too literal interpretations of their cut-off scores, together with the assumption that scores are only influenced by the disorder whose name is on the scale. Diagnostic skills also involve learning to recognize that older adults can have diagnoses other than depression and dementia, and that comorbid diagnoses (whether psychiatric or a combination of the physical and psychiatric) are common in later life.

In terms of assessment, useful skills to acquire in order to work well with older clients include knowing when to go beyond a simplistic referral (is this dementia?), learning how not to over-test (often over-testing is a way to manage anxiety in trainee psychologists), and becoming skilled at conveying the results of testing to the client, their family, and other health professionals in a way that helps all parties understand what is happening and what options going forward might include. One of the most common questions that occur during supervision with respect to testing, as well as during lectures, is whether to tell clients they have dementia and how this information should be conveyed. NP, personally, cannot understand why withholding diagnostic information from a patient is a good idea and often asks a class to consider whether their thinking on this matter changes if the diagnosis of "breast cancer" is substituted for "Alzheimer's disease." Of course, delivering such a diagnosis is often a difficult and sensitive task, but in general using simple language (augmented with line drawing of affected brain areas if warranted), coupled with patiently answering queries (and actually encouraging questions) is a good foundation to start from.

In therapy, essential skills in work with older clients include learning to interrupt older clients, handling client's repetition of stories, and guiding the session in therapeutic directions, as well as learning to confront older adults about issues within the therapy session. Therapists also need skills in actually promoting change-oriented therapy with older clients, and in learning to recognize when therapy is complete and the client is ready to terminate therapy.

The therapist's own age can become an issue during therapy with older clients and handling one's own age-related issues is a key skill in clinical geropsychology. One of the most common questions asked, both in supervision and during lectures on therapy with older adults, is how to handle questions about the therapist's age. Much of the impact of such questions comes from the therapist's anxiety about working with older adults and their own concerns about what they have to offer someone who is further along in the life cycle than they themselves are. The answer to this is that we have psychotherapeutic skills and process to offer. Older adults are generally quite used to relying on professionals of all sorts who are younger than themselves. BK often finds that what is really being asked is what stage of training the trainee is at. It is also worth noting that some clients ask about the therapist's age precisely because they suspect the question will make the therapist anxious and distract them from whatever was being discussed before the question is asked.

Middle-aged and older therapists are often overly convinced that their age will be an asset. In general, this is most often the case with those whose understanding of older clients is based entirely on their own clinical and personal experiences, not uncommon among therapists who age alongside their clients and referral sources. The supervision issues become more complicated if the older therapist being supervised has difficulty separating their own and their family's issues regarding aging, from those of their clients. In BK's experience, concurrent experience with major chronic illness and caregiving issues at home can render even therapists with considerable expertise and skill in aging issues paralyzed on the job.

The practice of geropsychology typically involves a high level of interaction with professionals from other disciplines. Getting some exposure to work with other disciplines while in graduate training is highly desirable. Discussing this experience is a great forum for helping trainees understand what strengths psychology brings to the table in interdisciplinary teamwork, and what we need to be able to comprehend from other disciplines. These discussions can also help the trainee understand the blind spots of other disciplines, as well as those common to psychologists. Learning to talk to other disciplines in ways that can be heard by them is an important skill that early exposure can help begin to build. BK often helps trainees understand the physician's reluctance to delve into emotional issues, and their need for brief and definite conclusions to consultations. He also tries to help students understand that doctoral-level psychologists and trainees are often perceived by people in the aging network of services (who have less education) as overly intellectual and conceited, and that finding ways to put them at their ease and communicate psychology consultations that they can and will use is helpful. NP uses a similar approach, but has begun to realize that unwittingly, field supervisors may be encouraging an aloofness and conceit in students through efforts to encourage "the correct way" to do things, because then students may come to believe that only psychologists understand this "right way." In her training program, NP is bringing field supervisors together to discuss such unintended outcomes of supervision.

Professional geropsychology also involves work in a variety of settings, and often takes the practitioner beyond the confines of the outpatient office. Providing early experience in working in more than one professional setting can help to instill this flexibility in the trainee early in their career. Depending on the resources available to the program this may include hospital and nursing home consultations, or home visits for therapy. Nursing home consultations and placements should be undertaken with care, because if the student is not adequately prepared, such experiences have been shown to cement, rather than dispel ageist attitudes on the part of trainees from a range of disciplines (Gatz & Pearson 1986).

A highly important conceptual skill is what we think of as the lifespan developmental psychology of everyday life. In the course of discussing day-to-day life (the supervisor's, the trainee's, and shared experiences in the program environment), it is very useful to weave the understanding of developmental aging, cohort effects, age-related social roles, and other aspects of lifespan thinking into discussions with mentees. BK commonly talks about ways in which his views are affected by being part of the Baby Boomer cohort, and also ways in which his professional life is affected by having been trained in the 1970s.

He encourages older trainees to think of where they stand in their career development based on when their career clock as a psychology trainee started running, rather than chronological age. NP often discusses aspects of her own aging in lectures and supervision to illustrate points about the aging process, and how individuals choose to cope (for example, contrasting a colleague's absolute resistance to wearing reading glasses, as opposed to her own growing collection of funky reading glasses, many strewn about her office at the university). Supervisors can also discuss examples of positive and negative ageism that arise in our conversations and in the program, in addition to those that come up in course and clinical work.

Considering the inputs for supervision

Traditionally, supervision has involved the person being supervised relating the contents and outcomes of an assessment evaluation or psychotherapy session to a supervisor. Tangible products resulting from the trainee's encounter with the supervisor, in the form of scored test protocols or videotapes are often used. Yet in many, perhaps most cases, the supervisor relies on verbal descriptions of what has transpired with a client. This could be because of time or resource pressures, or possibly because in the training setting audio- or videotaping is not allowed, or the client has not consented to it. In such situations, the supervisor must rely on the trainee's narrative of progress in the therapy. This narrative may or may not accurately reflect what is going on in this transaction with a client, even when related to the supervisor with all due care.

There are many ways in which a supervisor can gain insight into how their trainee is working with older clients. These include direct, real-time observation of skills in working with older adults (e.g., through a one-way mirror between consulting rooms or using "bug-in-the-ear" directed supervision), watching videotaped sessions, or observing interactions with standardized patients. All of these afford the supervisor data with which to discuss development of therapy and assessment skills, improve establishment of rapport, and facilitate case formulations and treatment planning. These data also provide information for the supervisor about the trainee's professional stance, interpersonal and organizational skills, and to some degree, attitudes and personal style. All of these may prove worthy of discussion in supervision.

In working with trainee psychologists, the geropsychology supervisor may find additional matters require discussion with the trainees, due to the nature of clients seen. Some of these issues may be *content-oriented*, for example pointing the trainee toward purpose-designed tests for older adults that the trainee may not have encountered before, or discussing how specific health concerns of an older adult may affect the therapy. Other elements may be more *process-oriented*, such as how elements of the CALTAP model as discussed in earlier chapters in this book (such as age, cohort effects, or counter-transference) may be relevant to a particular case. Finally, supervisors and trainees focus on gaining so-called metacompetence in the field—namely, being alert to what one does and does not know (Karel, Altman, Zweig, & Hinrichsen 2013).

Using standardized instruments in supervision

A valuable goal for clinical supervision in psychotherapy is one articulated by Duffy and Morales (1997), "Learning to 'meet the person' without being preoccupied with age differences and disability allows an intense 'personalized' psychological relationship that is necessary in being therapeutic with any client" (p. 375). Later in the same paragraph they note that "Without this, the 'differentness' and related stress of the geriatric practicum experience can have the effect of alienating and discouraging trainees" (p. 375). How are we doing as a field in clinical geropsychology with supervision?

The simple answer is that we do not know. There is simply no empirical work evaluating clinical supervision in cases involving older adults. In this we lag behind other areas of professional psychology, primarily in the quantitative sense. Reviews of the clinical supervision literature more generally are very critical of methods (e.g., an extensive reliance on self-report measures and the satisfaction of the participants in supervision with the experience) and what is really known, especially with regard to the seemingly key question of how supervision affects client outcomes (Bernard & Goodyear 2009; Falendar & Shafranske 2004).

Lambert et al. (2001) set out a program of research examining expected recovery curves in psychotherapy patients over time, and the construction of a system for tracking patient progress and feeding that progress back to the treating clinician. The instrument they use to measure patient outcomes is a standardized self-report instrument, the Outcome Questionnaire-45 (OQ-45; Lambert et al. 1996). Changes in outcomes as measured by the OQ-45 cover three domains: symptomatic functioning, interpersonal problems, and social role performance. The instrument takes about 5 minutes to administer and is meant to be given before each therapy session; thus, it was designed for repeat administrations. The authors of the instrument have devised a standard method of classifying the degree of response to treatment by individual patients, as well as developing standard recovery curves to use in identifying patients who are not making adequate progress (Lambert et al. 2001a,b).

In order to provide detailed feedback to clinicians, the OQ-45 provides color-coded graphic response descriptions about patient progress, as well as recommendations for what actions the therapist might consider taking, such as altering the treatment plan by intensifying treatment, shifting intervention strategies, or addressing the therapeutic alliance (Lambert et al. 2001b; Whipple et al. 2003). Such detailed feedback on patient progress offers a different perspective on the process of therapy over and above feedback reports from the patient.

What might be the effects of providing this information to clinicians? The ability to gauge whether clients are deteriorating in treatment is a difficult judgment for clinicians, even experienced practitioners, to make (Grove et al. 2000). Clinical researchers (e.g., Garb & Schramke 1996) have also suggested that practitioners lack accurate feedback about their practice, and that this may interfere with judgments about whether or not changes in direction or approach are required in therapy. In a study examining the effects of providing feedback on progress to therapists, Lambert et al. (2001a,b) report that clinicians receiving feedback about cases where the therapy was proceeding less well than could be expected had 26% of such clients manifest clinically significant or reliable change, whereas only 16% of patients in the no-feedback condition achieved such change. Furthermore, clinicians receiving feedback had 6% of cases where progress was identified as suboptimal deteriorate further, whereas 23% of clients of therapists not receiving such feedback deteriorated.

Lambert and colleagues have continued to collect data and refine their therapist feedback instruments. What are the implications for supervision? In the clinical psychology training program where NP is Director of Clinical Training, the OQ-45 is used routinely in supervision in the training clinic. Use of this standardized tool augments our feedback to the trainees and allows them to more closely monitor their patients, both to understand progress in therapy and to have an empirical basis to explore therapy directions and potential changes with their supervisor. Both supervisors and trainees can better track the progress of cases over time. The OQ-45 also provides an empirical tool to assist in determining a projected final therapy session. It has allowed NP's clinic to compare training data with other training programs in the area, allowing for reflection on our training procedures and processes. Reese et al. (2009) suggest that the use of such data may help make supervision more effective by allowing an empirical means of prioritizing cases for discussion. Lambert and Hawkins (2001) suggest that such feedback may also help the supervisor and trainee to insure that clients are not harmed by the interventions implemented.

NP's positive experiences in using the OQ-45 continuous assessment tool are mirrored in formal research. Reese et al. (2009) randomly assigned 28 trainees into a feedback or no-feedback condition in a clinical training setting; the instrument used in providing feedback was the Outcome Rating Scale (ORS; Miller & Duncan 2000), which is similar to the OQ-45. The students receiving feedback had more positive client outcomes, and displayed a stronger relationship between self-reported self-efficacy and client outcomes, than did students in the no-feedback condition. Reese et al. (2009) state that "When asked about the supervisory process after the study, supervisors explained that using the continuous assessment data in supervision made providing critical feedback easier and served as a starting point for providing more specific feedback" (p. 164). The supervisors in our training clinic have given us similar feedback, and use of the tool has been well-accepted by our clients.

There is currently no version of such a continuous assessment tool specifically targeting older adults, but this could be a useful future development. Younger trainees often feel unsure of themselves when working with older adults; perhaps continuous feedback on how older clients are doing might influence efficacy. Reese et al. (2009) found a positive link between such feedback and trainee self-efficacy. Moreover, older adults often present with complex issues, and it is possible that such feedback could insure adequate treatment dose in clinical settings. Finally, older adults may appreciate being able to provide such feedback to the therapist, given the fact that at least the current cohort of older clients may be relatively more unfamiliar with psychotherapy than later born cohorts. More research in the area of continuous feedback instruments when used with trainees seeing older clients is warranted.

In common with much of the field, there has been relatively little attention to the gatekeeper functions of supervision in geriatric mental health. In part, this is driven by a desire to see more people working with older adults, but greater concern with the monitoring roles of clinical supervision with regard to both client care and with whether the trainee has really become competent to work with older adults is in order. In the language of clinical supervision trainers, clinical geropsychology has tended to be more focused on the formative evaluation of trainees than on summative evaluation (Bernard & Goodyear 2009; Falendar & Shafranske 2004). Our observation is that while we are by no means unique in this (Bernard & Goodyear 2009, discuss this issue for the whole field), we have tended to avoid discussion of gatekeeping, much less to act on it. With an expanding public focus on psychological services for older adults, greater attention is needed with regard to the quality of such services for the older adult consumer of psychotherapy.

Consultation

As noted at the beginning of this chapter, in many ways peer consultation with colleagues is similar to supervision with trainees, assuming that the colleague is asking for assistance with an older adult case. Of course, since the consultation is peer to peer, it is often a one-time conversation, rather than an ongoing interaction, and the consultant is in an advisory position, rather than an evaluative one as is true with trainees. Regardless of one's stance in treating trainees with respect and as junior colleagues, there is a power differential, which the trainee is unlikely to forget even if the supervisor is genuinely not very focused on it. The absence of an ongoing relationship and the evaluative nature of supervision tends to put more emphasis during peer to peer consultations on diplomacy and persuasion.

The one-time nature of the consultation also means that the consultant has to be strategic in deciding how much can be imparted about the case in one contact and how to balance what seems most important for good case outcome, and what the therapist is most likely to take on board and use. Alternate diagnostic suggestions or revisions of case formulations can be relatively quick and likely to stick in the clinician's mind. Suggestions to use specific therapy techniques or to alter an interaction style are likely to be more complex, and perhaps more challenging for the therapist to hear. Remedies of sizable knowledge deficits and changes in attitudes are unlikely to result from a single consultation. However, if the need is critical enough, it may be necessary to point out such issues as kindly as possible with suggestions for readings or other experiences that might be helpful.

In Australia, it is a requirement of maintaining registration (licensure) to engage in documented peer supervision (minimum 10 hours per year). Many psychologists in Australia belong to informal peer supervision groups, whether in the public sector or in private practice; at their best, these groups serve as a forum to discuss new clinical research findings, and provide a supportive environment for new graduates in the workforce, as well as for experienced practitioners who may be moving into new areas such as geropsychology.

As the field begins to address the need for training in clinical geropsychology competencies for those who enter the field years after licensure as a psychologist, building resources for ongoing consultation relationships to facilitate the acquisition of attitude, skills, and knowledge competencies is a key training issue.

Summary

Supervision and peer consultation concerning working with older adults are an essential part of improving mental health care for older clients. The field of clinical geropsychology has grown tremendously since the 1970s, but the global population of older adults has grown faster. We need more psychologists working with older adults who have psychological problems in late life, and we need them to be competent in the work that they do. Specific attention to training in geropsychology competency is important in the wider context of providing the necessary mental health workforce to meet the needs of changing demographics. The development of particular tools such as the Pikes Peak Geropsychology Competency Assessment tool is important in a training and continuing professional development context (Karel et al. 2010b). As noted in this chapter, supervision and peer consultation are the main methods for imparting skill and attitude competencies, and can be used to increase knowledge competency as well. As noted throughout this book, working with older adults involves addressing challenging professional and personal issues surrounding interactions of medical and psychological disorders, the effects of the dementias on the affected persons and their families, handling bereavement, and understanding the changes of aging, as well as the ways in which older adults are affected by their cohort and cultural identities, and by their social environment.

References

Abbey, J., Piller, N., De Bellis, A., Esterman, A., Parker, D., Giles, L., and Lowcay, B. (2004) The Abbey pain scale: A 1 minute numerical indicator for people with end-stage dementia. International Journal of Palliative Nursing, **10**(1), 6–13.

Abdulla, A., Adams, N., Bone, M., Elliott, A.M., Gaffin, J., Jones, D., et al. (2013). Guidance on the management of pain in older people. Age and Ageing, **42**(Suppl 1), i1–57.

Abrams, D., Eller, A., and Bryant, J. (2006) An age apart: The effects of intergenerational contact and stereotype threat on performance and intergroup bias. Psychology and Aging, **21**, 691–702.

Abrams, R.C. (1991) The aging personality (editorial) International Journal of Geriatric Psychiatry, **6**, 1–3.

Abrams, R.C., and Horowitz, S.V. (1999) Personality disorders after age 50: A meta-analytic review. In E. Rosowsky, R. C. Abrams, and R. A. Zweig (Eds), Personality disorders in older adults: Emerging issues in diagnosis and treatment (pp. 55–68) Mahwah, NJ: Lawrence Erlbaum.

Access Economics. (2009) Keeping dementia front of mind: Incidence and prevalence 2009–2050. Retrieved from <http://www.alzheimers.org.au/common/files/NAT/20090800_Nat__AE_FullKeepDemFrontMind.pdf>

Adams, K. (2001) Depressive symptoms, depletion, or developmental change? Withdrawal, apathy, or lack of vigor in the Geriatric Depression Scale. Gerontologist, **41**, 768–777.

Agency for Health Care Research and Quality. (2010) Hospitalizations for medication and illicit drug-related conditions on the rise among Americans ages 45 and older. Retrieved from <http://archive.ahrq.gov/news/newsroom/press-releases/2010/hospmed.html>

Agronin, M.E., and Maletta, G. (2000) Personality disorders in late life. Understanding and overcoming the gap in research. American Journal of Geriatric Psychiatry, **8**, 4–18.

Aldwin, C.M., Yancura, L.A., and Boeninger, D.K. (2007) Coping, health, and aging. In C. M. Aldwin, C. L., Park, and A, Spiro, III (Eds), Handbook of health psychology and aging (pp. 210–226) New York: Guilford.

Alexopoulos, G. S., Abrams, R. C., Young, R. C., and Shamoian, C. A. (1988) Cornell Scale for Depression in Dementia. Biological Psychiatry, **23**(3), 271–284.

Almeida, O. P. and Almeida, S. A. (1999) Short versions of the geriatric depression scale: A study of their validity for the diagnosis of a major depressive episode according to ICD-10 and DSM-IV. International Journal of Geriatric Psychiatry, **14**(10), 858–865.

Almeida, O.P. and Fenner, S. (2002) Bipolar disorder: Similarities and differences between patients with illness onset before and after 65 years of age. International Psychogeriatrics, **14**, 311–322.

Almeida, O.P., Lautenschlager, N.T., Stocks, N., Alfonso, H., Pfaff, J.J., Pirkis, J., et al. (2012) A randomized trial to reduce the prevalence of depression and self-harm behavior in older primary care patients. Annals of Family Medicine, **10**(4), 347–356.

Alzheimer's Association. (2012) Alzheimer's Disease facts and figures. Alzheimer's and Dementia (Vol. 8) Chicago, IL: Alzheimer's Association.

Alzheimer's Association, Thies, B., and Bleiler, L. (2011) 2011 Alzheimer's disease facts and figures. Alzheimer's Dementia, 7(2), 208–244.

American Psychiatric Association (APA). (1980) DSM-III: Diagnostic and statistical manual of mental disorders. Washington, DC: American Psychiatric Association.

American Psychiatric Association (APA). (1994) DSM-IV: Diagnostic and statistical manual of mental disorders. Washington, DC: American Psychiatric Association.

American Psychiatric Association. (2000) DSM-IV-TR: Diagnostic and statistical manual of mental disorders. Washington, DC: American Psychiatric Association.

American Psychiatric Association. (2013) DSM 5: Diagnostic and statistical manual of mental disorders. Washington, DC: American Psychiatric Association.

American Psychological Association. (August, 2002) Guidelines on multicultural education, training, research, practice, and organizational change for psychologists. Retrieved from: <http://www.apa.org/pi/oema/resources/policy/multicultural-guidelines.aspx>, (accessed 28 December 2012).

American Psychological Association Taskforce on Dementia Assessment. (2012) Guidelines for the evaluation of dementia and age-related cognitive change. American Psychologist, 67(1), 1–9.

Ancoli-Israel, S. (2000) Insomnia in the elderly: A review for the primary care practitioner. Sleep, 23, S23–S30.

Anderson, R.J., Freedland, K. E., Clouse, R.E., and Lustman, P.J. (2001) The prevalence of comorbid depression in adults with diabetes: A meta-analysis. Diabetes Care, 24(6), 1069–1078.

Anderson, G. and Horvath, J. (2002) Chronic conditions: Making the case for ongoing care. Princeton, NJ: Robert Wood Johnson Foundation's Partnership for Solutions.

Andreescu, C., Reynolds, C.F., Lenze, E.J., Dew, M.A., Begley, A.E., Mulsant, B.H., et al. (2007) Effect of comorbid anxiety on treatment response and relapse risk in late-life depression: Controlled study. British Journal of Psychiatry, 190(4), 344–349.

Angst, J. (1988) European long-term studies of schizophrenia. Schizophrenia Bulletin, 14, 501–513.

Angst, F., Stassen, H.H., Clayton, P.J., and Angst, J. (2002) Mortality of patients with mood disorders: follow-up over 34–38 years. Journal of Affective Disorders, 68(2–3), 167–181.

Aparasu, R.R., Mort, J.R., and Brandt, H. (2003) Psychotropic prescription use by community-dwelling elderly in the United States. Journal of the American Geriatrics Society, 51, 671–677.

Apostolova, L.G. and Cummings, J.L. (2008) Neuropsychiatric manifestations in mild cognitive impairment: A systematic review. Dementia and Geriatric Cognitive Disorders, 25, 115–126.

Arens, E.A., Stopsack, M., Spitzer, C., Appel, K., Dudeck, M., Volzke, H., et al. (2013) Borderline personality disorder in four different age groups: A cross-sectional study of community residents in Germany. Journal of Personality Disorders, 27(2), 196–207.

Arfken, C.L., Lach, H.W., Birge, S.J., and Miller, J.P. (1994) The prevalence and correlates of fear of falling in elderly persons living in the community. American Journal of Public Health, 84, 565–570.

Atkinson, R.M., Tolson, R.L., and Turner, J.A. (1990) Late versus early onset problem drinking in older men. Alcoholism: Clinical and Experimental Research 14, 574–579.

Atkinson, T.M., Halabi, S., Bennett, A.V., Rogak, L., Sit, L., Li, Y., et al. (2012) Measurement of affective and activity pain interference using the Brief Pain Inventory (BPI): Cancer and Leukemia Group B 70903. Pain Medicine, **13**, 1417–1424.

Attix, D.K. and Welsh-Bohmer, K.A. (2006) Geriatric neuropsychology: Assessment and intervention. New York, NY: Guilford Press.

Australian Bureau of Statistics (ABS). (2006) National Health Survey: Summary of results 2004–2005. Canberra, Australia: ABS.

Australian Institute of Health and Welfare (AIHW). (2013) Depression in residential aged care 2008–2012. Aged Care Statistics Series No. 39, Cat. no. AGE 73. Canberra, Australia: AIHW.

Babor, T.F., Higgins-Biddle, J.C., and Monteiro, M.G. (2001). The Alcohol Use Disorders Identification Test: Guidelines for use in primary care (2nd edn). Geneva: WHO (Department of Mental Health and Substance dependence).

Bagby, R.M., Ryder, A.G., Schuller, D.R., and Marshall, M.B. (2004) The Hamilton Depression Rating Scale: Has the gold standard become a lead weight? American Journal of Psychiatry, **161**(12), 2163–2177.

Balsis, S., Carpenter, B.D., and Storandt, M. (2005) Personality change precedes clinical diagnosis of dementia of the Alzheimer type. Journals of Gerontology. Series B, Psychological Sciences and Social Sciences, **60**(2), P98–P101.

Balsis, S., Gleason, M.E.J., Woods, C.M., and Oltmanns, T.F. (2007) An item response theory analysis of DSM-IV personality disorder criteria across younger and older age groups. Psychology and Aging, **22**, 171–185.

Balsis, S., Segal, D.L., and Donahue, C. (2009) Revising the personality disorder diagnostic criteria for the Diagnostic and Statistical Manual of Mental Disorders-Fifth Edition (DSM-V): Consider the later life context. American Journal of Orthopsychiatry, **79**(4), 452–460.

Baltes, P.B. (1991) The many faces of human ageing: Toward a psychological culture of old age. Psychological Medicine, **21**, 837–854.

Bandura, A. (1989) Perceived self-efficacy. In V. Mays, G. Albee, and S. Schneider, (Eds), Prevention of AIDS: Psychological approaches (pp. 128–141). Newbury Park, CA: InSage.

Barbar, S.I., Enright, P.L., Boyle, P., Foley, D., Sharp, D. S., Petrovitch, H., et al. (2000) Sleep disturbances and their correlates in elderly Japanese American men residing in Hawaii. Journals of Gerontology. Series A, Biological sciences and medical sciences, **55**(7), M406–M411.

Bark, N., Florida, D., Gera, N., Varardi, R., Harghel, L., and Adlington, K. (2011) Evaluation of the routine clinical use of the Brief Psychiatric Rating Scale (BPRS) and the Abnormal Involuntary Movement Scale (AIMS) Journal of Psychiatric Practice, **17**, 300–303.

Barlow, J., Wright, C., Sheasby, J., Turner, A., and Hainsworth, J. (2002) Self-management approaches for people with chronic conditions: A review. Patient Education and Counseling, **48**(2), 177–187.

Barry, K.L. (1997) Alcohol and Drug Abuse. In M. Mengel and W. Holleman (Eds), Fundamentals of clinical practice: A textbook on the patient, doctor, and society (pp. 689–715). New York: Plenum.

Barry, K.L., and Blow, F.C. (2010) Screening, assessing and intervening for alcohol and medication misuse in older adults (pp. 307-330). In P. Lichtenberg (Ed.), Handbook of assessment in clinical gerontology (2nd ed.). New York: Wiley.

Barry, K.L., and Blow, F.C. (2014) Substance use, misuse, and abuse: Special issues for older adults. In N. A. Pachana and K. Laidlaw (Eds), Oxford handbook of clinical geropsychology (pp. 549–570). Oxford: Oxford University Press.

Bartels, S.J. (2002) Quality, costs, and effectiveness of services for older adults with mental disorders: A selective overview of recent advances in geriatric mental health services research. Current Opinion in Psychiatry, **15**, 411–416.

Bartels, S.J. (2003) Improving the system of care for older adults with mental illness in the United States. American Journal of Geriatric Psychiatry, **11**(5), 486–497.

Bartels, S. J., Forester, B., Miles, M.K., and Joyce, T. (2000) Mental health service use by elderly patients with bipolar disorder and unipolar major depression. American Journal of Geriatric Psychiatry, **8**, 160–166.

Bartels, S.J., Mueser, K.T., and Miles, K.M. (1997) Functional impairments in elderly patients with schizophrenia and major affective illness in the community: Social skills, living skills, and behavior problems. Behavior Therapy, **28**, 43–63.

Bauer, M.S. and McBride, L. (2003) Structured group psychotherapy for bipolar disorder (2nd edn). New York, NY: Springer.

Baxter, A.J., Scott, K.M., Vos, T., and Whiteford, H.A. (2013) Global prevalence of anxiety disorders: A systematic review and meta-regression. Psychological Medicine, **43**, 897–910

Beattie, E.R.A., and Pachana, N.A. (2010) Double jeopardy: Co-morbid anxiety and depression in late life. Research in Gerontological Nursing, **3**(3), 209–220.

Beaudreau, S.A., and O'Hara, R. (2008) Late-life anxiety and cognitive impairment: A review. American Journal of Geriatric Psychiatry, **16**, 790–803.

Bech, P., Rafaelsen, O.J., Kramp, P. and Bolwig, T.G. (1978) The Mania Rating Scale: Scale construction and interobserver agreement. Neuropsychopharmacology, **17**(6), 430–431.

Beck, A.T., Epstein, N., Brown, G., and Steer, R.A. (1988) An inventory for measuring clinical anxiety: Psychometric properties. Journal of Consulting and Clinical Psychology, **56**, 893–897.

Beck, A.T., Steer, R.A., and Brown, G.K. (1996) BDI-II, Beck Depression Inventory: Manual (2nd edn). Boston, MA: Harcourt Brace.

Beekman, A.T., Bremmer, M.A., Deeg, D.J., van Balkom, A.J., Smit, J.H., de Beurs, E., et al. (1998) Anxiety disorders in later life: A report from the Longitudinal Aging Study Amsterdam. International Journal of Geriatric Psychiatry, **13**(10), 717–726

Beekman, A., van Balkom, A., Deeg, D., van Dyck. R., and van Tilburg, W. (2000) Anxiety and depression in later life: Co-occurrence and communality of risk factors. American Journal of Psychiatry, **157**(1), 89–95.

Bennett-Levy, J., Klein-Boonschate, M.A., Batchelor, J., and McCarter, R. (1994) Encounters with Anna Thompson: The consumer's experience of neuropsychological assessment. Clinical Neuropsychologist, **8**, 219–238.

Ben-Porath, Y. (2012) Interpreting the MMPI-2-RF. Minneapolis, MN: University of Minnesota Press.

Berk, M., Berk, L. and Castle, D. (2004) A collaborative approach to the treatment alliance in bipolar disorder. Bipolar Disorder, **6**, 504–518.

Bernard, J.M., and Goodyear, R.K. (2009) Fundamentals of clinical supervision (4th edn). Upper Saddle River, NJ: Merrill.

Berrios, G.E., and Bakshi, N. (1991) Manic and depressive symptoms in the elderly: their relationships to treatment outcome, cognition and motor symptoms. Psychopathology, **24**, 31–38.

Bjelland, I., Dahl, A.A., Haug, T.T., and Neckelmann, D. (2002) The validity of the Hospital Anxiety and Depression Scale. Journal of Psychosomatic Research, **52**(2), 69–77

Black, D.A. (1990) Changing patterns and consequences of alcohol abuse in old age. Geriatric Medicine, **20**, 19–20.

Blackburn, J., Loudon, J., and Ashworth, C. (1977) A new scale for measuring mania. Psychological Medicine, **7**, 453–458.

Blazer, D.G. (1994) Dysthymia in community and clinical samples of older adults. American Journal of Psychiatry, **151**, 1567–1569.

Blazer, D.G. (2003a) Depression in late life: Review and commentary. Journal of Gerontology: Medical Sciences, **58A**(3), 249–265.

Blazer, D.G. (2003b) Geriatric psychiatry. In R. E. Hales and S. C. Yudofsky (Eds) The American psychiatric publishing textbook of clinical psychiatry (pp. 1535–1550). Washington, DC: APA.

Bliwise, D.L. (1993) Sleep in normal aging and dementia. Sleep, **16**, 40–81.

Blogg, L.C., Suzuki, N., Roberts, M., and Clifford, R.M. (2012) Prescribing benzodiazepines in residential aged care facilities. Journal of Pharmacy Practice and Research, **42**(4), 287–290.

Blow, F.C. (1998) Substance abuse among older Americans (DHHS No (SMA) 98–3179). Washington, D.C.: US Government Printing Office.

Blow, F.C., and Barry, K.L. (2012) Alcohol and substance misuse in older adults. Current Psychiatry Reports, **14**(4), 310–319.

Blow, F.C., Brockmann, L.M., and Barry, K.L. (2004) The role of alcohol in late-life suicide. Alcoholism: Clinical and Experimental Research, **28**(5S), 48S–56S.

Blow, F.C., Brower, K.J., Schulenberg, J.E., Demo-Dananberg, L.M., Young, J.P., and Beresford, T.P. (1992) The Michigan Alcoholism Screening Test—Geriatric Version (MAST-G): A new elderly-specific screening instrument. Alcoholism: Clinical and Experimental Research, **16**, 372.

Blow, F.C., Walton, M.A., Chermack, S.T., Mudd, S.A., Brower, K.J., and Comstock, M.A. (2000) Older adult treatment outcome following elder-specific inpatient alcoholism treatment. Journal of Substance Abuse Treatment, **19**(1), 67–75.

Bootzin, R.R., and Epstein, D.R. (2000) Stimulus control. In K. L. Lichstein and C. M. Morin (Eds), Treatment of late life insomnia (pp. 167–184). Thousand Oaks, CA: Sage Publications.

Bowling, A. (2005) Ageing well: Quality of life in old age. Maidenhead, United Kingdom: Open University Press.

Bowling, A., Fleissig, A., Gabriel, Z., Banister, D., Dykes, J., Dowding, L.M., et al. (2003) Let's ask them: A national survey of definitions of quality of life and its enhancement among people aged 65 and over. International Journal of Aging and Human Development, **56**(4), 269–306.

Brassington, G.S., King, A.C., and Bliwise, D.L. (2000) Sleep problems as a risk factor for falls in a sample of community-dwelling adults aged 64–99 years. Journal of the American Geriatrics Society, **48**, 1234–1240.

Broadhead, J. and Jacoby, R. (1990) Mania in old age: A first prospective study. International Journal of Geriatric Psychiatry, **5**, 215–222.

Brodaty, H., Luscombe, G., Parker, G., Wilhelm, K., Hickie, I., Austin, M.P., et al. (2001) Early and late onset depression in old age: Different aetiologies, same phenomenology. Journal of Affective Disorders, **66**(2–3), 225–236.

Brodaty, H., Pond, D., Kemp, N.M., Luscombe, G., Harding, L., Berman, K., et al. (2002) The GPCOG: A new screening test for dementia designed for general practice. Journal of the American Geriatrics Society, **50**(3), 530–534.

Brodaty, H., Sachdev, P., Koschera, A., Monk, D., and Cullen, B. (2003) Long-term outcome of late-onset schizophrenia: 5-year follow-up study. British Journal of Psychiatry, **183**, 213–219.

Brown, R.G., Dittner, A., Findley, L., and Wessely, S.C. (2005) The Parkinson Fatigue Scale. Parkinsonism and Related Disorders, **11**(1), 49–55.

Brown, S.T., Kirkpatrick, M.K., Swanson, M.S., and McKenzie, I.L. (2011) Pain experience of the elderly. Pain Management Nursing, **12**(4), 190–196.

Brown, K.W., Levy, A.R., Rosberger, Z., and Edgar, L. (2003) Psychological distress and cancer survival: A follow-up 10 years after diagnosis. Psychosomatic Medicine **65**(4), 636–643.

Brown, L.M., and Schinka, J.A. (2005) Development and initial validation of a 15-item informant version of the Geriatric Depression Scale. International Journal of Geriatric Psychiatry, **20**, 911–918.

Bruce, M. (2010) Subsyndromal depression and services delivery: At a crossroad? American Journal of Geriatric Psychiatry, **18**(3), 189–191.

Bryant, C. (2010) Anxiety and depression in old age: Challenges in recognition and diagnosis. International Psychogeriatrics, **22**, 511–513.

Bryant, C., Jackson, H., and Ames, D. (2008) The prevalence of anxiety in older adults: Methodological issues and a review of the literature. Journal of Affective Disorders, **109**, 233–250.

Buchsbaum, D.G., Buchanan, R.G., Welsh, J., Centor, R.M., and Schnoll, S.H. (1992) Screening for drinking disorders in the elderly using the CAGE questionnaire. Journal of the American Geriatrics Society, **40**(7), 662–665.

Burns, A., Lawlor, B., and Craig, S. (2004) Assessment scales in old age psychiatry (2nd edn). London, UK: CRC Press.

Burroughs, T.E., Desikan, R., Waterman, B.M., Gilin, D., and McGill, J. (2004) Development and validation of the Diabetes Quality of Life Brief Clinical Inventory. Diabetes Spectrum, **17**(1), 41–49.

Butler, R. (1963) The life review: An interpretation of reminiscence in the aged. Psychiatry, **26**, 65–76.

Butters, M.A., Bhalla, R.K., Andreescu, C., Wetherell, J.L., Mantella, R., Begley, A.E., et al. (2011) Changes in neuropsychological functioning following treatment for late-life generalised anxiety disorder. British Journal of Psychiatry, **199**, 211–218.

Butters, M.A., Pollock, B.G., Reynolds, R.C.F., Becker, J.T., Whyte, E.M., Nebes, R.D., et al. (2004) The nature and determinants of neuropsychological functioning in late-life depression. Archives of General Psychiatry, **61**(6), 587–595.

Buysse, D.J. (2004) Insomnia, depression and aging: Assessing sleep and mood interactions in older adults. Geriatrics, **59**(2), 47–51.

Buysse, D.J., Angst, J., Gamma, A., Ajdacic, V., Eich, D., and Rössler, W. (2008) Prevalence, course, and comorbidity of insomnia and depression in young adults. Sleep, 31(4), 473–480.

Buysse, D.J., and Reynolds, C.F., 3rd (2000) Pharmacologic treatment. In K. L. Lichstein and C. M. Morin (Eds), Treatment of late life insomnia (pp. 231–270) Thousand Oaks, CA: Sage Publications.

Buysse, D.J., Reynolds, C.F. 3rd, Monk, T.H., Berman, S.R., and Kupfer, D.J. (1989) The Pittsburgh Sleep Quality Index: A new instrument for psychiatric practice and research. Psychiatric Research, 28(2), 193–213.

Byrne, G.J.A., and Pachana, N.A. (2011) Development and validation of a short form of the Geriatric Anxiety Inventory—the GAI-SF. International Psychogeriatrics, 23(1), 125–131.

Byrne, G.J., Pachana, N.A., Goncalves, D.C., Arnold, E., King, R., and Khoo, S.K. (2010) Psychometric properties and health correlates of the Geriatric Anxiety Inventory in Australian community-residing older women. Aging and Mental Health, 14(3), 247–254.

Camp, C.J. (2006) Spaced retrieval: A case in dissemination of a cognitive intervention for persons with dementia. In D. K. Attix and K. A. Welsh-Bohmer (Eds), Geriatric neuropsychological assessment and intervention (pp. 275–292). New York: Guilford Press.

Carney, C.E., Buysse, D.J., Ancoli-Israel, S., Edinger, J.D., Krystal, A.D., Lichstein, K.L., et al. (2012) The consensus sleep diary: Standardizing prospective sleep self-monitoring. Sleep, 35, 287–302.

Casey, D.A., Rodriguez, M., Northcoot, C., Vickar, G., and Shihabuddin, L. (2011) Schizophrenia: Medical illness, mortality, and aging. International Journal of Psychiatry in Medicine, 41(3), 245–251.

Cassidy, F., and Carroll, B.J. (2002) Vascular risk factors in late-onset mania. Psychological Medicine, 32, 359–362.

Cassidy, E.L., Lauderdale, S., and Sheikh, J.I. (2005) Mixed anxiety and depression in older adults: Clinical characteristics and management. Journal of Geriatric Psychiatry and Neurology, 18, 83–88.

Center for Substance Abuse Treatment. (1998) Substance abuse among older adults. Treatment Improvement Protocol (TIP) Series, No. 26 (HHS Publication No. (SMA) 12-3918). Rockville, MD: Substance Abuse and Mental Health Services Administration.

Center for Substance Abuse Treatment. (2005) Substance abuse relapse prevention for older adults: A group treatment approach (DHHS Publication No. (SMA) 05-4053). Rockville, MD: Substance Abuse and Mental Health Services Administration.

Charles, S.T. (2011) Emotional experience and emotion regulation in later life. In K. W. Schaie and S. L. Willis (Eds), Handbook of the psychology of aging (7th edn, pp. 295–310). San Diego: Academic Press.

Chattat, R., Ellena, L., Cucinotta, D., Savorani, G., and Mucciarelli, G. (2001) A study on the validity of different short versions of the geriatric depression scale. Archives of Gerontology and Geriatrics, Suppl. 7, 81–86.

Cheavens, J.S., and Lynch, T.R. (2008) Dialectical behavior therapy for personality disorders in older adults. In D. Gallagher-Thompson, A. M. Steffen, and L. W. Thompson (Eds), Handbook of behavioral and cognitive therapies with older adults (pp. 187–199). New York: Springer.

Chermack, S.T., Blow, F.C., and Hill, E.M. (1996) The relationship between alcohol symptoms and consumption among older drinkers. Alcoholism: Clinical and Experimental Research, 20, 1153–1158.

Choi, N.G., and Gonzalez, J.M. (2005) Barriers and contributors to minority older adults' access to mental health treatment. Journal of Gerontological Social Work, **44**(3), 115–135.

Chu, D., Gildengers, A.G., Houck, P.R., Anderson, S.J., Mulsant, B.H., Reynolds, R.C.F., et al. (2010) Does age at onset have clinical significance in older adults with bipolar disorder? International Journal of Geriatric Psychiatry, **25**(12), 1266.

Chunyu, L.M.M., Friendman, B., Conwell, Y., and Fiscella, K. (2007) Validity of the Patient Health Questionnaire 2 (PHQ-2) in identifying major depression in older people. Journal of the American Geriatrics Society, **55**(4), 596–602.

Clare, L., and Giblin, S. (2008) Late onset psychosis. In R. Woods and L. Clare (Eds), Handbook of the clinical psychology of ageing (pp. 133–144). West Sussex, UK: John Wiley and Sons.

Clayton, P.J. (1983) The prevalence and course of the affective disorders. In J. M. Davis and J. W. Maas, (Eds), The affective disorders (pp. 93–201). Washington, D.C., American Psychiatric Association Press.

Cohen, C.I. (1993) Age-related correlations in patient symptom management strategies in schizophrenia: An exploratory study. International Journal of Geriatric Psychiatry, **8**, 211–213.

Cohen, C.I., Hassamal, S.K., and Begum, N. (2011) General coping strategies and their impact on quality of life in older adults with schizophrenia. Schizophrenia Research, **127**(1–3), 223–228.

Cohen, C.I., Shamoian, C., Cohen, G.D., Blank, K., Gaitz, C., Katz, I.R., et al. (2000) Schizophrenia and older adults. An overview: Directions for research and policy. American Journal of Geriatric Psychiatry: Official Journal of the American Association for Geriatric Psychiatry, **8**(1), 19.

Cohen, C.I., Talavera, N., and Hartung, R. (1996) Depression among older persons with schizophrenia who live in the community. Psychiatric Service, **47**, 601–607.

Cohen, C.I., Talavera, N., and Hartung, R. (1997) Predictors of subjective well-being among older persons with schizophrenia living in the community. American Journal of Geriatric Psychiatry, **5**, 145–155.

Cohen-Mansfield, J., Marx, M.S., and Rosenthal, A.S. (1989) A description of agitation in a nursing home. Journal of Gerontology: Medical Sciences, **44**(3), M77–M84.

Colenda, C.C., Mickus, M.A., Marcus, S.C., Tanielian, T.L., and Pincus, H.A. (2002) Comparison of adult and geriatric psychiatric practice patterns: Findings from the American Psychiatric Association's Practice Research Network. American Journal of Geriatric Psychiatry **10**, 609–617.

Collin, C., Wade, D.T., Davies, S., and Horne, V. (1988) The Barthel ADL Index: A reliability study. International Disability Studies, **10**, 61–63.

Conigliaro, J., Kraemer, K., and McNeil, M. (2000) Screening and identification of older adults with alcohol problems in primary care. Journal of Geriatric Psychiatry and Neurology, **13**(3), 106–114.

Connor, D.J., Sabbagh, M.N., and Cummings, J.L. (2008) Comment on administration and scoring of the Neuropsychiatric Inventory (NPI) in clinical trials. Alzheimer's Dementia, **4**(6), 390–394.

Conwell, Y. (1991) Suicide in elderly patients. In L. S. Schneider, C. F. Reynolds, B. D. Lebowitz, and A. J. Friedhoff (Eds), Diagnosis and treatment of depression in late life (pp. 397–418). Washington, DC: American Psychiatric Press.

Conwell, Y., and Thompson, C. (2008) Suicidal behavior in elders. Psychiatric Clinics of North America, **31**, 333–356.

Copeland, J.R.M., Kelleher, M.J., Kellett, J.M., Gourlay, A.J., Gurland, B.J., Fleiss, J.L., et al. (1976) A semi-structured clinical interview for the assessment of diagnosis and mental state in the elderly: The Geriatric Mental State Schedule I: Development and reliability. Psychological Medicine, **6**, 439–449.

Craig, D., Passmore, A.P., Fullerton, K.J., Beringer, T.R.O., Gilmore, D.H., Crawford, V.L.S., et al. (2003) Factors influencing prescription of CNS medications in different elderly populations. Pharmacoepidemiology and drug safety, **12**(5), 383–387.

Crowley, K. (2011) Sleep and sleep disorders in older adults. Neuropsychological Review, **21**, 41–53.

Crum, R.M., Anthony, J.C., Bassett, S.S., and Folstein, M.F. (1993) Population based norms for the Mini-Mental State Examination by age and educational level. Journal of the American Medical Association, **269**, 2386–2391.

Cuijpers, P., Sijbrandij, M., Koole, S., Huibers, M., Berking, M., and Andersson, G. (2014) Psychological treatment of generalized anxiety disorder: A meta-analysis. Clinical Psychology Review, **34**(2), 130–140.

Cullen, B., O'Neill, B., Evans, J.J., Coen, R.F., and Lawlor, B.A. (2007) A review of screening tests for cognitive impairment. Journal of Neurology, Neurosurgery, and Psychiatry, **78**, 790–799.

Culpepper, L. (2004) Effective recognition and treatment of generalized anxiety disorder in primary care. Primary Care Companion to the Journal of Clinical Psychiatry, **6**(1), 34–43.

Cummings, J.L. (1992) Neuropsychiatric complications of drug treatment in Parkinson's disease. In J. L. Cummings (Ed.), Parkinson's disease: Neurobehavioral aspects (pp. 313–327). New York, New York: Oxford University Press.

Cummings, S.M., Bride, B., Cassie, K.M., and Rawlins-Shaw, A. (2008) Substance abuse. Journal of Gerontological Social Work, **50**, 215–241.

Cummings, J.L., Mega, M., Gray, K., Rosenberg-Thompson, S., Carusi, D.A., and Gornbein, J. (1994) The Neuropsychiatric Inventory: Comprehensive assessment of psychopathology in dementia. Neurology, **44**(12), 2308–2314.

Curran, H.V., Collins, R., Fletcher, S., Kee, S.C.Y., Woods, B., and Iliffe, S. (2003) Older adults and withdrawal from benzodiazepine hypnotics in general practice: Effects on cognitive functioning, sleep, mood, and quality of life. Psychological Medicine, **33**(7), 1223–1237.

Davidson, M., Frecska, E., Harvey, P.D., Powchik, P., Parrella, M., White, L., et al. (1995) Severity of symptoms in chronically institutionalized geriatric schizophrenic patients. American Journal of Psychiatry, **152**(2), 197.

Dalrymple-Alford, J.C., Wells, S., Porter, R.J., Watts, R., Anderson, T.J., MacAskill, M.R., et al. (2010) The MoCA: well-suited screen for cognitive impairment in Parkinson disease. Neurology, **75**(19), 1717–1725.

Deimling, G.T., Bowman, K.F., Sterns, S., Wagner, L.J., and Kahana, B. (2006) Cancer-related health worries and psychological distress among older adult, long-term cancer survivors. Psycho-Oncology, **15**(4), 306–320.

Dennis, R.E., Boddington, S.J., and Funnell, N.J. (2007) Self-report measures of anxiety: Are they suitable for older adults? Aging and Mental Health, **11**, 668–677.

Dennis, M., Kadri, A., and Coffey, J. (2012) Depression in older people in the general hospital: A systematic review of screening instruments. Age and Ageing, **41**(2), 148–154.

Depp, C.A., Davis, C.E., Mittal, D., Patterson, T.L., and Jeste, D.V. (2006) Health-related quality of life and functioning of middle-aged and elderly adults with bipolar disorder. Journal of Clinical Psychiatry, **67**(2), 215–221.

Depp, C.A., and Jeste, D.V. (2004) Bipolar disorder in older adults: A critical review. Bipolar Disorders, **6**, 343–367.

Devanand, D.P., Turret, N., Moody, B.J., Fitzsimons, L., Peyser, S., Mickle, K., et al. (2000) Personality disorders in elderly patients with dysthymic disorder. American Journal of Geriatric Psychiatry: Official Journal of the American Association for Geriatric Psychiatry, **8**(3), 188–195.

Dew, M.A., Hoch, C.C., Buysse, D.J., Monk, T.H., Begley, A.E., Houck, P.R., et al. (2003) Healthy older adults' sleep predicts all-cause mortality at 4 to 19 years of follow-up. Psychosomatic Medicine, **65**(1), 63–73.

Dew, M.A., Reynolds, C.F, Monk, T.H., Buysse, D.J., Hoch, C.C., Jennings, J.R., et al. (1994) Psychosocial correlates and sequelae of electroencephalographic sleep in health elders. Journals of Gerontology, **49**, P8–P18.

Diefenbach, G.J., Tolin, D.F., Meunier, S.A., and Gilliam, C.M. (2009) Assessment of anxiety in older home care recipients. The Gerontologist, **49**(2), 141–153.

Dillon, H.R., Wetzler, R.G., and Lichstein, K.L. (2012) Evidence-based treatments for insomnia in older adults. In F. Scogin and A. Shah (Eds), Making evidence-based psychological treatments work with older adults (pp. 47–86). Washington, DC: American Psychological Association.

Dolan-Sewell, R.G., Krueger, R.F., and Shea, M.T. (2001) Co-occurrence with syndrome disorders. In W. J. Livesley (Ed.), Handbook of personality disorders (pp. 84–104). New York: Guilford Press.

Donders, J., and Hunter, S.J. (2010) Principles and practice of lifespan developmental neuropsychology. Cambridge: Cambridge University Press.

Douglass, A.B., Bornstein, R., Nino-Murcia, G., Keenan, S., Miles, L., Zarcone, V.P., et al. (1994) The Sleep Disorders Questionnaire I: Creation and multivariate structure of SDQ. Sleep, **17**(2), 160–167.

Dowrick, C. (2006) The chronic disease strategy for Australia. Medical Journal of Australia, **185**(2), 61–62.

Draper, B., Brodaty, H., Low, L.F., Richards, V., Paton, H., and Lie, D. (2002) Self-destructive behaviors in nursing home residents. Journal of the American Geriatrics Society, **50**, 354–358.

Drew, S.M., Wilkins, K.M., and Trevisan, L.A. (2010) Managing medication and alcohol misuse by your older patients. Current Psychiatry, **9**(2), 21–41.

Driscoll, H.C., Nebes, R.D., Miller, M.D., Reynolds, R.C.F., Serody, L., Patrick, S., et al. (2008) Sleeping well, aging well: A descriptive and cross-sectional study of sleep in "successful agers" 75 and older. American Journal of Geriatric Psychiatry: Official Journal of the American Association for Geriatric Psychiatry, **16**(1), 74–82.

Duffy, M., and Morales, P. (1997) Supervision of psychotherapy with older patients. In C. E. Watkins (Ed.), Handbook of psychotherapy supervision (pp. 366–380). New York: John Wiley and Sons.

Dupree, L.W., Schonfeld, L., Dearborn-Harshman, K.O., and Lynn, N. (2008) A relapse prevention model for older alcohol abusers. In D. Gallagher-Thompson, A. M. Steffen, and L. W. Thompson (Eds), Handbook of behavioral and cognitive therapies with older adults (pp. 61–75). New York, New York: Springer.

Eaton, W., Armenian, H., Gallo, J., Pratt, L., and Ford, D. (1996) Depression and risk for onset of type II diabetes. A prospective population-based study. Diabetes Care **19**, 1097–1102.

Ebrahim, I.O., Shapiro, C.M., Williams, A.J., and Fenwick, P.B. (2013) Alcohol and sleep I: Effects on normal sleep. Alcoholism: Clinical and Experimental Research, **37**(4), 539–549.

Edelstein, B.A., Heisel, M.J., McKee, D.R., Martin, R.R., Koven, L.P., Duberstein, P.R., et al. (2009) Development and psychometric evaluation of the Reasons for Living— Older Adults Scale: A suicide risk assessment inventory. Gerontologist, **49**(6), 736–745.

Edelstein, B.A., and Segal, D.L. (2011) Assessment of emotional and personality disorders in older adults. In K. W. Schaie and S. L. Willis (Eds), Handbook of the psychology of aging (7th edn, pp. 325–337). San Diego: Academic Press.

Edelstein, B.A., and Semenchuk, E.M. (1996) Interviewing older adults. In L. Carstensen, B. Edelstein and L. Dornbrand (Eds), The practical handbook of clinical gerontology (pp. 153–173). Thousand Oaks, CA: Sage.

Edelstein, B.A., Woodhead, E.L., Segal, D.L., Heisel, M.J., Bower, E.H., and Lowery, A.J. (2007) Older adult psychological assessment: Current instrument status and related considerations. Clinical Gerontologist, **31**, 1–35.

Efros, R.B. (2009) The immunological theory of aging revisited. In V. L. Bengtson, D. Gans, N. M. Putney, and M. Silverstein (Eds), Handbook of theories of aging (2nd edn, pp. 163–178). New York: Springer.

Elson, P. (2006) Do older adults presenting with memory complaints wish to be told if later diagnosed with Alzheimer's disease? International Journal of Geriatric Psychiatry, **21**, 419–425.

Ewing, J.A. (1984) Detecting alcoholism. The CAGE questionnaire. JAMA: Journal of the American Medical Association, **252**(14), 1905–1907.

Extermann, M., and Hurria, A. (2007) Comprehensive geriatric assessment for older patients with cancer. Journal of Clinical Oncology, **25**, 1824–1831.

Fallendar, C.A., and Shafranske, E.P. (2004) Clinical supervision: A competency-based approach. Washington, DC: American Psychological Association.

Fann, J.R. (2000) The epidemiology of delirium: A review of studies and methodological issues. Seminars in Clinical Neuropsychiatry, **5**, 64–74.

Farias, S.T., Mungas, D., Reed, B.R., Harvey, D., and DeCarli, C. (2009) Progression of mild cognitive impairment to dementia in clinic- vs community-based cohorts. Archives of Neurology, **66**(9), 1151–1157.

Farmer, R.F. (2000) Issues in the assessment and conceptualization of personality disorders. Clinical Psychology Review, **20**, 823—851.

Farrell, K.R., and Ganzini, L. (1995) Misdiagnosing delirium as depression in medically ill elderly patients. Archives of Internal Medicine, **155**, 2459–2464.

Ferretti, L., McCurry, S.M., Logsdon, R., Gibbons, L., and Teri, L. (2001) Anxiety and Alzheimer's disease. Journal of Geriatric Psychiatry and Neurology, **14**, 52–58.

Fiellin, D.A., Reid, C., and O'Connor, P.G. (2000) Screening for alcohol problems in primary care: A systematic review. Archives of Internal Medicine, **160**(13), 1977–1989.

Finch, C.E. and Morgan, D. (1987). Aging and schizophrenia: A hypothesis relating asynchrony in neural aging processes to the manifestations of schizophrenia and other neurologic diseases with age. In N. E. Miller and G. D. Cohen (Eds), *Schizophrenia and aging.* (pp. 97–108). New York: Guilford Press.

Finkel, S. (2000) Introduction to behavioural and psychological symptoms of dementia (BPSD) International Journal of Geriatric Psychiatry, **15**(S1), S2–S4.

Finn, S.E. (2007) In our client's shoes: Theory and techniques of therapeutic assessment. Manwah NJ: Lawrence Erlbaum Associates.

First, M., Gibbon, M., Spitzer, R.L., Williams, J.B.W., and Benjamin, L.S. (1996a) Structured clinical interview for DSM-IV Axis II personality disorders (SCID-II). Washington, D.C.: American Psychiatric Press.

First, M., Gibbon, M., Spitzer, R.L., Williams, J.B.W., and Benjamin, L.S. (1997) User's guide for the Structured Clinical Interview for DSM–IV Axis II personality disorders. Washington, DC: American Psychiatric Press.

First, M.B., Spitzer, R.L., Gibbon, M., and Williams, J.B.W. (1996b) Structured Clinical Interview for DSM-IV Axis I disorders: Non-patient edition (SCID-NP, v. 2.0). New York: New York State Psychiatric Institute.

Fischer, C.T., and Finn, S.E. (2008) Developing life meaning from psychological test data: Collaborative and therapeutic approaches. In R. P. Archer and S. R. Smith (Eds), Personality assessment (pp. 379–404). New York: Routledge.

Fiske, A., Wetherell, J., and Gatz, M. (2009) Depression in older adults. Annual Review of Clinical Psychology, **5**, 363–389.

Flint, A.J., and Rifat, S.L. (1996a) The effect of sequential antidepressant treatment on geriatric depression. Journal of Affective Disorders, **36**(3), 95–105.

Flint, A.J., and Rifat, S.L. (1996b) Validation of the Hospital Anxiety and Depression Scale as a measure of severity of geriatric depression. International Journal of Geriatric Psychiatry, **11**(11), 991–994.

Foley, D.J., Ancoli-Israel, S., Britz, P., and Walsh, J. (2004) Sleep disturbances and chronic disease in older adults: Results of the 2003 National Sleep Foundation Sleep in America survey. Journal of Psychosomatic Research, **56**(5), 497–502.

Folstein, M.F., Folstein, S.E., and McHugh, P.R. (1975) "Mini-mental state." A practical method for grading the cognitive state of patients for the clinician. Journal of Psychiatric Research, **12**(13), 189–198.

Frances, A.J. (1980) The DSM-III personality disorders section: A commentary. American Journal of Psychiatry, **137**, 1050–1054.

Frank, D., DeBenedetti, A.F., Volk, R.J., Williams, E.C., Kivlahan, D.R., and Bradley, K.A. (2008) Effectiveness of the AUDIT-C as a screening test for alcohol misuse in three race/ethnic groups. Journal of General Internal Medicine, **23**(6), 781–787.

Frasure-Smith, N., and Lesperance, F. (2010) Depression and cardiac risk: Present status and future directions. Postgraduate Medical Journal, **86**(1014), 193–196.

Fratiglioni, L., and Rocca, W.A. (2001) Epidemiology of dementia. In F. Boller and S. F. Cappa (Eds), Aging and dementia: Handbook of neuropsychology (2nd edn, pp. 193–215). Amsterdam: Elsevier.

Fremouw, W., McCoy, K., Tyner, E.A., and Musick, R. (2009) Suicidal Older Adult Protocol—SOAP. In J. A. Allen, E. Wolf, and L. VandeCreek (Eds), Innovations in clinical practice: A 21st century sourcebook (pp. 203–212). Sarasota, FL: Professional Resource Press/Professional Resource Exchange.

Friedman, B., Heisel, M.J., and Delavan, R.L. (2005) Psychometric properties of the 15-item geriatric depression scale in functionally impaired, cognitively intact, community-dwelling elderly primary care patients. Journal of the American Geriatric Society, 53(9), 1570–1576.

Fröjdh, K., Håkansson, A., Karlsson, I., Institute of Clinical Neurosciences, S. o. P., Göteborgs, u., Institutionen för klinisk neurovetenskap, S. f. p., et al. (2004) The Hopkins Symptom Checklist-25 is a sensitive case-finder of clinically important depressive states in elderly people in primary care. International Journal of Geriatric Psychiatry, 19(4), 386–390.

Gabryelewicz, T., Barcikowska, M., Styczynska, M., Luczywek, E., Barczak, A., Pfeffer, A., et al. (2007) The rate of conversion of mild cognitive impairment to dementia: Predictive role of depression. International Journal of Geriatric Psychiatry, 22(6), 563–567.

Gagnon, L.M., and Patten, S.B. (2002) Major depression and its association with long-term medical conditions. Canadian Journal of Psychiatry, 47, 149–152.

Gallagher, D., Coen, R., Kilroy, D., Belinski, K., Bruce, I., Coakley, D., et al. (2011) Anxiety and behavioural disturbance as markers of prodromal Alzheimer's disease in patients with mild cognitive impairment. International Journal of Geriatric Psychiatry, 26(2), 166–172.

Gallo, J., Rabins, P., and Lyketsos, C. (1994) Depression without sadness: Functional outcomes of nondysphoric depression in later life. Journal of the American Geriatrics Society, 45, 570–578.

Garb, H.B., and Schramke, C.J. (1996) Judgment research and neuropsychological assessment: A narrative review and meta-analysis. Psychological Bulletin, 120, 140–153.

Gass, C.S., and Brown, M.C. (1992) Neuropsychological test feedback to patients with brain dysfunction. Psychological Assessment, 4, 272–277.

Gatz, M., Fiske, A., Fox, L., Kaskie, B., Kasl-Godley, J., McCallum T.J., et al. (1998). Empirically validated psychological treatments of older adults. Journal of Mental Health and Aging, 4, 9–46.

Gatz, M., and Pearson, C.G. (1986) Training clinical psychology students in aging. Gerontology and Geriatrics Education, 6, 15–25.

Gellis, Z.D. (2006) Mental health and emotional disorders among older adults. In B. Berkman (Ed.), Oxford handbook of social work in health and aging (pp. 129–139). New York: Oxford University Press.

Germans, S., Van Heck, G.L., Masthoff, E.D., Trompenaars, F.J.W.M., and Hodiamont, P.P.G. (2010) Diagnostic efficiency among psychiatric outpatients of a self-report version of a subset of screen items of the Structured Clinical Interview for DSM-IV-TR personality disorders (SCID-II) Psychological Assessment, 22(4), 945–952.

Gijsen, R., Hoeymans, N., Schellevis, F.G., Ruwaard, D., Satariano, W.A., and van den Bos, G. A. (2001) Causes and consequences of comorbidity: A review. Journal of Clinical Epidemiology, 54, 661–674.

Gildengers, A.G., Butters, M.A., Chisholm, D., Anderson, S.J., Begley, A., Holm, M., et al. (2012) Cognition in older adults with bipolar disorder versus major depressive disorder. Bipolar disorders, 14(2), 198–205.

Glass, J., Lanctot, K.L., Herrmann, N., Spoule, B.A., and Busto, U.E. (2005) Sedative hypnotics in older people with insomnia: Meta-analysis of risks and benefits. British Medical Journal, **331**, 1169.

Gloster, A.T., Rhoades, H.M., Novy, D., Klotsche, J., Senior, A., Kunik, M., et al. (2008) Psychometric properties of the Depression Anxiety and Stress Scale-21 in older primary care patients. Journal of Affective Disorders, **110**(3), 248–259.

Goldberg, R., Morris, P., Christian, F., Badger, J., Chabot, S., and Edlund, M. (1990) Panic disorder in cardiac outpatients. Psychosomatics, **31**(2), 168–173.

Golden, C.J., and Freshwater, S.M. (2001) Luria-Nebraska Neuropsychological Battery. In W. I. Dorfmann and M. Hersen (Eds), Understanding psychological assessment: Perspectives on individual differences (pp. 59–75). New York: Kluwer Academic/Plenum Publishers.

Gonidakis, S., and Longo, V.D. (2009) Programmed longevity and programmed aging theories. In V. L. Bengtson, D. Gans, N. M. Putney, and M. Silverstein (Eds), Handbook of theories of aging (2nd edn, pp. 215–228). New York: Springer.

Goodwin, F., and Jamison, K. (1990) Manic-depressive illness. Oxford: Oxford University Press.

Gooneratne, N.S., Gehrman, P.R., Nkwuo, J.E., Bellamy, S.L., Schutte-Rodin, S., Dinges, D.F., et al. (2006) Consequences of comorbid insomnia symptoms and sleep-related breathing disorder in elderly subjects. Archives of Internal Medicine, **166**(16), 1732–1738.

Gorske, T.T. (2008) Therapeutic neuropsychological assessment: A humanistic model and case example. Journal of Humanistic Psychology, **48**(3), 320–339.

Gorske, T.T., and Smith, S.R. (2009) Collaborative therapeutic neuropsychological assessment. New York, NY: Springer.

Gradman, T.J., Thompson, L.W., and Gallagher-Thompson, D. (1999) Personality disorders and treatment outcome. In E. Rosowsky, R. C. Abrams, and R. A. Zweig (Eds), Personality disorders in older adults: Emerging issues in diagnosis and treatment (pp. 69–94). Mahwah, NJ: Lawrence Erlbaum.

Graf, C. (2008) The Lawton Instrumental Activities of Daily Living Scale. American Journal of Nursing, **108**(4), 52–62.

Graham, J.R. (2006) MMPI 2: Assessing personality and psychopathology (4th edn). New York, NY: Oxford University Press.

Gray, S.L., LaCroix, A.Z., Hanlon, J.T., Penninx, B.W.J.H., Blough, D.K., Leveille, S.G., et al. (2006) Benzodiazepine use and physical disability in community-dwelling older adults. Journal of the American Geriatrics Society, **54**(2), 224–230.

Green, J. (2006) Feedback. In D. K. Affix and K. A. Welch-Bohmer (Eds), Geriatric neuropsychology: Assessment and intervention (pp. 223–236). New York, NY: Guilford Press.

Grove, W.M., Zald, D.H., Lebow, B.S., Snitz, B.E., and Nelson, C. (2000) Clinical versus mechanical prediction: A meta-analysis. Psychological Assessment, **12**, 19–30.

Gunderson, E.W., Haughey, H.M., Ait-Daoud, N., Joshi, A.S., and Hart, C.L. (2012) "Spice" and "K2" herbal highs: A case series and systematic review of the clinical effects and biopsychosocial implications of synthetic cannabinoid use in humans. American Journal of Addictions, **21**(4), 320–326.

Gureje, O., Loadeji, B.D., Abiona, T., Makanjuola, V., and Esan, O. (2011) The natural history of insomnia in the Ibadan Study of Ageing. Sleep, **34**(7), 965–973.

Hadjistavropoulos, T., Lynn Beattie, B., Chibnall, J.T., Craig, K.D., Ferrell, B., Ferrell, B., et al. (2007) An interdisciplinary expert consensus statement on assessment of pain in older persons. Clinical Journal of Pain, 23 Suppl. 1(1 Suppl.), S1–S43.

Halvorsrud, L., Kalfoss, M., Diseth, A., and Kirkevold, M. (2012) Quality of life in older Norwegian adults living at home: A cross-sectional survey. Journal of Research in Nursing, 17(1), 12–29.

Ham, R., Sloane, D., and Warshaw, G. (2002) Primary care geriatrics: A case-based approach (pp 32–33). St Louis, MO: Mosby.

Hamilton, M. (1960) A rating scale for depression. Journal of Neurology, Neurosurgery and Psychiatry, 23, 56–62.

Harris, Y. (2007) Depression as a risk factor for nursing home admission among older individuals. Journal of the American Directors Association, 8(1), 14–20.

Harvey, P.D., Howanitz, E., Parrella, M., White, L., Davidson, M., Mohs, R.C., et al. (1998) Symptoms, cognitive functioning, and adaptive skills in geriatric patients with lifelong schizophrenia: A comparison across treatment sites. American Journal of Psychiatry, 155(8), 1080.

Hausdorff, J.M., Rios, D.A., and Edelber, H.K. (2001) Gait variability and fall risk in community–living older adults: A 1-year prospective study. Archives of Physical Medicine and Rehabilitation, 82(8), 1050–1056.

Haley, W. (1996) The medical context of psychotherapy with the elderly. In: S. H. Zarit and B. G. Knight (Eds.) A guide to psychotherapy and ageing: Effective clinical interventions in a life-stage context. (pp. 221–239). American Psychological Association, Washington, DC.

Haywood, K., Garratt, A., Schmidt, L., Mackintosh, A., and Fitzpatrick, R. (2004) Health status and quality of life in older people: A review. Report from the Patient-reported Health Instruments Group to the Department of Health.

Heisel, M.J., and Duberstein, P.R. (2005) Suicide prevention in older adults. Clinical Psychology: Science and Practice, 12(3), 242–259.

Heisel, M.J., and Flett, G.L. (2006) The development and initial validation of the geriatric suicide ideation scale. American Journal of Geriatric Psychiatry, 14(9), 742–751.

Helme, R.D., and Gibson, S.J. (2001) The epidemiology of pain in elderly people. Clinics in Geriatric Medicine, 17, 417–431.

Hertzog, C., Van Alstine, J., Usala, P.D., Hultsch, D.F., and Dixon, R. (1990) Measurement properties of the Center for Epidemiological Studies Depression Scale (CES-D) in older populations. Psychological Assessment, 2(1), 64–72.

Hess, T.M., Auman, C., Colcombe, S.J., and Rahhal, T.A. (2003) The impact of stereotype threat on age differences in memory performance. Journal of Gerontology: Psychological Sciences, 58(1), 3–11.

Hess, T.M., and Hinson, J.T. (2006) Age-related variation in the influences of aging stereotypes on memory in adulthood. Psychology and Aging, 21, 621–625.

Hesse, M., and Moran, P. (2010) Screening for personality disorder with the Standardised Assessment of Personality: Abbreviated Scale (SAPAS): Further evidence of concurrent validity. BMC psychiatry, 10(1), 10–10.

Hickey, A.M., Bury, G., O'Boyle, C.A., Bradley, F., O'Kelly, F.D., and Shannon, W. (1996) A new short form individual quality of life measure (SEIQOL-DW): Application in a cohort of individuals with HIV/AIDS. British Medical Journal (Clinical Research Ed.), **313**, 29–33.

Hinrichsen, G.A., Zeiss, A.M., Karel, M.J., and Molinari, V.A. (2010) Competency-based geropsychology training in doctoral internships and postdoctoral fellowships. Training and Education in Professional Psychology, **4**(2), 91–98.

Hirschfield, R.M.A. (2002) The Mood Disorder Questionnaire: A simple, patient-rated screening instrument for bipolar disorder. Journal of Clinical Psychiatry Primary Care Companion, **4**, 9–11.

Hirschfeld, R.M., Calabrese, J.R., Weissman, M.M., Reed, M., Davies, M.A., Frye, M.A., et al. (2003a) Screening for bipolar disorder in the community. Journal of Clinical Psychiatry, **64**, 53–59.

Hirschfeld, R.M., Holzer, C., Calabrese, J.R., Weissman, M., Reed, M., and Davies, M. (2003b) Validity of the Mood Disorder Questionnaire: A general population study. American Journal of Psychiatry, **160**, 178–180.

Hirschfeld, R.M., Rapport, D.J., Russell, J.M., Sachs, G.S., Zajecka, J., Williams, J.B., et al. (2000) Development and validation of a screening instrument for bipolar spectrum disorder: The Mood Disorder Questionnaire. American Journal of Psychiatry, **157**(11), 1873–1875.

Holden, J.D., Hughes, I.M., and Tree, A. (1994) Benzodiazepine prescribing and withdrawal for 3234 patients in 15 general practices. Family Practice, **11**, 358–362.

Holmes, C., Cairns, N., Lantos, P., and Mann, A. (1999) Validity of current clinical criteria for Alzheimer's disease, vascular dementia and dementia with Lewy bodies. British Journal of Psychiatry, **174**, 45–50.

Hopko, D.R., Stanley, M.A., Reas, D.L., Loebach Wetherell, J., Gayle Beck, J., Novy, DM., et al. (2003) Assessing worry in older adults: Confirmatory factor analysis of the Penn State Worry Questionnaire and psychometric properties of an abbreviated model. Psychological Assessment, **15**(2), 173–183.

Hu, H.C. (1944) The Chinese concept of "face." American Anthropologist, **46**, 45–64.

Hubbard, G., Cook, A., Tester, S., and Downs, M. (2002) Beyond words: Older people with dementia using and interpreting nonverbal behavior. Journal of Aging Studies, **16**, 155–167.

Inouye, S.K. (2003) The Confusion Assessment Method (CAM): Training Manual and Coding Guide. New Haven: Yale University School of Medicine.

Inouye, S.K., van Dyck, C.H., Alessi, C.A., Balkin, S., Siegal, A.P., and Horwitz, R.I. (1990) Clarifying confusion: The Confusion Assessment Method. A new method for detection of delirium. Annals of Internal Medicine, **113**(12), 941–948.

International Psychogeriatric Association (IPA) (2002) BPSD: Introduction to behavioural and psychological symptoms of dementia. Retrieved from <http://www.ipa-online.org>

Ismail, Z., Rajji, T.K., and Shulman, K.I. (2010) Brief cognitive screening instruments: An update. International Journal of Geriatric Psychiatry, **25**(2), 111–120.

Izal, M., Montorio, I., Nuevo, R., Perez-Rojo, G., and Cabrera, I. (2010) Optimising the diagnostic performance of the Geriatric Depression Scale. Psychiatry Research, **178**(1), 142–146.

James, I.A. (2008) Schemas and schema-focused approaches with older people. In K. Laidlaw and B. Knight (Eds), Handbook of emotional disorders in later life: Assessment and treatment (pp. 117–140). Oxford: Oxford University Press.

James, I. A., Postma, K., and Mackenzie, L. (2003) Using an IPT conceptualization to treat a depressed person with dementia. Behavioural and Cognitive Psychotherapy, **31**(4), 451–456.

James, J.W., and Haley, W.E. (1995) Age and health bias in practicing clinical psychologists. Psychology and Aging, **10**(4), 610–616.

James, M.A., Golden, C.J., Ariel, R., and Gustavson, J.L. (1983) Interpretation of the Luria–Nebraska Neuropsychological Battery (Vol. 1). New York: Grune and Stratton.

Jean-Louis, G., Zizi, F., Casimir, G., and Compas, J.C. (2007) Sleep in America: Is race or culture an important factor? In D. Léger and S. R. Pandi-Perumal (Eds), Sleep disorders: Their impact on public health. (pp. 49–58). Abingdon: Informa Healthcare.

Jeste, D.V., Blazer, D., Casey, D., Meeks, T., Salzman, C., Schneider, L., et al. (2008) ACNP White Paper: Update on use of antipsychotic drugs in elderly persons with dementia. Neuropsychopharmacology, **33**(5), 957–970.

Jeste, D.V., Blazer, D.G., and First, M. (2005) Aging-related diagnostic variations: Need for diagnostic criteria appropriate for elderly psychiatric patients. Biological Psychiatry, **58**, 165–271.

Jeste, D.V., Blazer, D.G., and First, M.B. (2007) Aging-related diagnostic variations: Need for diagnostic criteria appropriate for elderly patients. In W. E. Narrow, M. B. First, P. J. Sirovatka, and D. A. Regier (Eds), Age and gender considerations in psychiatric diagnosis: A research agenda for DSM-V (pp. 273–288). Arlington, VA: American Psychiatric Publishing, Inc.

Jeste, N.D., Hays, J.C., and Steffens, D.C. (2006) Clinical correlates of anxious depression among elderly patients with depression. Journal of Affective Disorders, **90**(1), 37–41.

Jeste, D.V., Reynolds III, C.F., Lebowitz, B.D., Alexopoulos, G.S., Bartels, S.J., Cummings, J.L., et al. (1999) Consensus statement on the upcoming crisis in geriatric mental health: Research agenda for the next 2 decades. Archives of General Psychiatry, **56**(9), 848–853.

Jeste, D.V., Wolkowitz, O.M., and Palmer, B.W. (2011) Divergent trajectories of physical, cognitive, and psychosocial aging in schizophrenia. Schizophrenia Bulletin, **37**(3), 451–455.

Jimenez, D.E., Alegria, M., Chen, C., Chan, D., and Laderman, M. (2010) Prevalence of psychiatric illnesses among ethnic minority elderly. Journal of the American Geriatrics Society, **58**(2), 256–264.

Jiménez-Martín, S., Labeaga, J.M., and Martínez Granado, M. (1999) Health status and retirement decisions for older European couples. IRISS Working Paper No. 1999–1901. Luxembourg, Integrated Research Infrastructure in Social Sciences.

Johansson, P., Alehagen, U., Svanborg, E., Dahlstrom, U., and Brostrom, A. (2009) Sleep disordered breathing in an elderly community-living population: Relationship to cardiac function, insomnia symptoms and daytime sleepiness. Sleep Medicine, **10**, 1005–1011.

Johns, M.W. (1991) A new method for measuring daytime sleepiness: The Epworth Sleepiness Scale. Sleep, **14**(6), 540–545.

Johnson, K.G., and Johnson, D.C. (2010) Frequency of sleep apnea in stroke and TIA patients: A meta-analysis. Journal of Clinical Sleep Medicine, **6**, 131–137.

Jongenelis, K., Pot, A.M., Eisses, A.M., Gerritsen, D.L., Derksen, M., Beekman, A.T., et al. (2005) Diagnostic accuracy of the original 30-item and shortened versions of the Geriatric Depression Scale in nursing home patients. International Journal of Geriatric Psychiatry, **20**(11), 1067–1074.

Jorm, A.F. (1994) A short form of the Informant Questionnaire on Cognitive Decline in the Elderly (IQCODE): Development and cross-validation. Psychological Medicine, **24**(1), 145–153.

Jorm, A.F., and Jacomb, P.A. (1989) The Informant Questionnaire on Cognitive Decline in the Elderly (IQCODE): Socio-demographic correlates, reliability, validity and some norms. Psychological Medicine, **19**(4), 1015–1022.

Joseph, C.L., Ganzini, L., and Atkinson, R.M. (1995) Screening for alcohol use disorders in the nursing home. Journal of the American Geriatrics Society, **43**(4), 368–373.

Judd, T. (1999) Neuropsychotherapy community integration: Brain illness, emotions, and behavior. New York: Kluwer Academic Publishers.

Kane, R.L. (2000) Choosing and using an assessment tool. In R. L. Kane (Ed.), Assessing older persons: Measures, meaning and practical applications (pp. 1–13). New York, NY: Oxford University Press.

Kane, J.M., Jeste, D.V., Barnes, T.R.E., and Members of the Task Force (1992) Tardive dyskinesia: A Task Force Report of the American Psychiatric Association. Washington, DC: American Psychiatric Association.

Kane F.J., Strohlein J., and Harper R.G. (1993) Nonulcer dyspepsia associated with psychiatric disorder. Southern Medical Journal, **86**, 641–646.

Kaplan, E. (1988) The process approach to neuropsychological assessment. Aphasiology, **2**(3–4), 309–312.

Karel, M.J., Altman, A.N., Zweig, R.A., and Hinrichsen, G.A. (2014) Supervision in professional geropsychology training: Perspectives of supervisors and supervisees. Training and Education in Professional Psychology, **8**(1), 43–50.

Karel, M. J., Emery, E.E., and Molinari, V. (2010) Development of a tool to evaluate geropsychology knowledge and skill competencies. International Psychogeriatrics, **22**(6), 886–896.

Karel, M.J., Holley, C.K., Whitbourne, S.K., Segal, D.L., Tazeau, Y.N., Emery, E.E., et al. (2012) Preliminary validation of a tool to assess competencies for professional geropsychology practice. Professional Psychology: Research and Practice, **43**, 110—117.

Karel, M.J., Knight, B.G., Duffy, M., Hinrichsen, G.A., and Zeiss, A.M. (2010) Attitude, knowledge and skill competencies for practice in professional geropsychology: Implications for training and building a geropsychology workforce. Training and Education in Professional Psychology, **4**(2), 75–84.

Karim, S. and Byrne, E.J. (2005) Treatment of psychosis in elderly people. Advances in Psychiatric Treatment, **11**, 286–296.

Kathol, R.G., Turner, R., and Delahunt, J.W. (1986) Depression and anxiety associated with hyperthyroidism: Response to antithyroid therapy. Psychosomatics, **27**, 501–505.

Katon, W.J. (2003) Clinical and health services relationships between major depression, depressive symptoms, and general medical illness. Biological Psychiatry, **54**, 216–226.

Kawakami, N., Takatsuka, N., Shimizu, H., and Ishibashi, H. (1999) Depressive symptoms and occurrence of type II diabetes among Japanese men. Diabetes Care, **22**, 1071–1076.

Kazantzis, N., Pachana, N.A., and Secker, D.L. (2003) Cognitive-behavioral therapy for older adults: Practical guidelines for the use of homework assignments. Cognitive and Behavioral Practice, **10**, 324–332.

Keefe, F.J., Abernethy, A.P., and Campbell, L.C. (2005) Psychological approaches to understanding and treating disease-related pain. Annual Review of Psychology, **56**, 601–630.

Keith, S., Regier, D., and Rae, D. (1991) Schizophrenic disorders. In L. Robins and D. Regier (Eds), Psychiatric disorders in America: The Epidemiological Catchment Area Study (pp. 33–52). New York, NY: Free Press.

Keller, S., Bann, C.M., Dodd, S.L., Schein, J., Mendoza, T.R., and Cleeland, C.S. (2004) Validity of the Brief Pain Inventory for use in documenting the outcomes of patients with noncancer pain. Clinical Journal of Pain, **20**(5), 309–318.

Kenan, M.M., Kendjelic, E.M., Molinari, V.A., Williams, W., Norris, M., and Kunik, M.E. (2000) Age-related differences in the frequency of personality disorders among inpatient veterans. International Journal of Geriatric Psychiatry, **15**, 831–837.

Kessing, L.V., and Andersen, P.K. (2004) Does the risk of developing dementia increase with the number of episodes in patients with depressive disorder and in patients with bipolar disorder? Journal of Neurology, Neurosurgery and Psychiatry, **75**, 1662–1666.

Kessler, R.C., Berglund, P., Demler, O., Jin, R., Merikangas, K.R., and Walters, E.E. (2005a) Lifetime prevalence and age-of-onset distributions of DSM-IV disorders in the National Comorbidity Survey Replication. Archives of General Psychiatry, **62**(6), 593–602.

Kessler, R.C., Demler, O., Frank, R.G., Olfson, M., Pincus, H.A., Walters, E.E., et al. (2005b) Prevalence and treatment of mental disorders, 1990 to 2003. The New England Journal of Medicine, **352**(24), 2515–2523.

Kessler, R.C., McGonagle, K.A., Zhao, S., Nelson, C.B., Hughes, M., Eshleman, S., et al. (1994) Lifetime and 12-month prevalence of DSM-III-R psychiatric disorders in the United States. Results from the National Comorbidity Survey. Archives of General Psychiatry, **51**(1), 8–19.

Kimmel, D. (2014) Lesbian, gay, bisexual and transgender aging concerns. Clinical Gerontologist, **37**(1), 49–63.

Kingdon, D., Swelam, M., and Granholm, E. (2008) Cognitive therapy for older people with psychoses. In D. Gallagher-Thompson, A. M Steffen, and L. W. Thompson (Eds), Handbook of behavioral and cognitive therapies with older adults (pp. 151–170). New York: Springer.

Klein, W.C., and Jess, C. (2002) One last pleasure? Alcohol use among elderly people in nursing homes. Health and Social Work, **27**(3), 193–203.

Klerman, E.B., Davis, J.B., Duffy, J.F., Dijk, D.J., and Kronauer, R.E. (2004) Older people awaken more frequently but fall back asleep at the same rate as younger people. Sleep, **27**(4), 793–798.

Klonsky, E.D., Oltmanns, T.F., and Turkheimer, E. (2002) Informant reports of personality disorder: Relation to self-reports and future research directions. Clinical Psychology: Science and Practice, **9**, 300–311.

Knight, B.G. (2010) Clinical supervision for psychotherapy with older adults. In N. Pachana, K. Laidlaw, and B. G. Knight (Eds), Casebook of clinical geropsychology (pp. 107–118). Oxford: Oxford University Press.

Knight, B.G., Karel, M.J., Hinrichsen, G.A., Qualls, S.H., and Duffy, M. (2009) Pikes Peak Model for training in professional geropsychology. American Psychologist, **64**, 205–214.

Knight, B.G., and Lee, L.O. (2008) Contextual adult life span theory for adapting psychotherapy. In K. Laidlaw and B. G. Knight (Eds), Handbook of emotional disorders in late life: Assessment and treatment (pp. 59–88). Oxford: Oxford University Press.

Knight, B.G., and Poon, C. (2008) The socio-cultural context in understanding older adults: Contextual adult life span theory for adapting psychotherapy. In B. Woods (Ed.), The handbook of the clinical psychology of ageing (pp. 439–456). Chichester: Wiley.

Knight, R.G. (1992) The neuropsychology of degenerative brain diseases. Hillsdale, NJ: Lawrence Erlbaum Associates.

Knopman, D.S., and Roberts, R.O. (2011) Estimating the number of persons with frontotemporal lobar degeneration in the US population. Journal of Molecular Neuroscience, **45**, 330–335.

Koder, D.A., and Helmes, E. (2006) Clinical psychologists in aged care in Australia: A question of attitude or training? Australian Psychologist, **41**(3), 179–185.

Koenig, H.G., George, L.K., and Schneider, R. (1994) Mental health care for older adults in the year 2020: A dangerous and avoided topic. Gerontologist, **34**, 674–679.

Köhler, S., Thomas, A.J., Barnett, N.A., and O'Brien, J.T. (2010) The pattern and course of cognitive impairment in late-life depression. Psychological Medicine, **40**(4), 591–602.

Konnert, C., Dobson, K., and Stelmach, L. (2009) The prevention of depression in nursing home residents: A randomized clinical trial of cognitive-behavioral therapy. Aging and Mental Health, **13**(2), 288–299.

Kraemer, K.L., Mayo-Smith, M.F., and Calkins, D.R. (1997) Impact of age on the severity, course, and complications of alcohol withdrawal. Archives of Internal Medicine, **157**(19), 2234–2241.

Kroenke, K., Spitzer, R.L., and Williams, J.B. (2001) The PHQ-9: Validity of a brief depression severity measure. Journal of General Internal Medicine, **16**(9), 606–613.

Kroenke, K., Spitzer, R.L., Williams, J.B.W., and Lowe, B. (2010) The Patient Health Questionnaire Somatic, Anxiety, and Depressive Symptom Scales: A systematic review. General Hospital Psychiatry, **32**(4), 345–359.

Kushida, C.A., Chang, A., Gadkary, C., Guilleminault, C., Carrillo, O., and Dement W.C. (2001) Comparison of actigraphic, polysomnographic, and the subjective assessment of sleep parameters in sleep disordered patients. Sleep Medicine, **2**, 389–396.

Labouvie-Vief, G., and Diehl, M. (2000) Cognitive complexity and cognitive-affective integration: Related or separate domains of adult development? Psychology and Aging, **15**, 490–504.

Labouvie-Vief, G., and Medler, M. (2002) Affect optimization and affect complexity: Modes and styles of regulation in adulthood. Psychology and Aging, **17**(4), 571–587.

Lacro, J.P., and Jeste, D.V. (1997) Geriatric psychosis. Psychiatric Quarterly, **68**, 247–260.

Laidlaw, K., and Pachana, N.A. (2009) Aging, mental health, and demographic change: Challenges for psychotherapists. Professional Psychology: Research and Practice, **40**(6), 601–608.

Lambert, M.J., Hansen, N.B., and Finch, A.E. (2001a) Patient-focused research: Using patient outcome data to enhance treatment effects. Journal of Consulting and Clinical Psychology, **69**(2), 159–172.

Lambert, M.J., Hansen, N.B., Umphress, V., Lunnen, K., Okiishi, J., Burlingame, G., et al. (1996) Administration and scoring manual for the Outcome Questionnaire (OQ-45). Wilmington, DE: American Professional Credentialing Services.

Lambert, M.J., and Hawkins, E.I. (2001) Using information about patient progress in supervision: Are outcomes enhanced? Australian Psychologist, **36**, 131–138.

Lambert, M.J., Whipple, J.L., Smart, D.W., Vermeersch, D.A., Nielsen, S.L., and Hawkins, E.J. (2001b) The effects of providing therapists with feedback on patient progress during psychotherapy: Are outcomes enhanced? Psychotherapy Research, 11, 49–68.

Langbehn, D.R., Links, P., Pfohl, B.M., Reynolds, S., Clark, L.A., Battaglia, M., et al. (1999) The Iowa Personality Disorder Screen: development and preliminary validation of a brief screening interview. Journal of Personality Disorders, 13(1), 75–89.

Lawton, M.P. (1980) Environment and aging. Belmont, CA: Brooks/Cole.

Lawton, M.P., and Brody, E.M. (1969) Assessment of older people: Self-maintaining and instrumental activities of daily living. The Gerontologist, 9(3), 179–186.

Lecrubier, Y. (2001) The burden of depression and anxiety in general medicine. Journal of Clinical Psychiatry, 62, 4–9.

Lecrubier, Y., Sheehan, D.V., Weiller, E., Amorim, P., Bonora, I., Harnett Sheehan, K., et al. (1997) The Mini International Neuropsychiatric Interview (MINI) a short diagnostic structured interview: Reliability and validity according to the CIDI. European Psychiatry, 12(5), 224–231.

Lee, Y.A. (2011) Vascular dementia. Chonnam Medical Journal, 47(2), 66–71.

Lemke, S.P., and Schaefer, J.A. (2010) Recent changes in the prevalence of psychiatric disorders among VA nursing home residents. Psychiatric Services, 61(4), 356–363.

Lenze, E.J., Karp, J.F., Mulsant, B.H., Blank, S., Shear, M.K., Houck, P.R., et al. (2005) Somatic symptoms in late-life anxiety: Treatment issues. Journal of Geriatric Psychiatry and Neurology, 18(2), 89–96.

Lenze, E.J., Mulsant, B.H., Dew, M.A., Shear, M.K., Houck, P.R., Pollock, B.G., et al. (2003) Good treatment outcomes in late-life depression with co-morbid anxiety. Journal of Affective Disorders, 77, 247–254.

Lenze, E.J., Mulsant, B.H., Shear, M.K., Schulberg, H.C., Dew, M.A., Begley, A.E., et al. (2000) Comorbid anxiety disorders in depressed elderly patients. American Journal of Psychiatry, 157(5), 722–728.

Lenze, E.J., and Wetherell, J.L. (2009) Bringing the bedside to the bench and then to the community: A prospectus for intervention research in late-life anxiety disorders. International Journal of Geriatric Psychiatry, 24, 1–14.

Leon, C., Gerretsen, P., Uchida, H., Suzuki, T., Rajji, T., and Mamo, D.C. (2010) Sensitivity to antipsychotic drugs in older adults. Current Psychiatry Reports, 12, 28–33.

Le Roux, H., Gatz, M., and Wetherell, J.L. (2005) Age at onset of generalized anxiety disorder in older adults. American Journal of Geriatric Psychiatry, 13(1), 23–30.

Levenson, R.W., Carstensen, L.L., Friesen, W.V., and Ekman, P. (1991) Emotion, physiology, and expression in old age. Psychology and Emotion, 6, 28–35.

Leverenz, J.B., and McKeith, I.G. (2002) Dementia with Lewy bodies. Medical Clinics of North America, 86, 519–535.

Levkoff, S.E., Rowe, J., Evans, D.A., Liptzin, B., Cleary, P.D., Lipsitz, L.A., et al. (1992) Delirium. The occurrence and persistence of symptoms among elderly hospitalized patients. Archives of Internal Medicine, 152(2), 334–340.

Levy, B., Conway, K., Brommelhoff, J., and Merikengas, K. (2003) Intergenerational differences in the reporting of elders' anxiety. Journal of Mental Health and Aging, 9(4), 233–241.

Li, G., Wang, L.Y., Shofer, J.B., Thompson, M.L., Peskind, E.R., McCormick, W., et al. (2011) Temporal relationship between depression and dementia: findings from a large community-based 15-year follow-up study. Archives of General Psychiatry, **68**(9), 970–977.

Lichstein, K.L., Durrence, H.H., Taylor, D.J., Bush, A.J., and Riedel, B.W. (2003) Quantitative criteria for insomnia. Behaviour Research and Therapy, **41**(4), 427–445.

Lichstein, K.L., Riedel, B.W., Lester, K.W., and Aguillard, R.N. (1999) Occult sleep apnea in a recruited sample of older adults with insomnia. Journal of Consulting and Clinical Psychology, **67**(3), 405–410.

Lichstein, K.L., Stone, K.C., Donaldson, J., Nau, S.D., Soeffing, J.P., Murray, D., et al. (2006) Actigraphy validation with insomnia. Sleep, **29**(2), 232–239.

Lichtenberg, P.A. (2010) Handbook of Assessment in Clinical Gerontology (2nd edn). New York, NY: Academic Press.

Lichtenberg, P.A., Marcopulos, B.A., Steiner, D.A., and Tabscott, J.A. (1992) Comparison of the Hamilton Depression Rating Scale and the Geriatric Depression Scale: Detection of depression in dementia patients. Psychological Reports, **70**, 515–521.

Lindesay, J., Stewart, R., and Bisla, J. (2012) Anxiety disorders in older people. Reviews in Clinical Gerontology, **22**, 204–217.

Lindsey, P.L. (2009) Psychotropic medication use among older adults: What all nurses need to know. Journal of Gerontological Nursing, **35**(9), 28–38.

Little, M.O., and Morley, A. (2013) Reducing polypharmacy: Evidence from a simple quality improvement initiative. Journal of the American Medical Directors Association, **14**(3), 152–156.

Llorente, M.D., David, D., Golden, A.G., and Silverman, M.A. (2000) Defining patterns of benzodiazepine use in older adults. Journal of Geriatric Psychiatry and Neurology, **13**(3), 150–160.

Logsdon, R.G., McCurry, S.M., and Teri, L. (2007) Evidence-based psychological treatments for disruptive behaviors in individuals with dementia. Psychology and Aging, **22**(1), 28–36.

Lovibond, P.F., and Lovibond, S.H. (1995) The structure of negative emotional states: Comparison of the Depression Anxiety Stress Scales (DASS) with the Beck Depression and Anxiety Inventories. Behaviour Research and Therapy, **33**, 335–343.

Mackinnon, A., and Mulligan, R. (1998) Combining cognitive testing and informant report to increase accuracy in screening for dementia. American Journal of Psychiatry, **155**, 1529–1535.

Maher, P. (1999) A review of "traditional" Aboriginal health beliefs. Australian Journal of Rural Health, **7**(4), 229–236.

Mann, A.H., Jenkins, R., Cutting, J.C., and Cowen, P.J. (1981) The development and use of a standardized assessment of abnormal personality. Psychological Medicine, **11**(4), 839–847.

Masand, P.S. (2000) Atypical antipsychotics for elderly patients with neurodegenerative disorders and medical conditions. Psychiatric Annals, **30**, 203–208.

Mascolo, M.P., and Fischer, K.W. (2010) The dynamic development of thinking, feeling, and acting over the life span. In W. F. O. R. M. Lerner (Ed.), The handbook of lifespan development, Vol 1: Cognition, biology, and methods (pp. 149–194). Hoboken, NJ: John Wiley and Sons Inc.

Massie, M.J. (2004) Prevalence of depression in patients with cancer. Journal of the National Cancer Institutes Monograph, **32**, 57–71.

McAiney, C.A., Stolee, P., Hillier, L.M., Harris, D., Hamilton, P., Kessler, L., et al. (2007) Evaluation of the sustained implementation of a mental health learning initiative in long-term care. International Psychogeriatrics, 19(5), 842–858.

McCarthy, M., Mueser, K.T., and Pratt, S.I. (2008) Integrated psychosocial rehabilitation and health care for older people with serious mental illness. In D. Gallagher-Thompson, A. M. Steffen, and L. W. Thompson (Eds), Handbook of behavioral and cognitive therapies with older adults (pp. 118–134). New York, NY: Springer.

McCrae, R.R. (2009) The five-factor model of personality traits: Consensus and controversy. In P. J. Corr and G. Matthews (Eds), Cambridge handbook of personality psychology (pp. 148–161). New York: Cambridge University Press.

McCrae, R.R., Barbaranelli, C., Chae, J-H., Piedmont, R.L., Costa, P.T., Pedroso de Lima, M., et al. (1999) Age differences in personality across the adult life span: Parallels in five cultures. Developmental Psychology, 35(2), 466–477.

McCrae, C.S., Rowe, M.A., Tierney, C.G., Cautovich, N.D., DeFinis, A.L., and McNamara, J.P.H. (2005) Sleep complaints, subjective and objective sleep patterns, health, psychological adjustment, and daytime functioning in community-dwelling older adults. Journal of Gerontology: Psychological Sciences, 60(4), 182–189.

McCurry, S.M., Reynolds, C.F., Ancoli-Israel, S., Teri, L., and Vitiello, M.V. (2000) Treatment of sleep disturbance in Alzheimer's disease. Sleep Medicine Reviews, 4(6), 603–628

McDonald, R.J., and Spielberger, C.D. (1981) Measuring anxiety in hospitalized geriatric patients. In C. D. Spielberger and R. Diaz-Guerrero (Eds), Cross-cultural anxiety (vol. 2). New York, NY: Hemisphere Publishing Co.

McGlashan, T.H. (1988) A selective review of recent North American long-term follow-up studies of schizophrenia. Schizophrenia Bulletin, 14, 515–542.

McGlashan, T.H., and Fenton, W.S. (1992) The positive-negative distinction in schizophrenia: Review of natural history validators. Archives of General Psychiatry, 49, 63–72.

McKeith, I.G., Galasko, D., Kosaka, K., Perry, E.K., Dickson, D.W., Hansen, L.A., et al. (1996) Consensus guidelines for the clinical and pathological diagnosis of dementia with Lewy bodies (DLB): Report of the consortium on DLB International workshop. Neurology, 47, 1113–1124.

McKhann, G., Kopman, D., Chertkow, H., Hyman, B., Jack, C., Kawas, C., et al. (2011) The diagnosis of dementia due to Alzheimer's disease: Recommendations from the National Institute on Aging—Alzheimer's Association Workgroups on diagnostic guidelines for Alzheimer's disease. Alzheimer's and Dementia, 7(3), 263–269.

McLennan, S., Mathias, J., Brennan, L., and Stewart, S. (2011) Validity of the Montreal Cognitive Assessment (MoCA) as a screening test for mild cognitive impairment (MCI) in a cardiovascular population. Journal of Geriatrics Psychiatry, 24, 33–38.

McQuaid, J.R., Granholm, E., McClure, F.S., Roepke, S., Pedrelli, P., Patterson, T.L., et al. (2000) Development of an integrated cognitive-behavioral and social skills training intervention for older patients with schizophrenia. Journal of Psychotherapy Practice and Research, 9, 149–156.

Meeks, S. (1999) Bipolar disorder in the latter half of life: Symptom presentation, global functioning and age of onset. Journal of Affective Disorders, 52, 161–167.

Meeks, S., Carstesen, L.L., Stafford, P.B., Brenner, L.L., Weathers, F., Welch, R., et al. (1990) Mental health needs of the chronically mentally ill elderly. Psychology and Aging, 5, 63–71.

Menken, M. (2000) The Global Burden of Disease Study: Implications for neurology. Archives of Neurology, 57, 418–420.

Menninger, J.A. (2002) Assessment and treatment of alcoholism and substance-related disorders in the elderly. Bulletin of the Menninger Clinic, 66, 166–183.

Merckelbach, H., Jelicic, M., and Jonker, C. (2012) Planting a misdiagnosis of Alzheimer's disease in a person's mind. Acta Neuropsychiatrica, 24, 60–62.

Meyer, T., Miller, M., Metzger, R., and Borkovec, T.D. (1990) Development and validation of the Penn State Worry Scale. Behaviour Research and Therapy, 28, 487–495.

Meyers, B.S., and Greenberg, R. (1986) Late-life delusional depression. Journal of Affective Disorders, 11(2), 133–137.

Mezuk, B., Eaton, W.W., Albrecht, S., and Golden, S.H. (2008) Depression and type 2 diabetes over the lifespan. A meta-analysis. Diabetes Care, 31(12), 2383–2390.

Miles, L. (1982) Stanford Sleep Questionnaire and Assessment of Wakefulness (SQAW) (Appendix I) In: C. Guilleminault (Ed.), Sleeping and waking disorders: Indications and techniques (pp. 384–413). Menlo Park, CA: Addison-Wesley.

Miller, S.D., and Duncan, B.L. (2000) The Outcome Rating Scale. Chicago: Author.

Miller, W.R. and Rollnick, S. (2002) Motivational interviewing: Preparing people for change (2nd edn). New York, NY: Guilford Press.

Millon, T., Millon, C., and Davis, R. (1997) MCMI-III manual (2nd edn). Minneapolis, MN: National Computer Systems.

Miloyan, B., Suddendorf T., and Pachana, N.A. (2014) The future is here: A review of foresight systems in anxiety and depression. Cognition and Emotion, 28(5), 795–810.

Mitchell, A.J., Bird, V., Rizzo, M., and Meader, N. (2010) Diagnostic validity and added value of the geriatric depression scale for depression in primary care: A meta-analysis of GDS30 and GDS15. Journal of Affective Disorders, 125(1–3), 10–17.

Mitchell, A.J., and Shiri-Feshki, M. (2009) Rate of progression of mild cognitive impairment to dementia—meta-analysis of 41 robust inception cohort studies. Acta Psychiatrica Scandinavia, 119(4), 252–265.

Moak, G. (1990) Characteristics of demented and non-demented geriatric admissions to a state hospital. Hospital and Community Psychiatry, 41, 799–801.

Mohlman, J., Sirota, K.G., Papp, L.A., Staples, A.M., King, A., and Gorenstein, E.E. (2012) Clinical interviewing with older adults. Cognitive and Behavioral Practice, 19, 89–100.

Monastero, R., Mangialasche, F., Camarda, C., Ercolani, S., and Camarda, R. (2009) A systematic review of neuropsychiatric symptoms in mild cognitive impairment. Journal of Alzheimer's Disease, 18(1), 11–30.

Mondolo, F., Jahanshahi, M., Grana, A., Biasutti, E., Cacciatori, E., and Benedetto, P. (2006) The validity of the Hospital Anxiety and Depression Scale and the Geriatric Depression Scale in Parkinson's disease. Behavioral Neurology, 17(2), 109–115.

Monk, T.H. (2005) Aging human circadian rhythms: Conventional wisdom may not always be right. Journal of Biological Rhythms, 20(4), 366–374.

Monk, T.H., Buysse, D.J., Hall, M., Nofzinger, E.A., Thompson, W.K., Mazumdar, S.A., et al. (2006) Age-related differences in the lifestyle regularity of seniors experiencing bereavement, care-giving, insomnia, and advancement into old-old age. Chronobiology International, 23(4), 831–841.

Moore, R.D., Bone, L.R., Geller, G., Mamon, J.A., Stokes, E.J., and Levine, D.M. (1989) Prevention, detection and treatment of alcoholism in hospitalized patients. Journal of the American Medical Association, **261**, 403–407.

Moran, P., Walsh, E., Tyrer, P., Burns, T., Creed, F., and Fahy, T. (2003) Standardised Assessment of Personality—Abbreviated Scale (SAPAS): Preliminary validation of a brief screen for personality disorder. British Journal of Psychiatry, **183**, 228–232.

Morgan, K. (2000) Sleep and aging. In K. L. Lichstein and C. M. Morin (Eds), Treatment of late life insomnia (pp. 3–36). Thousand Oaks, CA: Sage Publications.

Morin, C.M. (1993) Insomnia: Psychological assessment and management. New York, NY: Guilford Press.

Morin, C.M., Blais, F.C., and Savard, J. (2002) Are changes in beliefs and attitudes about sleep related to sleep improvements in the treatment of insomnia? Behaviour Research and Therapy, **40**, 741–752.

Morin, C.M., and Espie, C.A. (2003) Insomnia: A clinical guide to assessment and treatment. New York, NY: Kluwer Academic/Plenum Publishers.

Morin, C.M., Savard, J., and Blais, F.C. (2000) Cognitive therapy. In K. L. Lichstein and C. M. Morin (Eds), Treatment of late life insomnia (pp. 207–230). Thousand Oaks, CA: Sage Publications.

Morin, C.M., Stone, J., Trinkle, D., Mercer, J., and Remsberg, S. (1993) Dysfunctional beliefs and attitudes about sleep among older adults with and without insomnia complaints. Psychology and Aging, **8**(3), 463–467.

Morin, C.M., Vallères, A., and Ivers, H. (2007) Dysfunctional Beliefs and Attitudes about Sleep (DBAS): Validation of a brief version (DBAS-16). Sleep, **30**, 1547–1554.

Morley, J.E. (2004) The top 10 hot topics in aging. Journals of Gerontology A: Biological Science and Medical Science, **59**, 24–33.

Morris, J.C. (1997) Clinical dementia rating: A reliable and valid diagnostic and staging measure for dementia of the Alzheimer Type. International Psychogeriatrics, **9**(Suppl. S1), 173–176.

Morris, J.C. (2012) Revised criteria for mild cognitive impairment may compromise the diagnosis of Alzheimer disease dementia. Archives of Neurology, **69**, 700–708.

Morris, R.G., Worsley, C., and Matthews, D. (2000) Neuropsychological assessment in older people: Old principles and new directions. Advances in Psychiatric Treatment, **6**, 362–372.

Morton, J.L., Jones, T.V., and Manganaro, M.A. (1996) Performance of alcoholism screening questionnaires in elderly veterans. American Journal of Medicine, **101**(2), 153–159.

Moye, J., Marson, D.C., and Edelstein, B. (2013) Assessment of capacity in an aging society. American Psychologist, **68**(3), 158–171.

Mroczek, D.K., Spiro III, A., and Griffin, P.W. (2006) Personality and aging. In J. E. Birren and K. W. Schaie (Eds), Handbook of the psychology of aging (6th edn, pp. 363–377). San Diego: Elsevier Academic Press.

Nasreddine, Z.S., Phillips, N.A., Bedirian, V., Charbonneau, S., Whitehead, V., Collin, I., et al. (2005) The Montreal Cognitive Assessment, MoCA: A brief screening tool for mild cognitive impairment. Journal of the American Geriatrics Society, **53**(4), 695–699.

Nemiroff, R.A., and Colarusso, C.A. (1985) The race against time: Psychotherapy and psychoanalysis in the second half of life. New York: Plenum Press.

Neutel, C.I., Perry, S., and Maxwell, C. (2002) Medication use and risk of falls. Pharmacoepidemiology and Drug Safety, **11**(2), 97–104.

Nobili, A., Garattini, S., and Mannucci, P.M. (2011) Multiple diseases and polypharmacy in the elderly: Challenges for the internist of the third millennium. Journal of Co-Morbidity, **1**(1), 28–44.

Novak, M., Mucsi, I., Shapiro, C.M., Rethelyi, J., and Koop, M.S. (2004) Increased utilization of health services by insomniacs—an epidemiological perspective. Journal of Psychosomatic Research, **56**(5), 527–536.

O'Boyle, C.A., McGee, H.M., Hickey, A., Joyce, C.R.B., Browne, J., O'Malley, K., et al. (1993) The Schedule for the Evaluation of Individual Quality of Life (SEIQoL): Administration manual. Dublin: Royal College of Surgeons in Ireland.

O'Boyle, C.A., McGee, H.M., Hickey, A., O'Malley, K., and Joyce, C.R.B. (1992) Individual quality of life in patients undergoing hip replacement. Lancet, **339**, 1088–1091.

Ohayon, M.M. (2004) Interactions between sleep normative data and sociocultural characteristics in the elderly. Journal of Psychosomatic Research, **56**(5), 479–486.

Ohayon, M.M., Carskadon, M.A., Guilleminault, C., and Vitiello, M.V. (2004) Meta-analysis of quantitative sleep parameters from childhood to old age in healthy individuals: Developing normative sleep values across the human lifespan. Sleep, **27**(7), 1255–1273.

Ohayon, M.M., Zulley, J., Guilleminault, C., Smirne, S., and Priest, R.G. (2001) How age and daytime activities are related to insomnia in the general population: Consequences for older people. Journal of the American Geriatrics Society, **49**(4), 360–366.

Okazaki, S., Kallivayalil, D., and Sue, S. (2002) Clinical personality assessment with Asian Americans. In J. T. Butcher (Ed.), Clinical personality assessment: Practical approaches (2nd edn, pp. 135–153). London: Oxford University Press.

Oltmanns, T.F., and Balsis, S. (2011) Personality disorders in later life: Questions about the measurement, course, and impact of disorders. Annual Review of Clinical Psychology, **27**(7), 321–349.

O'Riley, A.A., Segal, D.L., and Coolidge, F.I. (2005) Convergent and discriminant validity of the BDI-II among older adults. Poster presented at the annual meeting of the American Psychological Association, Washington, DC.

Ormel, J., Rijsdij, K.F., Sullivan, M., Van Sonderan, E., and Kempen, G. (2002) Temporal and reciprocal relationship between IADL (ADL disability) and depressive symptoms in late life. Journals of Gerontology B: Psychological Science, Social Science, **57**, 338–347.

Oslin, D.W., Streim, J.E., Parmalee, P., Boyce, A.A., and Katz, I.R. (1997) Alcohol abuse: A source of reversible functional disability among residents of a VA nursing home. International Journal of Geriatric Psychiatry, **12**(8), 825–832.

Overall, J.E., and Gorham, D.R. (1962) The Brief Psychiatric Rating Scale. Psychological Reports, **10**, 799–812.

Owens, K.M.B., Hadjistavropoulos, T., and Asmundson, G.J.G. (2000) Addressing the need for appropriate norms when measuring anxiety in seniors. Aging and Mental Health, **4**, 309–314.

Pachana, N.A., and Byrne, G.J. (2012) The Geriatric Anxiety Inventory: International use and future directions. Australian Psychologist, **47**(1), 33–38.

Pachana, N.A., Byrne, G.J., Siddle, H., Koloski, N., Harley. E., and Arnold, E. (2007) Development and validation of the Geriatric Anxiety Inventory. International Psychogeriatrics, **19**, 103–114.

Pachana, N.A., Gallagher-Thompson, D., and Thompson, L.W. (1994) Assessment of depression. In M. P. Lawton and J. Teresi (Eds), Annual review of gerontology and geriatrics (Vol. 14): Assessment techniques (pp. 234–256). New York: Springer Publishing.

Pachana, N.A., Helmes, E., Byrne, G.J.A., Edelstein, B.A., Konnert, C.A., and Pot, A.M. (2010a) Screening for mental disorders in residential aged care facilities. International Psychogeriatrics, **22**(7), 1107–1120.

Pachana, N.A., Paton, H., and Squelch, N. (2010b) The importance of feedback and communication strategies with older adults: Therapeutic and ethical considerations. In N. A. Pachana, K. Laidlaw, and B. G. Knight (Eds), Casebook of clinical geropsychology: International perspectives on practice (pp. 155–177). Oxford: Oxford University Press.

Pachana, N.A., Thompson, L.W., Marcopulos, B.A., and Yoash-Gantz, R. (2004) California Older Adult Stroop Test (COAST): A Stroop test for older adults. Clinical Gerontologist, **27**, 3–22.

Palmer, K., Berger, A.K., Monastero, R., Winblad, B., Bäckman, L., and Fratiglioni, L. (2007) Predictors of progression from mild cognitive impairment to Alzheimer disease. Neurology, **68**, 1596–1602.

Paranthaman, R., Burns, A.S., Cruickshank, J.K., Jackson, A., Scott, M.L.J., and Baldwin, R.C. (2012) Age at onset and vascular pathology in late-life depression. American Journal of Geriatric Psychiatry: Official Journal of the American Association for Geriatric Psychiatry, **20**(6), 524.

Paris, J. (2003) Personality disorders over time: Precourse, course and outcome. Journal of Personality Disorders, **17**, 479–488.

Paris J., and Zweig-Frank, H. (2001) A 27-year follow-up of patients with borderline personality disorder. Comprehensive Psychiatry, **42**, 782–787

Park, H.L., O'Connell, J.E., and Thomson, R.G. (2003) A systematic review of cognitive decline in the general elderly population. International Journal of Geriatric Psychiatry, **18**(12), 1121–1134.

Parker, G., and Hadzi-Pavlovic, D. (1996) Melancholia: A disorder of movement and mood. New York, NY: Cambridge University Press.

Patterson, T.L., Mausbach, B.T., McKibbin, C., Goldman, S., Bucardo, J., and Jeste, D.V. (2006) Functional Adaptation Skills Training (FAST): A randomized trial of a psychosocial intervention for middle-aged and older patients with chronic psychotic disorders. Schizophrenia Research, **86**, 291–299.

Patterson, T.L., McKibbin, C., Taylor, M., Goldman, S., Davila-Fraga, W., Bucardo, J., et al. (2003) Functional adaptation skills training (FAST): A pilot psychosocial intervention study in middle-aged and older patients with chronic psychotic disorders. American Journal of Geriatric Psychiatry, **11**(1), 17–23.

Petersen, R.C. (2004) Mild cognitive impairment as a diagnostic entity. Journal of Internal Medicine, **256**(3), 183–194.

Pfohl, B., Blum, N., and Zimmerman, M. (1997) Structured interview for DSM-IV personality (SIDP-IV). Washington D.C.: American Psychiatric Press.

Phelps, J.R., and Ghaemi, S.N. (2006) Improving the diagnosis of bipolar disorder: Predictive value of screening tests. Journal of Affective Disorders, **92**, 141–148.

Phillips, N., Chertkow, H., Nasreddine, N., Whitehead, V., Bishundayal, S., and McHenry, C. (2011) Validation of alternate forms for the Montreal Cognitive

Assessment (MoCA). Presented at the 39th International Neuropsychological Society Meeting in Boston February 2–5.

P.I.E.C.E.S. Canada (2008) Putting the P.I.E.C.E.S together: A learning resource for providers caring for older adults with complex physical and cognitive/mental health needs and behavioural changes. Ontario: P.I.E.C.E.S..

Pinkahana, J., Happell, B., and Keks, N. (2003) Suicide and schizophrenia: A review of literature for the decade (1990-1999) and implications for mental health nursing. Issues in Mental Health Nursing, 24, 27–43.

Pinquart, M., and Duberstein, P.R. (2007) Treatment of anxiety disorders in older adults: A meta-analytic comparison behavioral and pharmacological interventions. American Journal of Geriatric Psychiatry, 15(8), 639–651.

Pinquart, M., Duberstein, P.R., and Lyness, J.M. (2006) Treatments for late-life depressive conditions: A meta-analytic comparison of pharmacotherapy and psychotherapy. American Journal of Psychiatry, 163(9), 1493–1501.

Pinquart, M., and Sörensen, S. (2006) Helping caregivers of persons with dementia: Which interventions work and how large are their effects? International Psychogeriatrics, 18(4), 577–595.

Pinsker, D.M., Stone, V.E., Pachana, N.A., and Greenspan, S. (2006) Social vulnerability scale for older adults: A validation study. Clinical Psychologist, 10, 109–119.

Pinto-Meza, A., Serrano-Blanco, A., Peñarrubia, M.T., Blanco, E., and Haro, J.M. (2005) Assessing depression in primary care with the PHQ-9: Can it be carried out over the telephone? Journal of General Internal Medicine, 20(8), 738–742.

Pollak, C.P., Perlick, D., Linsner, J.P., Wenston, J., and Hsieh, F. (1990) Sleep problems in the community elderly as predictors of death and nursing home placement. Journal of Community Health, 15(2), 123–135.

Pope, K.S. (1992) Responsibilities in providing psychological test feedback to clients. Psychological Assessment, 4(3), 268–271.

Postal, K., and Armstrong, K. (2013) Feedback that sticks: The art of effectively communicating neuropsychological assessment results. New York, NY: Oxford University Press.

Poulsen, E.E., Sibbritt, D., McLaughlin, D., Adams, J., and Pachana, N.A. (2013) Predictors of Complimentary and Alternative Medicine (CAM) use in two cohorts of Australian women. International Psychogeriatrics, 25(1), 168–170.

Prince, M., Bryce, R., Albanese, E., Wimo, A., Ribeiro, W., and Ferri, C.P. (2013) The global prevalence of dementia: A systematic review and meta-analysis. Alzheimer's Dementia, 9(1), 63–72.

Psychiatric Rehabilitation Consultants. (1991) Modules in the UCLA Social and Independent Living Skill Series. Camarillo, CA: Psychiatric Rehabilitation Consultants.

Pusey, H., and Richards, D.A. (2001) A systematic review of the effectiveness of psychosocial interventions for carers of people with dementia. Aging and Mental Health, 5(2), 107–119.

Qualls, S.H., Duffy, M., and Crose, R. (1995) Clinical supervision and practicum placements in graduate training. In B. G. Knight, L. Teri, J. Santos and P. Wohlford (Eds), Mental health services for older adults: Implications for training and practice in geropsychology (pp. 119–128). Washington, DC: American Psychological Association.

Qualls, S.H., and Noecker, T.L. (2009) Caregiver family therapy for conflicted families. In S. H. Qualls and S. H. Zarit (Eds), Aging families and caregiving (pp. 155–188). New Jersey: John Wiley and Sons.

Quinn, T.J., Langhorne, P., and Stott, D.J. (2011) Barthel index for stroke trials: development, properties and application. Stroke, **42**, 1146–1151.

Rahhal, T.A., Hasher, L., and Colcombe, S.J. (2001) Instructional manipulations and age differences in memory: Now you see them, now you don't. Psychology and Aging, **16**, 697–706.

Ratnavalli, E., Brayne, C., Dawson, K., and Hodges, J.R. (2002) The prevalence of frontotemporal dementia. Neurology, **58**, 1615–1621.

Ray, W., Thapa, P., and Gideon, P. (2000) Benzodiazepines and the risk of falls in nursing home residents. Journal of the American Geriatrics Society, **48**, 682–685.

Ready, R.E., Carvalho, J.O., and Weinberger, M.I. (2008) Emotional complexity in younger, midlife, and older adults. Psychology and Aging, **23**(4), 928–933.

Reese, R.J., Usher, E.L., Bowman, D.C., Norsworthy, L.A., Halstead, J.L., Rowlands, S.R., et al. (2009) Using client feedback in psychotherapy training: An analysis of its influence on supervision and counsellor self-efficacy. Training and Education in Professional Psychology, **3**(3), 157–168.

Reid, K.J., Glazer Baron, K., Lu, B., Naylor, E., Wolfe, L., and Zee, P.C. (2010) Aerobic exercise improves self-reported sleep and quality of life in older adults with insomnia. Sleep Medicine, **11**(9), 934–940.

Reinert, D.F., and Allen, J.P. (2002) The Alcohol Use Disorders Identification Test (AUDIT): A review of recent research. Alcoholism: Clinical and Experimental Research, **26**(2), 272–279.

Reynolds, C.F., and Redline, S. (2010) The DSM5 sleep-wake disorders nosology: An update and an invitation to the sleep community. Sleep, **33**(1), 10–11.

Reynolds, C.R., Richmond, B.O., and Lowe, P.A. (2003) The Adult Manifest Anxiety Scale–Elderly Version (AMAS-E). Los Angeles: Western Psychological Services.

Reynolds, T., Thornicroft, G., Abas, M., Woods, B., Hoe, J., Leese, M., et al. (2000) Camberwell Assessment of Need for the Elderly (CANE): development, validity, and reliability. British Journal of Psychiatry, **176**, 444–452.

Ricklefs, R.E., and Finch, C.E. (1995) Aging: A natural history. New York: Scientific American Library.

Riedel, B. (2000) Sleep hygiene. In K. L. Lichstein and C. M. Morin (Eds), Treatment of late life insomnia (pp. 125–146). Thousand Oaks, CA: Sage Publications.

Riedel, B.W., and Lichstein, K.L. (2000) Insomnia and daytime functioning. Sleep Medicine Reviews, **4**(3), 277–298.

Riedel, B.W., Winfield, C.F., and Lichstein, K.L. (2001) First night effect and reverse first night effect in older adults with primary insomnia: Does anxiety play a role? Sleep Medicine, **2**(2), 125–133.

Ripich, D.N., Wykle, M., and Niles, S. (1995) Alzheimer's disease caregivers: The FOCUSED program: A communication skills training program helps nursing assistants to give better care to patients with Alzheimer's disease. Geriatric Nursing, **16**(1), 15–19.

Robb, C., Haley, W.E., Becker, M.A., Polivka, L.A., and Chwa, H.J. (2003) Attitudes towards mental health care in younger and older adults: Similarities and differences. Aging and Mental Health, **7**, 142–152.

Rodolfa. E., Bent, R., Eisman, E., Nelson, P., Rehm, L., and Ritchie, P. (2005) A cube model for competency development: Implications for psychology educators and regulators. Professional Psychology: Research and Practice, **36**, 347–354.

Rokke, P.D., and Scogin, F. (1995) Depression treatment preferences in younger and older adults. Journal of Clinical Geropsychology, **1**, 243–257.

Rose, M.K., Soares, H.H., and Joseph, C. (1992) Frail elderly clients with personality disorders: A challenge for social work. Journal of Gerontological Social Work, **19**(3–4), 153–165.

Rosowsky, E., and Gurian, B. (1992) Impact of borderline personality disorder in late life on systems of care. Hospital and Community Psychiatry, **43**, 386–389.

Roux, F.J., and Kryger, M.H. (2010) Medication effects on sleep. Clinics in Chest Medicine, **31**(2), 397–405.

Ruff, R. (2003) A friendly critique of neuropsychology: Facing the challenges of our future. Archives of Clinical Neuropsychology, **18**(8), 847–864.

Rugulies, R. (2002) Depression as a predictor for coronary heart disease: A review and meta-analysis. American Journal of Preventative Medicine, **23**, 51–61.

Ruiter Petrov, M.E., Vander Wal, G.S., and Lichstein, K.L. (2014) Late-life insomnia. N. A. Pachana and K. Laidlaw (Eds), Oxford Handbook of Clinical Geropsychology (pp. 527–548). Oxford: Oxford University Press.

Sajatovic, M., Bingham, C.R., Campbell, E.A., and Fletcher, D.F. (2005a) Bipolar disorder in older adult inpatients. Journal of Nervous and Mental Disorders, **193**(6), 417–419.

Sajatovic, M., Blow, F.C., Ignacio, R.V., and Kales, H.C. (2004) Bipolar disorder in the Veterans Health Administration: Age-related modifiers of clinical presentation and health services use. Psychiatric Services, **55**(9), 1014–1021.

Sajatovic, M., Blow, F.C., Ignacio, R.V., and Kales, H.C. (2005b) New-onset bipolar disorder in later life. American Journal of Geriatric Psychiatry, **13**(4), 282–289.

Sakauye K. (2012) Cultural psychiatry considerations in older adults. American Journal of Geriatric Psychiatry, **20**(11), 911–914.

Salthouse, T. (2010) Selective review of cognitive aging. Journal of the International Neuropsychological Society, **16**(5), 754–760.

Sartorius, N., Ustun, T.B., Lecrubier, Y., and Wittchen, H. (1996) Depression co-morbid with anxiety: Results from the WHO study on psychological disorders in primary care. British Journal of Psychology, **168**, 38–43.

Satre, D.D. (2013) Treatment of older adults. In B. S. McCrady and E. E. Epstein (Eds), Addictions: A comprehensive guidebook (pp. 742–757). New York: Oxford University Press.

Satre, D.D., Chi, F.W., Mertens, J.R., and Weisner, C.M. (2012) Effects of age and life transitions on alcohol and drug treatment outcomes over nine years. Journal of Studies on Alcohol and Drugs, **73**, 459–468.

Satre, D.D., Sterling, S.A., Mackin, R.S., and Weisner, C. (2011) Patterns of alcohol and drug use among depressed older adults seeking outpatient psychiatric services. American Journal of Geriatric Psychiatry, **19**, 695–703.

Saunders, P.A., Copeland, J.R., Dewey, M.E., Davidson, I.A., McWilliam, C., Sharma, V., et al. (1991) Heavy drinking as a risk factor for depression and dementia in elderly men. Findings from the Liverpool longitudinal community study. British Journal of Psychiatry, **159**, 213–216.

Sayegh, P., and Knight, B.G. (2013) Cross-cultural differences in dementia: the Sociocultural Health Belief Model. International Psychogeriatrics/IPA, **25**(4), 517.

Schaie, K.W. (2013) Developmental influences on adult intellectual development: The Seattle Longitudinal Study. New York: Oxford University Press.

Scherder, E.J.A. and Bouma, A. (2000) Visual analogue scales for pain assessment in Alzheimer's disease. Gerontology **46**, 47–53.

Schieber, F. (2006) Vision and aging. In J. E. Birren and K. W. Schaie (Eds), Handbook of the Psychology of Aging (6th edn, pp. 129–161). Burlington, MA: Elsevier.

Schonfeld, L., and Dupree, L.W. (1991) Antecedents of drinking for early- and late-onset elderly alcohol abusers. Journal of Studies on Alcohol **52**, 587–592.

Schonfeld, L., King-Kallimanis, B.L., Duchene, D.M., Etheridge, R.L., Herrera, J.R., Barry, K.L., et al. (2010) Screening and brief intervention for substance misuse among older adults: The Florida BRITE project. American Journal of Public Health, **100**(1), 108–114.

Schroeter, M.L. (2012) Considering the frontomedian cortex in revised criteria for behavioural variant frontotemporal dementia. Brain, **135**(4), e213.

Schroeter, M.L., Vogt, B., Frisch, S., Becker, G., Barthel, H., Mueller, K., et al. (2012) Executive deficits are related to the inferior frontal junction in early dementia. Brain, **135**, 201–215.

Schurhoff, F., Bellivier, F., Jouvent, R., Mouren-Simeoni, M.C., Bouvard, M., Allilaire, J.F. et al. (2000) Early and late onset bipolar disorders: two different forms of manic-depressive illness? Journal of Affective Disorders, **58**, 215–221.

Schuster, J-P., Hoertel, N., Le Strat, Y., Manetti, A., and Limosin, F. (2013) Personality disorders in older adults: Findings from the national epidemiological survey on alcohol and related conditions. American Journal of Geriatric Psychiatry, **21**, 757–768.

Scogin, F., Floyd, M., and Forde, J. (2000) Anxiety in older adults. In S. K. Whitbourne (Eds), Psychopathology in later adulthood (pp. 117–140). New York: John Wiley and Sons.

Secker, D.L., Kazantzis, N., and Pachana, N.A. (2004) Cognitive behavior therapy for older adults: Practical guidelines for adapting therapy structure. Journal of Rational-Emotive and Cognitive Behavior Therapy, **22**, 93–109.

Segal, D.L., and Coolidge, F.L. (2001) Personality disorders. In B. Edelstein (Ed.), Clinical geropsychology (vol. 7, pp. 267–289). Amsterdam: Pergamon.

Segal, D.L., and Coolidge, F.L. (2003) Structured interviewing and DSM classification. In M. Hersen and S. Turner (Eds), Adult psychopathology and diagnosis (4th edn, pp. 72–103). New York: Wiley.

Segal, D.L., Coolidge, F.L., and Rosowsky, E. (2006) Personality disorders and older adults: Diagnosis, assessment and treatment. Hoboken, NJ: Wiley.

Segal, D.L., June, A., Payne, M., Coolidge, F.L., and Yochim, B. (2010) Development and initial validation of a self-report assessment tool for anxiety among older adults: the Geriatric Anxiety Scale. Journal of Anxiety Disorders, **24**(7), 709–714.

Series, H., and Esiri, M. (2012) Vascular dementia: a pragmatic review. Advances in Psychiatric Treatment, **18**(5), 372–380.

Shah, A., Scogin, F., and Floyd, M. (2012) Evidence-based psychological treatments for geriatric depression. In F. Scogin and A. Shah (Eds), Making evidenced-based psychological treatments work with older adults (pp. 87–130). Washington, DC: American Psychological Association.

Shankar, K.K., Walker, M., Frost, D., and Orrell, M.W. (1999) The development of a valid and reliable scale for rating anxiety in dementia (RAID) Aging and Mental Health, 3(1), 39–49.

Sheehan, D.V., Lecrubier, Y., Sheehan, K.H., Amorim, P., Janavs, J., Weiller, E., et al. (1998) The Mini-International Neuropsychiatric Interview (M.I.N.I.): The development and validation of a structured diagnostic psychiatric interview for DSM-IV and ICD-10. Journal of Clinical Psychiatry, **59**(Suppl 20), 22–33.

Shepherd, S., Depp, C.A., Harris, G., Halpain, M., Palinkas, L.A., and Jeste, D.V. (2012) Perspectives on schizophrenia over the lifespan: A qualitative study. Schizophrenia Bulletin, **38**(2), 295–303.

Shringarpure, R., and Davies, K.J.A. (2009) Free radicals and oxidative stress in aging. In V. L. Bengtson, D. Gans, N. M. Putney, and M. Silverstein (Eds), Handbook of theories of aging (2nd edn, pp. 229–244). New York: Springer.

Siberski, J. (2012) Dementia and DSM-5: Changes, cost, and confusion. Aging Well, **5**, 12.

Simoni-Wastila, L., and Yang, H.K. (2006) Psychoactive drug abuse in older adults. American Journal of Geriatric Pharmacotherapy, **4**(4), 380–394.

Sinoff, G., Ore, L., Zlotogorsky, D., and Tamir, A. (1999) Short Anxiety Screening Test—a brief instrument for detecting anxiety in the elderly. International Journal of Geriatric Psychiatry, **14**, 1062–1071.

Skevington, S.M., Lofty, M., O'Connell, K.A., and the WHOQOL Group. (2004) The World Health Organization's WHOQOL-BREF quality of life assessment: Psychometric properties and results of the international field trial. A report from the WHOQOL group. Quality of Life Research, **13**(2), 299–310.

Smith, S.S. (2010) Treating late life insomnia: A case study. In N. A. Pachana, K. Laidlaw, and B. G. Knight (Eds), Casebook of clinical geropsychology: International perspectives on practice. (pp. 179–194). Oxford: Oxford University Press.

Smith, M.T., and Haythornthwaite, J.A. (2004) How do sleep disturbance and chronic pain inter-relate? Insights from the longitudinal and cognitive-behavioral clinical trials literature. Sleep Medicine Reviews, **8**(2), 119–132.

Smith, S.S., Horswill, M.S., Chambers, B., and Wetton, M. (2009) Hazard perception in novice and experienced drivers: The effects of sleepiness. Accident Analysis and Prevention, **41**(4), 729–733.

Smith, S.R., Wiggins, C.M., and Gorske, T.T. (2007) A survey of psychological assessment feedback practices. Assessment, **14**(3), 310–319.

Smits, I.A.M., Dolan, C.V., Vorst, H.C.M., Wicherts, J.M., and Timmerman, M.E. (2011) Cohort differences in big five personality factors over a period of 25 years. Journal of Personality and Social Psychology, **100**(6), 1124–1138.

Snow, A.L. and Jacobs, M.L. (2014) Pain in persons with dementia and communication impairment. In N. A. Pachana and K. Laidlaw (Eds), Oxford Handbook of Clinical Geropsychology (pp. 876–908). Oxford: Oxford University Press.

Snow, A.L., Petersen, N.J., Stanley, M.A., Huddleston, C., Robinson, C., Kunik, M.E., et al. (2012) Psychometric properties of a structured interview guide for the rating for anxiety in dementia. Aging and Mental Health, **16**(5), 592–602.

Spalletta, G., Caltagirone, C., Palmer, K., Musicco, M., Padovani, A., Rozzini, L., et al. (2010) Neuropsychiatric symptoms and syndromes in a large cohort of newly diagnosed, untreated patients with Alzheimer disease. American Journal of Geriatric Psychiatry:

Official Journal of the American Association for Geriatric Psychiatry, **18**(11), 1026–1035.

Spector, A., Orrell, M., Lattimer, M., Hoe, J., King, M., Harwood, K., et al. (2012) Cognitive behavioural therapy (CBT) for anxiety in people with dementia: study protocol for a randomised controlled trial. Trials, **13**(1), 197–197.

Spielberger, C.D. (1983) Manual for the State-Trait Anxiety Inventory. Palo Alto, CA: Consulting Psychologists Press.

Spiers, N., Bebbington, P., McManus, S., Brugha, T.S., Jenkins, R., and Meltzer, H. (2011) Age and birth cohort differences in the prevalence of common mental disorder in England: National Psychiatric Morbidity Surveys 1993–2007. British Journal of Psychiatry, **198**, 479–484.

Spinhoven, P., Ormel, J., Sloekers, P.P., Kempen, G.I., Speckens, A.E., and Van Hemert, A.M. (1997) A validation study of the Hospital Anxiety and Depression Scale (HADS) in different groups of Dutch subjects. Psychological Medicine, **27**(2), 363–370.

Stanley, M.A., Novy, D.M., Bourland, S.L., Beck, J.G., and Averill, P.M. (2001) Assessing older adults with generalized anxiety: A replication and extension. Behaviour Research and Therapy, **39**, 221–235.

Stepanski, E.J., and Wyatt, J.K. (2003) Use of sleep hygiene in the treatment of insomnia. Sleep Medicine Reviews, **7**(3), 215–225.

Stevens, J.A., and Dellinger, A.M. (2002) Motor vehicle and fall related deaths among older Americans 1990–1998: Sex, race, and ethnic disparities. Injury Prevention, **8**, 272–275.

Stevenson, J., Meares, R., and Comerford, A. (2003) Diminished impulsivity in older patients with borderline personality disorder. American Journal of Psychiatry, **160**, 165–166.

Storey, J., Rowland, J., Basic, D., Conforti, D., and Dickson, H. (2004) The Rowland Universal Dementia Assessment Scale (RUDAS): A Multicultural Cognitive Assessment Scale. International Psychogeriatrics, **16**(1), 13–31.

Stroebe, M., and Schut, H. (1999) The dual process model of coping with bereavement: Rationale and description. Death Studies, **23**, 197–224.

Sue, S., Cheng, J.K.Y., Saad, C.S., and Chu, J.P. (2012) Asian American mental health: A call to action. American Psychologist, **67**(7), 532–544.

Swafford, K.L., Miller, L.L., Tsai, P-F., Herr, K.A., and Ersek, M. (2009) Improving the process of pain care in nursing homes: A literature synthesis. Journal of the American Geriatrics Society, **57**(6), 1080–1087.

Targum, S.D. (2001) Treating psychotic symptoms in elderly patients. Primary Care Companion Journal of Clinical Psychiatry, **3**, 156–163.

Targum, S.D., and Abbott, J.L. (1999) Psychosis in the elderly: a spectrum of disorders. Journal of Clinical Psychiatry, **60**(Suppl. 8), 4–10.

Tariot, P.N., Schneider, L.S., Mintzer, J.E., Cutler, A.J., Cunningham, M.R., Thomas, J.W. et al. (2001) Safety and tolerability of divalproex sodium in the treatment of signs and symptoms of mania in elderly patients with dementia: Results of a double-blind, placebo-controlled trial. Current Therapies Research, **62**, 51–67.

Teng, E.L., and Chui, H.C. (1987) The Modified Mini-Mental State (3MS) examination. Journal of Clinical Psychiatry, **48**(8), 314–318.

Therrien, Z., and Hunsley, J. (2012) Assessment of anxiety in older adults: A systematic review of commonly used measures. Aging and Mental Health, **16**(1), 1–16.

Thorp, L. (1997) The treatment of psychotic disorders in later life. Canadian Journal of Psychiatry, **42**(Suppl. 1), 19S–27S.

Todaro, J.F., Shen, B-J., Raffa, S.D., Tilkemeier, P.L., and Niaura, R. (2007) Prevalence of anxiety disorders in men and women with established coronary heart disease. Journal of Cardiopulmonary Rehabilitation and Prevention, **27**(2), 86–91.

Tombaugh, T.N., McDowell, I., Kristjansson, B., and Hubley, A. (1996) Mini-Mental State Examination (MMSE) and the Modified MMSE (3MS): A psychometric comparison and normative data. Psychological Assessment, **8**, 54–59.

Towsley, G., Neradilek, M.B., Snow, A.L., and Ersek, M. (2012). Evaluating the Cornell Scale for Depression in Dementia as a proxy measure in nursing home residents with and without dementia. Aging and Mental Health, **16**, 892–901.

Triebwasser, J. and Shea, M.T. (1996) Personality change resulting from another mental disorder. In T. A. Widiger, A. J. Frances, H. A. Pincus, R. Ross, M. B. First, and W. W. Davis (Eds), DSM–IV sourcebook (Vol. 2, pp. 861–868). Washington, DC: American Psychiatric Association.

Troxel, W.M., Buysse, D.J., Monk, T.H., Begley, A., and Hall, M. (2010) Does social support differentially affect sleep in older adults with versus without insomnia? Journal of Psychosomatic Research, **69**(5), 459–466.

Tsai, S., Kuo, C., Chen, C., and Lee, H. (2002) Risk factors for completed suicide in bipolar disorder. Journal of Clinical Psychiatry, **63**, 469–476.

Twiss, J., Jones, S., and Anderson, I. (2008) Validation of the Mood Disorder Questionnaire for screening for bipolar disorder in a UK sample. Journal of Affective Disorders, **110**, 180–184.

US Department of Health and Human Services (USDHHS) (1999) Mental health: A report of the surgeon general. Rockville, MD: USDHHS.

van Alphen, S.P.J., Engelen, G.J.J.A., Kuin, Y., and Derksen, J.J.L. (2006a) The relevance of a geriatric sub-classification of personality disorders in the DSM-IV. International Journal of Geriatric Psychiatry, **21**, 205–209.

van Alphen, S.P.J., Engelen, G.J.J.A., Kuin, Y., Hoijtink, H.J.A., and Derksen, J.J.L. (2006b) A preliminary study of the diagnostic accuracy of the Gerontological Personality disorders Scale (GPS). International Journal of Geriatric Psychiatry, **21**, 862–868.

van Haastregt, J.C., Zijlstra, G.A., van Rossum, E., van Eijk, J.T., and Kempen, G.I. (2008) Feelings of anxiety and symptoms of depression in community-living older persons who avoid activity for fear of falling. American Journal of Geriatric Psychiatry, **16**, 186–193.

Van Horn, E., Manley, C., Leddy, D., Cicchetti, D., and Tyrer, P. (2000) Problems in developing an instrument for the rapid assessment of personality status. European Psychiatry, **15**(Suppl. 1), 29–33.

van Lennep, J.E., Westerveld, H.T., Erkelens, D.W., and van der Wall, E.E. (2002) Risk factors for coronary heart disease: Implications of gender. Cardiovascular Research, **53**, 538–549.

Ventura, J., Green, M.F., Shaner, A., and Liberman, R.P. (1993) Training and quality assurance with the Brief Psychiatric Rating Scale: "The Drift Busters." International Journal of Methods in Psychiatric Research, **3**, 221–224.

Vink, D., Aartsen, M.J., Comijs, H.C., Heymans, M.W., Penninx, B.W.J.H., Stek, M.L., et al. (2009) Onset of anxiety and depression in the aging population:

comparison of risk factors in a 9-year prospective study. The American Journal of Geriatric Psychiatry, **17**(8), 642.

Vink, D., Aartsen, M.J., and Schoevers, R.A. (2008) Risk factors for anxiety and depression in the elderly: A review. Journal of Affective Disorders, **1–2**, 29–44.

Wakisaka, Y., Furuta, A., Tanizaki, Y., Kiyohara, Y., Iida, M., and Iwaki, T. (2003) Age-associated prevalence and risk factors of Lewy body pathology in a general population: the Hisayama study. Acta Neuropathologica, **106**(4), 374–382.

Walker, D., and Clarke, M. (2001) Cognitive behavioral psychotherapy: A comparison between younger and older adults in two inner city mental health teams. Aging and Mental Health, **5**, 197–199.

Walters, K., Iliffe, S., Tai, S.S., and Orrell, M. (2000) Assessing needs from patient, carer, and professional perspectives: The Camberwell Assessment of Need for Elderly people in primary care. Age and Ageing, **29**(6), 505–510.

Ware, J.E., Kosinski, M., Turner-Bowker, D.M., and Gandek, B. (2002). How to score Version 2 of the SF-12® Health Survey (with a supplement documenting Version 1). Lincoln, RI: QualityMetric Incorporated.

Webster, J., and Grossberg, G.T. (1998) Late-life onset of psychotic symptoms. American Journal of Geriatric Psychiatry, **6**, 196–202.

Weinberger, M.I., Roth, A.J., and Nelson, C.J. (2009) Untangling the complexities of depression diagnosis in older cancer patients. The Oncologist, **14**, 60–66.

Weissman, M.M., Leaf, P.J., and Tischler, G.L. (1988). Affective disorders in five United States communities. Psychological Medicine, **18**, 141–153.

Werner, P., Cohen-Mansfield, J., Koroknay, V., and Braun J. (1994) The impact of a restraint-reduction program on nursing home residents. Geriatric Nursing, **15**(3), 142–146.

Wetherell, J.L., and Arean, P.A. (1997) Psychometric evaluation of the Beck Anxiety Inventory with older medical patients. Psychological Assessment, **9**, 136–144.

Wetherell, J.L., and Gatz, M. (2005) The Beck Anxiety Inventory in older adults with generalized anxiety disorder. Journal of Psychopathology and Behavior Assessment, **27**(1), 17–24.

Wetherell, J.L., Gatz, M., and Craske, M.G. (2003) Treatment of generalized anxiety disorder in older adults. Journal of Consulting and Clinical Psychology, **71**, 31–40.

Wetherell, J., Gatz, M., and Pedersen, N.L. (2001) Longitudinal analysis of anxiety and depressive symptoms. Psychology and Aging, **16**(2), 187–195

Wettergren, L., Kettis-Lindblad, A., Sprangers, M., Ring, L., Uppsala, U., Medicinska och farmaceutiska, V., et al. (2009) The use, feasibility and psychometric properties of an individualised quality-of-life instrument: A systematic review of the SEIQoL-DW. Quality of Life Research, **18**(6), 737–746.

Whipple, J.L., Lambert, M.J., Vermeersch, D.A., Smart, D.W., Nielsen, S.L., and Hawkins, E.J. (2003) Improving the effects of psychotherapy: The use of early identification of treatment failure and problem-solving strategies in routine practice. Journal of Counseling Psychology, **50**, 59–68.

Whitbourne, S.K., and Meeks, S. (2011) Psychopathology, bereavement, and aging. In K. W. Schaie and S. L. Willis (Eds), Handbook of the psychology of aging (7th edn, pp. 295–310). San Diego: Academic Press.

Whitlock, E.P., Green, C.A., Polen, M.R., Berg, A., Klein, J., Siu, A., et al. (2004) Behavioral counseling interventions in primary care to reduce risky/harmful alcohol use by adults: A summary of the evidence for the US Preventive Services Task Force. Annals of Internal Medicine, **140**, 557–568.

WHOQOL Group. (1995) The World Health Organization Quality of Life assessment (WHOQOL): Position paper from the World Health Organization. Social Science and Medicine, **41**, 1403–1409.

Widiger, T.A. (1998) Personality disorders. In D. F. Barone, M. Hersen, and V. B. Van Hasselt (Eds), Advanced personality (pp. 335–352). New York: Plenum Press.

Widiger, T.A. (2002) Personality disorders. In M. M. Antony and D. H. Barlow (Eds), Handbook of assessment, treatment planning, and outcome for psychological disorders (pp. 453–480). New York: Guilford Press.

Widiger, T.A., and Coker, L.A. (2002) Assessing personality disorders. In J. N. Butcher (Ed.), Clinical personality assessment. Practical approaches (2nd edn, pp. 407–434). New York, NY: Oxford University Press.

Widiger, T.A., and Samuel, D.B. (2005) Evidence-based assessment of personality disorders. Psychological Assessment, **17**(3), 278–287.

Williamson, J.D., and Fried, L.P. (1996) Characterization of older adults who attribute functional decrements to "old age." Journal of the American Geriatrics Society, **44**(2), 1429–1434.

Wisocki, P.A., Handen, B., and Morse, C.K. (1986) The Worry Scale as a measure of anxiety among homebound and community active elderly. The Behavior Therapist, **9**, 91–95.

Woerner, M.G., Mannuzza, S., and Kane, M. (1988) Anchoring the BPRS: An aid to improved reliability. Psychopharmacology Bulletin, **24**, 112–117.

Wolitzky-Taylor, K.B., Castriotta, N., Lenze, E.J., Stanley, M.A., and Craske, M.G. (2010) Anxiety disorders in older adults: A comprehensive review. Depression and Anxiety, **27**, 190–211.

Wolkove, N., Elkholy, O., Baltzan, M., and Palayew, M. (2007) Sleep and aging: 1. Sleep disorders commonly found in older people. Canadian Medical Association Journal, **176**(9), 1299–1304.

Wood, J.M., Garb, H.N., Lilienfeld, S.O., and Nezworski, M.T. (2002) Clinical assessment. Annual Review of Psychology, **53**, 519—543.

Woodhead, E.L., Emery, E.E., Pachana, N.A., Scott, T.L., Konnert, C.A., and Edelstein, B.A. (2013) Graduate students' geropsychology training opportunities and perceived competence in working with older adults. Professional Psychology: Research and Practice, **44**(5), 355–362.

Woodward, A.T., Taylor, R.J., Bullard, K.M., Aranda, M.P., Lincoln, K.D., and Chatters, L.M. (2012) Prevalence of lifetime DSM-IV affective disorders among older African Americans, Black Caribbeans, Latinos, Asians, and Non-Hispanic White people. International Journal of Geriatric Psychiatry, **27**(8), 816–827.

Woodward, R., and Pachana, N.A. (2009) Attitudes towards psychological treatment among older Australians. Australian Psychologist, **44**(2), 86–93.

Worden, J.W. (2008) Grief counseling and grief therapy (4th edn). New York: Springer Publishing Company.

World Health Organization (WHO). (2004) The global burden of disease: 2004 update. Geneva: WHO.

World Health Organization (WHO). (2010) Global status report on non-communicable diseases. Geneva: WHO.

Worthman, C.M. (2011) Developmental cultural ecology of sleep. In M. El-S (Ed.), Sleep and development (pp. 167–194). Oxford: Oxford University Press.

Wu, L., and Blazer, D.G. (2011) Illicit and nonmedical drug use among older adults: A review. Journal of Aging and Health, **23**, 481–504.

Yang, L. (2007) Application of mental illness stigma theory to Chinese societies: Synthesis and new directions. Singapore Medical Journal, **48**(11), 977–985.

Yassa, R., Nair, V., Nastase, C., Camile, Y., and Belzile, L. (1988) Prevalence of bipolar disorder in a psychogeriatric population. Journal of Affective Disorders, **14**, 197–201.

Yesavage, J.A., Brink, T.L., Rose, T.L., Lum, O., Huang, V., Adey, M., et al. (1982) Development and validation of a geriatric depression screening scale: A preliminary report. Journal of Psychiatric Research, **17**(1), 37–49.

Yeung, A., Chang, D., Gresham, R.L., Nierenberg, A.A., and Fava, M. (2004) Illness beliefs of depressed Chinese American patients in primary care. Journal of Nervous and Mental Disease, **192**(4), 324–327.

Yohannes, A., Baldwin, R., and Connolly, M. (2000) Depression and anxiety in elderly outpatients with chronic obstructive pulmonary disease: Prevalence, and validation of the BASDEC screening questionnaire. International Journal of Geriatric Psychiatry, **15**, 1090–1096.

Zammit, G.K., Weiner, J., Damato, N., Sillup, G.P., and McMillan, C.A. (1999) Quality of life in people with insomnia. Sleep, **22** (Suppl. 2), S379–S385.

Zarit, J.M., and Zarit, S.H. (2007) Mental disorders in older adults: Fundamentals of assessment and treatment. New York: Guilford Press.

Zeimer, H. (2008) Medications and falls in older people. Journal of Pharmacy Practice and Research, **38**(2), 148–151.

Zhang, B., and Wing, Y. (2006) Sex differences in insomnia: A meta-analysis. Sleep, **29**(1), 85–93.

Zinbarg, R.E., Craske, M.G., and Barlow, D.H. (2006) Mastery of your anxiety and worry (2nd edn). New York, NY: Oxford University Press.

Zoccolella, S., Savarese, M., Lamberti, P., Manni, R., Pacchetti, C., and Logroscino, G. (2010) Sleep disorders and the natural history of Parkinson's disease: The contribution of epidemiological studies. Sleep Medicine Review, **15**(1), 41–50.

Zung, W.W.K. and Zung, E.M. (1986), Use of the Zung Self-Rating Depression Scale in the elderly. Clinical Gerontologist, **5**(1–2), 137–148.

Zweig, R.A., and Hillman, J. (1999) Personality disorders in older adults: A review. In E. Rosowsky, R. C. Abrams, and R. A. Zweig (Eds), Personality disorders in older adults: Emerging issues in diagnosis and treatment (pp. 31–54). Mahwah, NJ: Lawrence Erlbaum.

Author Index

A
Abbey, J. 96, 97
Abbott, J.L. 177
Abdulla, A. 120
Abrams, D. 22
Abrams, R.C. 191, 193
Adams, K. 39
Agronin, M.E. 193
Aldwin, C.M. 201
Alexopolous, G.S. 27, 45, 91, 94
Allen, J.P. 142
Almeida, O.P. 43, 44, 46, 175
Altman, A.N. 218
Ameida, S.A. 43, 44
Ancoli-Israel, S. 154
Andersen, P.K. 175
Anderson, G. 112, 113
Andreescu, C. 63
Angst, F. 176, 182
Aparasu, R.R. 164
Apostolova, L.G. 33
Arean, P.A. 71
Arens, E.A. 201
Arfken, C.L. 68
Armstrong, K. 36
Atkinson, R.M. 121, 137
Attix, D.K. 25, 36

B
Babor, T.F. 141
Bagby, R.M. 46
Bakshi, N. 175
Balsis, S. 192, 193, 194, 200, 201
Baltes, P.B. 26
Bandura, A. 181
Barbar, S.I. 154
Bark, N. 179
Barlow, J. 139
Barry, K.L. 134, 135, 136, 138, 139, 144
Bartels, S.J. 172, 174, 175
Bauer, M.S. 181
Baxter, A.J. 62
Beattie, E.R.A. 63
Beaudreau, S.A. 86
Bech, P. 179
Beck, A.T. 44, 45, 70, 71
Beekman, A.T. 62, 63
Bennett-Levy, J. 36
Ben-Porath, Y. 179
Berk, M. 182
Bernard, J.M. 218, 220

Berrios, G.E. 175
Bjelland, I. 46, 70
Black, D.A. 135
Blackburn, J. 179
Blazer, D.G. 39, 40, 42, 66, 89, 133, 149
Bliwise, D.L. 155
Blogg, L.C. 135
Blow, F.C. 134, 137, 138, 139, 140, 141, 144
Bootzin, R.R. 165
Bouma, A. 96
Bowling, A. 119
Brassington, G.S. 154
Brodaty, H. 27, 39, 173
Brody, E.M. 118
Brown, G.K. 44
Brown, K.W. 38
Brown, L.M. 44
Brown, M.C. 36
Brown, R.G. 32
Brown, S.T. 120
Bruce, M. 40
Bryant, C. 62, 65
Buchsbaum, D.G. 141
Burns, A. 27, 87
Butler, R. 51
Butters, M.A. 86
Buysse, D.J. 153, 154, 159, 162
Byers 62
Byrne, E.J. 173
Byrne, G.J.A. 32, 33, 62, 69, 70, 162

C
Camp, C.J. 21
Carney, C.E. 160
Carroll, B.J. 175
Casey, D.A. 182
Cassidy, F. 63, 64, 175
Charles, S.T. 201, 202
Chattat, R. 43
Cheavens, J.S. 205
Chermack, S.T. 135
Choi, N.G. 42
Chu, D. 175
Chui, H.C. 43, 68, 90
Clare, L. 172
Clarke, M. 48
Clayton, P.J. 175
Clifford, R.M. 135
Cohen, C.I. 172, 173, 174, 182, 183
Cohen-Mansfield, J. 95, 97
Coker, L.A. 193, 196

Colarusso, C.A. 59
Colenda, C.C. 135
Collin, C. 117
Conigliaro, J. 141
Connor, D.J. 97
Conwell, Y. 47, 138
Coolidge, F.L. 194, 195, 196, 197, 198
Copeland, J.R.M. 70
Craig, D. 164
Crowley, K. 153, 154, 155
Crum, R.M. 90
Cuijpers, P. 73
Cullen, B. 90
Culpepper, L. 114, 115
Cummings, J.L. 27, 33, 41, 97, 98, 152, 179
Curran, H.V. 144

D
Dalrymple-Alford, J.C. 34
Davidson, M. 182
Deimling, G.T. 66
Dellinger, A.M. 67
Dennis, M. 46
Dennis, R.E. 24, 71
Depp, C.A. 175, 176, 183
Devanand, D.P. 199
Dew, M.A. 154, 155
Diefenbach, G.J. 70
Diehl, M. 26
Dillon, H.R. 165
Dolan-Sewell, R.G. 193
Donders, J. 19
Dorwick, C. 112
Douglass, A.B. 160
Draper, B. 47
Drew, S.M. 142
Driscoll, H.C. 154
Duberstein, P.R. 47, 73
Duffy, M. 207, 218
Duncan, B.L. 219
Dupree, L.W. 137, 152

E
Eaton, W. 113
Ebrahim, I.O. 156
Edelstein, B.A. 24, 47, 70, 90, 200
Efros, R.B. 121
Elson, P. 85
Epstein, D.R. 165
Espie, C.A. 154, 155, 157
Ewing, J.A. 140
Extermann, M. 116

F
Falendar, C.A. 218, 220
Fann, J.R. 95, 178
Farias, S.T. 83
Farmer, R.F. 191, 193

Farrell, K.R. 95
Fenner, S. 175
Fenton, W.S. 182
Ferretti, L. 86
Fiellin, D.A. 141
Finch, C.E. 121, 182
Finkel, S. 106
Finn, S.E. 22
First, M.B. 23, 139, 156, 197
Fischer, C.T. 22
Fischer, K.W. 26
Fiske, A. 38
Flett, G.L. 47
Flint, A.J. 46, 70
Foley, D.J. 155, 166
Folstein, M.F. 33, 90, 96
Frances, A.J. 191
Frank, D. 141
Frasure-Smith, N. 39
Fratiglioni, L. 85
Fremouw, W. 47
Freshwater, S.M. 21
Fried, L.P. 114
Friedman, B. 43
Fröjdh, K. 46

G
Gabryelewicz, T. 83
Gagnon, L.M. 114, 115
Gallagher, D. 86
Gallo, J. 39
Ganzini, L. 95
Garb, H.B. 219
Gass, C.S. 36
Gatz, M. 71, 98, 216
Gellis, Z.D. 63
Germans, S. 198, 199
Ghaemi, S.N. 179, 180
Giblin, S. 172
Gibson, S.J. 120
Gijsen, R. 113
Gildengers, A.G. 175
Glass, J. 164
Gloster, A.T. 46
Goldberg, R. 66
Golden, C.J. 21
Gonidakis, S. 121
Gonzalez, J.M. 42
Goodwin, F. 175
Goodyear, R.K. 218, 220
Gooneratne, N.S. 160
Gorham, D.R. 178
Gorske, T.T. 21, 22
Gradman, T.J. 204
Graham, J.R. 179
Gray, S.L. 67
Green, J. 37
Greenberg, R. 46

Grossberg, G.T. 177
Grove, W.M. 219
Gunderson, E.W. 133
Gureje, O. 155
Gurian, B. 193

H
Hadjistavropoulos, T. 96
Hadzi-Pavlovic, D. 39
Haley, W.E. 11, 66
Halvorsrud, L. 119
Ham, R. 113
Hamilton, M. 46
Harris, Y. 39
Harvey, P.D. 183
Hausdorff, J.M. 67
Hawkins, E.I. 219
Haythornthwaite, J.A. 155
Haywood, K. 119
Heisel, M.J. 47
Helme, R.D. 120
Helmes, E. 11
Hertzog, C. 45
Hess, M. 22
Hess, T.M. 22
Hesse, M. 199
Hickey, A.M. 119
Hillman, J. 201
Hinrichsen, G.A. 212, 218
Hinson, J.T. 22
Hirschfeld, R.M. 174, 180
Holden, J.D. 144
Holmes, C. 85
Hopko, D.R. 71
Horowitz, S.V. 191
Horvath, J. 112
Hu, H.C. 41
Hubbard, G. 99
Hunter, S.J. 19
Hurria, A. 116

I
Inouye, S.K. 96, 138, 178
Ismail, Z. 33
Izal, M. 43

J
Jacobs, M.L. 97
Jacomb, P.A. 91
James, I.A. 205
James, J.W. 11
James, M.A. 21, 99
Jamison, K. 175
Jean-Louis, G. 168
Jess, C. 148
Jeste, D.V. 40, 63, 97, 172, 174, 175, 176, 177, 182, 183
Jimenez, D.E. 79

Jiménez-Martin, S. 113
Johansson, P. 154
Johns, M.W. 159
Johnson, D.C. 154
Johnson, K.G. 154
Jorm, A.F. 91
Joseph, C.L. 147
Judd, T. 21

K
Kane, F.J. 66
Kane, J.M. 173, 197
Kaplan, E. 21
Karel, M.J. v–vi, 208, 209, 218, 222
Karim, S. 173
Kathol, R.G. 66
Katon, W.J. 115
Kawakami, N. 113
Kazantzis, N. 13, 29
Keefe, F.J. 139
Keith, S. 175
Keller, S. 120
Kenan, M.M. 193
Kessing, L.V. 175
Kessler, R.C. 12, 23, 62
Kimmel, D. 11
Kingdon, D. 189
Klein, W.C. 148
Klerman, E.B. 154
Klonsky, E.D. 197
Knight, B.G. v–vi, 3, 20, 110, 138, 208, 214
Knopman, D.S. 86
Koder, D.A. 11
Koenig, H.G. 12
Köhler, S. 86
Konnert, C. 99
Kraemer, K.L. 152
Kroenke, K. 46
Kryger, M.H. 164
Kushida, C.A. 164

L
Labouvie-Vief, G. 26
Lacro, J.P. 97, 177
Laidlaw, K. 19, 26
Lambert, M.J. 218, 219
Langbehn, D.R. 199
Lawton, M.P. 7, 118
Lecrubier, Y. 23, 24, 72, 139, 156, 178
Lee, Y.A. 3, 85
Lemke, S.P. 147
Lenze, E.J. 62, 63, 66, 68
Leon, C. 174, 182
Lesperance, F. 39
Levenson, R.W. 73
Leverenz, J.B. 86
Levkoff, S.E. 95
Levy, B. 63

Li, G. 40
Lichstein, K.L. 155, 159, 162, 164, 166
Lichtenberg, P.A. 36, 46
Lindesay, J. 73
Lindsey, P.L. 174
Little, M.O. 40
Llorente, M.D. 135
Logsdon, R.G. 98
Longo, V.D. 121
Lovibond, P.F. 46
Lovibond, S.H. 46
Lynch, T.R. 205

M
Mackinnon, A. 91
Maher, P. 127
Maletta, G. 193
Mann, A.H. 199
Masand, P.S. 97
Mascolo, M.P. 26
Massie, M.J. 116
McAiney, C.A. 106
McBride, L. 181
McCarthy, M. 189
McCrae, R.R. 12, 158, 204
McCurry, S.M. 154
McDonald, R.J. 71
McGlashan, T.H. 182
McKeith, I.G. 86, 97
McKhann, G. 84
McLennan, S. 34
McQuaid, J.R. 181
Medler, M. 26
Meeks, S. 172, 176, 183
Menken, M. 31
Menninger, J.A. 133, 134, 136, 144
Merckelbach, H. 29
Meyer, T. 41, 70, 71
Meyers, B.S. 46
Mezuk, B. 113
Miles, L. 160
Miller, S.D. 219
Miller, W.R. 181
Millon, T. 200
Miloyan, B. 74
Mitchell, A.J. 27, 44
Moak, G. 174
Mohlman, J. 41, 47, 65
Mondolo, F. 46
Monk, T.H. 156, 166
Moore, R.D. 134
Morales, P. 207, 218
Moran, P. 199
Morgan, K. 153, 166, 182
Morin, C.M. 154, 155, 157, 159, 165
Morley, A. 40, 116
Morris, J.C. 84, 88
Morris, R.G. 26
Morton, J.L. 141

Moye, J. 34
Mroczek, D.K. 204
Mulligan, R. 91

N
Nasreddine, Z.S. 32, 34, 42, 68, 90, 96
Nemiroff, R.A. 59
Neutel, C.I. 135, 164
Nobili, A. 113
Noecker, T.L. 99
Novak, M. 154

O
O'Boyle, C.A. 119
O'Hara, R. 86
Ohayon, M.M. 156, 166
Okazaki, S. 192
Oltmanns, T.F. 192, 193, 200
O'Reily, A.A. 45
Ormel, J. 113
Oslin, D.W. 147
Overall, J.E. 178
Owens, K.M.B. 25

P
Pachana, N. v–vi, 8, 19, 25, 26, 27, 32, 33, 39, 45, 62, 63, 69, 70, 90, 91, 162
Palmer, K. 87
Paranthaman, R. 40
Paris, J. 201
Parker, G. 39
Patten, S.B. 114, 115
Patterson, T.L. 181
Pearson, C.G. 216
Petersen, R.C. 83
Pfohl, B. 195, 198
Phelps, J.R. 179, 180
Phillips, N. 34
Pinkahana, J. 176
Pinquart, M. 48, 73, 99
Pinsker, D.M. 34
Pinto-Meza, A. 46
Pollak, C.P. 155
Poon, C. 3, 20
Pope, K.S. 36
Postal, K. 36
Poulsen, E.E. 69, 125
Prince, M. 83
Pusey, H. 99

Q
Qualls, S.H. 99, 207
Quinn, T.J. 117

R
Rahhal, T.A. 22
Ratnavelli, E. 85, 86
Ray, W. 67, 135
Ready, R.E. 26

Redline, S. 156
Reese, R.J. 207, 219, 220
Reid, K.J. 168
Reinert, D.F. 142
Reynolds, C.F. 153, 156
Reynolds, C.R. 70, 88
Richards, D.A. 99
Ricklefs, R.E. 121
Riedel, B.W. 154, 158, 162, 169
Rifat, S.L. 46, 70
Ripich, D.N. 107
Robb, C. 48
Roberts, M. 135
Roberts, R.O. 86
Rocca, W.A. 85
Rodolfa, E. 207
Rokke, P.D. 48
Rollnick, S. 181
Rose, M.K. 194
Rosowsky, E. 193
Roux, F.J. 164
Ruff, R. 21
Rugulies, R. 113

S

Sajatovic, M. 175, 176
Sakauye, K. 42
Salthouse, T. 75
Samuel, D.B. 192, 196
Sartorius, N. 64
Satre, D.D. 133, 138, 144, 145, 149, 150, 152
Saunders, P.A. 135
Sayegh, P. 110
Schaefer, J.A. 147
Schaie, K.W. 12
Scherder, E.J.A. 96
Schieber, F. 26
Schinka, J.A. 44
Schonfield, L. 137, 142
Schramke, C.J. 219
Schroeter, M.L. 86
Schurhoff, F. 175
Schuster, J-P. 191, 192, 201
Schut, H. 60
Scogin, F. 48, 63
Secker, D.L. 13
Segal, D.L. 70, 179, 194, 195, 196, 197, 198, 200, 201, 202
Semenchuk, E.M. 24
Shafranske, E.P. 218, 220
Shah, A. 48
Shankar, K.K. 91, 94
Shea, M.T. 195
Sheehan, D.V. 23
Shepherd, S. 173
Siberski, J. 84
Simoni-Wastila, L. 133, 134, 138, 144
Sinoff, G. 69
Skevington, S.M. 118

Smith, M.T. 155
Smith, S.R. 21, 22, 36
Smith, S.S. 153, 159
Smits, I.A.M. 12
Snow, A.L. 95, 97
Sörensen, S. 99
Spalletta, G. 95
Spector, A. 86, 99
Spielberger, C.D. 71
Spiers, N. 12
Spinhoven, P. 70
Stanley, M.A. 71
Steer, R.A. 44
Stepanski, E.J. 165
Stevens, J.A. 67
Stevenson, J. 201
Storey, J. 68, 90
Stroebe, M. 60
Sue, S. 79
Suzuki, N. 135
Swafford, K.L. 96

T

Targum, S.D. 98, 176, 177
Tariot, P.N. 179
Teng, E.L. 43, 68, 90
Thompson, C. 47
Thorp, L. 46
Todaro, J.F. 66
Tombaugh, T.N. 33
Towsley, G. 45, 94
Triebwasser, J. 195
Troxel, W.M. 154
Tsai, S. 176
Twiss, J. 179

V

van Alphen, S.P.J. 192, 194, 198
van Haastregt, J.C. 68
Van Horn, E. 198
van Lennep, J.E. 125
Ventura, J. 179
Vink, D. 63

W

Wakisaka, Y. 85
Walker, D. 48
Walters, D. 88
Ware, J.E. 192
Webster, J. 177
Weinberger, M.I. 116
Weissman, M.M. 174
Welsh-Bohmer, K.A. 25, 36
Werner, P. 95, 97
Wetherell, J.L. 63, 68
Wettergren, L. 120
Whitbourne, S.K. 172
Whitlock, E.P. 144
Widiger, T.A. 192, 193, 195, 196, 204

Williamson, J.D. 114
Wing, Y. 166
Wisocki, P.A. 70
Woerner, M.G. 179
Wolitzky-Taylor, K.B. 62, 63
Wolklove, N. 154
Wood, J.M. 195
Woodhead, E.L. 209
Woodward, R. 39, 79
Worden, J.W. 60
Worthman, C.M. 168
Wu, L. 133, 149
Wyatt, J.K. 165

Y
Yang, H.K. 133, 134, 138, 144
Yang, L. 41

Yassa, R. 174
Yesavage, J.A. 32, 43, 69, 91, 162, 195
Yeung, A. 41
Yohannes, A. 66

Z
Zammit, G.K. 154
Zarit, J.M. 41
Zarit, S.H. 41
Zeimer, H. 67
Zhang, B. 166
Zinbarg, R.E. 81
Zoccolella, S. 154
Zung, E.M. 45
Zung, W.W.K. 45
Zweig, R.A. 201, 218
Zweig-Frank, H. 201

Subject Index

A
actigraphy 164
activities of daily living (ADLs) 117
adherence to medical treatment 131
Adult Manifest Anxiety Scale–Elderly version (AMAS-E) 70
ageism 29
age-segregating environments 7–9
aging v–vi, 2
 attributions to 49–50
 developmental *see* developmental aging
agitation 95
alcohol misuse/abuse 133, 134
 assessment 135, 136
 clinical characteristics of early and late onset problem drinkers 137
 depression 134–35
 nursing home context 147–49
 pain 138–39
 sleep disorders 138–39
 sleep disturbance 156, 165
Alcohol Use Disorders Identification Test (AUDIT) 141–42
Alzheimer's disease 85–6, 87
analgesics 115
antibiotics 115
antihistamines 115
antihypertensives 115
antipsychotics 115
antisocial personality disorder 191, 192
anxiety 62–4, 82
 alcohol misuse/abuse 138
 assessment 64–72
 associated medical conditions 114
 associated medication 115
 clinical interview 64–9
 cohort differences 76–7
 comorbid with depression 45, 63–4
 cultural influences 77–9
 dementia 94–5
 developmental aging 73–4
 insomnia 162
 problems in therapy 79–81
 protective factors 63
 psychotherapy 72–81
 risk factors 63
 social context 75
 symptoms 69–71
anxiolytics 115
apnea during sleep 156
ASSIST tool for illicit drug abuse 142

assisted living 53
asthma 114
attitudes in geropsychology 209–12
avoidant personality disorder 192

B
Baby Boomers 12, 13
Bech–Rafaelson Mania Scale (BRMS) 179
Beck Anxiety Inventory (BAI) 45, 70–1
Beck Depression Inventory II (BDI-II) 44–5
Behavioral and Psychological Symptoms in Dementia (BPSD) 97, 106
 FOCUSED strategy 107
 PIECES framework 106
behavioral variant of fronto-temporal dementia (BVFTD) 86
benzodiazepines 67
 age-related withdrawal symptoms 144
 misuse/abuse 135, 138
 sleep disorders 162
bereavement 60
bipolar disorder 172, 190
 assessment 176–80
 clinical interview 177–78
 cohort effects 185–87
 cultural contexts 187–88
 developmental influences 182–85
 later life 174–76
 social contexts 185
 substance misuse/abuse 138
 symptoms 178–80
 therapy 181–90
 therapy issues 188–90
breath, shortness of 66
Brief Pain Inventory (BPI) 120–21
Brief Psychiatric Rating Scale (BPRS) 178

C
CAGE questionnaire 140–41, 143
California Older Adult Stroop Test 26
CALTAP assessment approaches and strategies 19–21, 37
 see also Contextual Adult Lifespan Theory for Adapting Psychology (CALTAP) model
 after assessment 35–6
 clinical interviews 23–4
 cognitive screens 33–4
 cohort differences 31
 complications 32–6
 cultural influences 31

CALTAP assessment approaches (*continued*)
  developmental aging 24–7
  illness 32–3
  research and practice imperatives 36–7
  sharing results and recommendations 36
  social context 27–31
Camberwell Assessment of Needs in the Elderly (CANE) 88–9
cancer drugs 115
cancers 114
cardiac disease 114
Center for Epidemiologic Studies Depression Scale (CES-D) 45–6
cerebrovascular disease (CVD) 85
challenges of later life 6–7
chronic obstructive pulmonary disease (COPD) 114
circadian rhythms 166, 168
Clinical Dementia Rating Scale (CDR) 88
clinical interviews 23–4
  anxiety 64–9
  bipolar disorder 177–78
  cognitive screening 89–92
  dementia 87–9
  depression 40–2
  psychosis 177–78
  schizophrenia 177–78
  sleep disorders 156–62
  substance misuse/abuse 139–40
cognitive behavioral therapy (CBT)
  anxiety 73
  dementia 99
  sleep disorders 159
cognitive complexity 26–7
cognitive screening 33–4
  dementia 89–92
  depression 42–3
Cohen Mansfield Agitation Inventory (CMAI) 95, 97
cohort influences 11–14
  anxiety 76–7
  bipolar disorder 185–87
  CALTAP assessment 31
  dementia 109
  depression 56–7
  issues affecting medical conditions 124–26
  personality disorders 204
  psychosis 185–87
  schizophrenia 185–87
  sleep disorders 168
  substance misuse/abuse 149–50
communication 129
  results and recommendations 36
community-based programs 10
competency in geropsychology 208–9
Composite International Diagnostic Interview (CIDI) 23
Confusional Assessment Method (CAM) 96

substance misuse/abuse 138
consultation in clinical geropsychology 208, 220–22
Contextual Adult Lifespan Theory for Adapting Psychology (CALTAP) model v, vii, 1–4, 17–18
  cohort influences 11–14
  cultural context 15–17
  developmental aging 4–6
  social contexts 7–11
  specific challenges of later life 6–7
  see also CALTAP assessment approaches and strategies
coordination of care 128, 130
Cornell Scale for Depression in Dementia 27, 45, 94
corticosteroids 115
Council of Professional Geropsychology Training Programs (CoPGTP) 208
cultural influences 15–17, 31
  anxiety 77–9
  bipolar disorder 187–88
  dementia 109–10
  depression 41, 57–9
  issues affecting medical conditions 127–28
  personality disorders 204
  psychosis 187–88
  schizophrenia 187–88
  sleep disorders 168
  substance misuse/abuse 150
culturally and linguistically diverse (CALD) backgrounds 31

D

daylight exposure 168
delirium 95–6
  substance misuse/abuse 137–38
dementia 83, 110
  agitation 95
  anxiety 94–5
  assessment 87–98
  attitudes towards dementia 99–100
  clinical interview 87–9
  cohort influences 109
  comorbidities 86–7
  cultural influences 109–10
  delirium 95–6
  depression 53–5, 93–4
  developmental influences 100–1
  DSM-5 classification 83–7
  end-stage dementia 105
  interventions 98–9
  issues 110
  pain 96–7
  psychotherapy 98–110
  psychotic symptoms 97–8
  social context 105–9
  subtypes 85–6

symptoms 92–3
working with caregivers 103–4
working with patients 103
Dementia Outcomes Management Suite (DOMS) 87
dependent personality disorder 192
depletion syndrome 39
depression 38–40, 61
  alcohol misuse/abuse 134–35, 138
  anxiety 63–4
  assessing symptoms 43–6
  assessment 40–8
  associated medical conditions 114
  associated medication 115
  attributions to aging 49–50
  bereavement and grief 60
  clinical interview 40–2
  cognitive screening 42–3
  cohort effects 56–7
  complications in therapy 59–60
  cultural differences 57–9
  dementia 93–4
  downs and ups of developmental aging 51
  late life problems 59–60
  late onset versus lifelong depression 49
  life expectancy as cognitive intervention 50–1
  psychotherapy 48–51
  psychotic symptoms 46
  social context 52–5
  suicidal ideation 47–8
  using client's history to change depressive thoughts 52–7
  without sadness 39
Depression Anxiety Stress Scale (DASS) 46
detoxification 152
developmental aging 4–6
  anxiety 73–5
  bipolar disorder 182–85
  CALTAP assessment 24–7
  depression 51
  issues affecting medical conditions 121–23
  personality disorders 201–2
  psychosis 182–85
  schizophrenia 182–85
  sleep disorders 166–67
digitalis 115
Disability-Adjusted Life Years 39
drug abuse *see* substance misuse and abuse
drug withdrawal 114
Dysfunctional Beliefs about Sleep (DBAS) scale 159
dysthymic disorder 39

E
education level as a cohort effect 124–25
emotional changes 5
emotional complexity 26–7

endocrine conditions 114
epilepsy 114
Epworth Sleepiness Scale (ESS) 159
estrogen 115
exercise 168

F
falls 67–8
family relationships
  age-segregating environments 9
  conflicts 14
  immigrant families 17
  structures 15
FOCUSED strategy 107
Functional Adaptations and Skills Training (FAST) 181
functional assessment 117–18

G
gastrointestinal conditions 114
gay individuals in old age 56
generalized anxiety disorder (GAD) 62, 71–2
genitourinary conditions 114
Geriatric Anxiety Inventory (GAI) 32, 45, 69–70
Geriatric Anxiety Scale (GAS) 70
Geriatric Depression Scale (GDS) 32, 43–4
Geriatric Mental Status Examination 70
Geriatric Suicidal Ideation Scale (GSIS) 47
Gerontological Personality Disorder Scale 198
geropsychology
  attitude competencies 209–12
  competency 208–9
  consultation 208, 220–21
  knowledge competencies 212–14
  skills competencies 214–17
  supervision 207–8, 217–20
grief 60
guilt 125

H
Hamilton Rating Scale for Depression (HAM-D) 46
Harmful Behaviors Scale (HBS) 48
health as part of self-concept during aging 122–23
histrionic personality disorder 191, 192
homosexuality in old age 57
Hopkins Symptom Checklist-25 (HSCL-25) 46
Hospital Anxiety and Depression Scale (HADS) 46, 70, 71

I
illnesses in later life 32–3
immigrant families 17
Informant Questionnaire on Cognitive Decline in the Elderly (IQCODE) 91

insomnia 138–39, 154
  assessment 155–56
  chronic 155
  clinical interview 156–59
  cohort and cultural effects 168
  developmental effects 166–67
  medication 164
  psychotherapy 164–70
  social context 167–68
  treatment issues 169–70
  see also sleep disorders
instrumental activities of daily living (IADLs) 118
insulin 115
interpersonal therapy (IPT) 99
interview, clinical *see* clinical interview
Iowa Personality Disorder Screen (IPDS) 199

K
knowledge base in geropsychology 212–14

L
late-onset depression 39–40
Lawton Instrumental Activities of Everyday Living Scale 118
Lewy bodies 86
life expectancy 50–1
Life Goals Program 181

M
major depressive disorder (MDD) 38
medical care settings 28–9
medical conditions affected by psychological issues 112–16
  assessment 116–21
  functional assessment 117–18
  illness associated with anxiety/depression 114
  medication associated with anxiety/depression 115
  pain assessment 120–21
  psychotherapy 121–31
  quality of life (QOL) assessment 118–20
Michigan Alcoholism Screening Test–Geriatric Version (MAST-G) 141, 143
mild cognitive impairment (MCI) 4, 23, 87
Millon Clinical Multiaxial Inventory–III (MCMI-III) 200–1
MINI International Neurophysiological Interview (MINI) 23–4
Mini-Mental State Exam (MMSE) 33
  dementia 90
minor depressions 39
MMPI 2 psychopathology assessment tool 179
Modified Manic State Scale (MMSS) 179
Modified Mini-Mental State Exam (3MS) 33–4
  anxiety 68
  dementia 90
  depression 43
Montreal Cognitive Assessment (MoCA) 32, 34
  anxiety 68
  dementia 90
  depression 42
Mood Disorder Questionnaire (MDQ) 179–80
muscle relaxation technique 79–80
musculoskeletal conditions 114

N
neurocognitive disorder (NCD) 6, 83–5
  subtypes 85–6
Neuropsychiatric Inventory (NPI) 27, 41, 97, 179
neuropsychotherapy approach of CALTAP 21–2
non-steroidal anti-inflammatory drugs (NSAIDs) 115

O
obsessive–compulsive disorder (OCD) 191, 192
older clients
  challenges of later life 6–7
  working with 1–4
Outcome Questionnaire-45 (OQ-45) 218–20
Outcome Rating Scale (ORS) 219–20
over the counter (OTC) medication misuse/abuse 133, 134

P
pain
  assessment 120–21
  dementia 96–7
  substance misuse/abuse 138–39
paranoid personality disorder 191, 192
Parkinson Fatigue Scale (PFS-16) 32
Patient Health Questionnaire (PHQ) 46
Penn State Worry Questionnaire (PSWQ) 70, 71
personality disorders 5, 191–95, 205–6
  age of onset 193
  assessment 195–201
  cohort and cultural influences 204
  developmental influences 201–2
  Gerontological Personality Disorder Scale 198
  social context 202–4
  therapy 201–6
  treatment issues 204–6
phobias 62
physical exercise 168
PIECES framework 106
Pikes Peak Model for Geropsychology Training 208–9

Pittsburgh Sleep Quality Index (PSQI) 159
polysomnography (PSG) 164
practice imperatives in geriatric
    assessment 36–7
prescription medication misuse/abuse 135
presenting problems of older adults 4
progressive relaxation 79–81
psychosis 172, 190
    assessment 176–80
    clinical interview 177–78
    cohort effects 185–87
    cultural contexts 187–88
    developmental influences 182–85
    differential diagnosis in later life 176
    later life 172–74
    risk factors in later life 177
    social contexts 185
    symptoms 178–80
    therapy 181–90
    therapy issues 188–90
psychotherapy for anxiety 72–82
    cohort differences 76–7
    cultural influences 77–9
    developmental aging 73–5
    problems in therapy 79–81
    social context 75
psychotherapy for bipolar disorder
        181–82
    cohort effects 185–87
    cultural contexts 187–88
    developmental influences 182–85
    social contexts 185
    therapy issues 188–90
psychotherapy for dementia sufferers and
    caregivers 98
    attitudes towards dementia 99–100
    cohort influences 109
    cultural influences 109–10
    developmental influences 100–1
    end-stage dementia 105
    interventions 98–9
    issues 110
    social context 105–9
    working with caregivers 103–4
    working with patients 103
psychotherapy for depression 48, 49
    attributions to aging 49–50
    bereavement and grief 60
    cohort effects 56–7
    complications 59–60
    cultural differences 57–9
    downs and ups of developmental aging 51
    late life problems 59–60
    life expectancy as cognitive
        intervention 50–1
    social context 52–5
    using client's history to change depressive
        thoughts 52–7

psychotherapy for issues affecting medical
        conditions 132
    cohort effects 124–26
    cultural influences 127–28
    developmental aging 121–23
    issues in psychotherapy 128–31
    social context 123–24
psychotherapy for personality disorders
    cohort and cultural influences 204
    developmental influences 201–2
    social context 202–4
    treatment issues 204–6
psychotherapy for schizophrenia 181–82
    cohort effects 185–87
    cultural contexts 187–88
    developmental influences 182–85
    social contexts 185
    therapy issues 188–90
psychotherapy for sleep disorders 164–66
    cohort and cultural effects 168
    developmental effects 166–67
    social context 167–68
    treatment issues 169–70
psychotherapy for substance misuse and
        abuse 144–45
    cohort and cultural effects 149–50
    developmental influences 145–46
    social context 146–49
    treatment issues 150–52
psychotic symptoms
    dementia 97–8
    depression 46

Q
quality of life (QOL) assessment 118–20

R
Rating Anxiety in Dementia (RAID) 94–5
Reasons for Living Scale–Older Adults
    (RFL-OA) 47
relaxation for anxiety 79–80
research imperatives in geriatric
    assessment 36–7
residential care 27–8
role of psychotherapist 129–30
Rowland Universal Dementia Assessment
    Scale (RUDAS) 68, 90–1

S
Schedule for the Evaluation of Individual
    Quality of Life (SEIQOL/SEIQOL-DW)
    118–19
schizoid personality disorder 191, 192
schizophrenia 172–74
    assessment 176–80
    clinical interview 177–78
    cohort effects 185–87
    cultural contexts 187–88

schizophrenia (*continued*)
  developmental influences 182–85
  social contexts 185
  therapy 181–90
  treatment issues 188–90
sharing results and recommendations 36
Short Anxiety Screening Test (SAST) 69
shortness of breath 66
side effects of medications 131
skills for geropsychology 214–17
sleep diaries 160
sleep disorders 153–55
  assessment 155–56
  clinical interview 156–59
  cohort and cultural effects 168
  developmental effects 166–67
  medication 164
  psychotherapy 164–70
  social context 167–68
  substance misuse/abuse 138–39
  treatment issues 169–70
Sleep Disorders Questionnaire (SDQ) 160
sleep hygiene 156, 165
  education 169
sleep onset latency (SOL) 155
smoking and medical conditions in later life 125
social contexts 7–11
  anxiety 75
  bipolar disorder 185
  CALTAP assessment 27–31
  dementia 105–9
  issues affecting medical conditions 123–24
  personality disorders 202–4
  psychosis 185
  psychotherapy for depression 52–5
  schizophrenia 185
  sleep disorders 167–68
  substance misuse/abuse 146–49
social networks 30–1
societal ageism 29
Standardized Assessment of Personality–Abbreviated Scale (SAPAS) 199

Standardized Assessment of Personality (SAP) 199
Stanford Sleep Questionnaire and Assessment of Wakefulness (SQAW) 160
State Trait Anxiety Inventory (STAI) 71
stress and physical health 126
Stroop test 26
Structured Clinical Interview (SCID) 23
substance misuse and abuse 133–35, 152
  assessment 135–37
  clinical interview and screening 139–40
  cohort and cultural effects 149–50
  comorbidities 137–39
  developmental influences 145–46
  psychotherapy 144–52
  social context 146–49
  specific screening tools for older adults 140–44
  treatment issues 150–52
suicidal ideation 47–8
Suicidal Older Adult Protocol (SOAP) 47
supervision in clinical geropsychology 207–8, 221–22
  inputs 217–18
  standardized instruments 218–20

T
tachycardia 66
tests 25–6
training in geropsychology 208–9
twelve-step substance abuse programs 151

V
vascular disorders 114

W
wake time after sleep (WASO) 155
withdrawal from drugs 114
Worry Scale 70

Z
Zung Depression Rating Scale (ZDRS) 45–6

The manufacturer's authorised representative in the EU for product safety is Oxford University Press España S.A. of el Parque Empresarial San Fernando de Henares, Avenida de Castilla, 2 – 28830 Madrid (www.oup.es/en or product.safety@oup.com). OUP España S.A. also acts as importer into Spain of products made by the manufacturer.

www.ingramcontent.com/pod-product-compliance
Ingram Content Group UK Ltd.
Pitfield, Milton Keynes, MK11 3LW, UK
UKHW021135240326
469240UK00020B/148